Prostate Brachytherapy
MADE COMPLICATED

SECOND EDITION

Prostate Brachytherapy
MADE COMPLICATED

SECOND EDITION

Kent Wallner
John C. Blasko
Michael Dattoli

SmartMedicine Press
Seattle, Washington

Second Edition

Library of Congress Catalog Card Number:
ISBN: 0-9648991-4-0

Published by SmartMedicine Press, Seattle, Washington
Printed by Sheridan Books, Ann Arbor, Michigan
Cover design by Deborah Rust

Dedicated to our patients—
pioneers in prostate brachytherapy

Acknowledgments

The following people share credit for this book. Their insightful comments and suggestions were invaluable:

Kas Badiozamani, MD
Jerry Barker, MD
Carl Bergsagel, MS
David Beyer, MD
William Cavanagh, MS
Brian Davis, PhD, MD
Jason, Dominitz, MD
Kathryn Elliott, MD
Benjamin Han, MD
Cory Hoffman, RN
Christine Jacobs
Ben Liem, MD

Gregory Merrick, MD
Felix Mick, PhD
Bradley Prestidge, MD
Mack Roach, MD
T. Tydings Robin, Jr. PhD, LLB
Stephen Smith, MD
Richard Stock, MD
Steven Sutlief, PhD
Lawrence True, MD
Joseph Walker
Anthony Zietman, MD

Kent Wallner, M.D.
Chief, Radiation Oncology
Puget Sound Health Care System, Veterans Administration
Associate Professor
Department of Radiation Oncology
University of Washington Medical Center
Seattle, Washington

John Blasko, M.D.
Seattle Prostate Institute
Clinical Professor
Department of Radiation Oncology
University of Washington Medical Center
Seattle, Washington

Michael Dattoli, M.D.
Physician in Chief
Dattoli Cancer Center and Brachytherapy Research Institute
Sarasota, Florida

Contents

1

Why a Second Edition

When we wrote the first edition of this book in 1996, prostate brachytherapy was in the midst of a rebirth, fueled by improvements in transrectal ultrasound, computer-planning, and the pioneering efforts of physicians and patients willing to question and defy traditional wisdom. By 2000, prostate brachytherapy had been reborn! It's become *conventional* therapy, and even the most diehard former critics have implemented prostate brachytherapy programs within their practices.

We wrote the first edition of this book primarily because no other comprehensive text for prostate brachytherapy was available at the time. There is now a rapidly

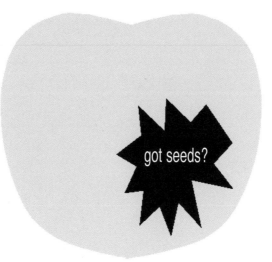

growing body of literature regarding prostate brachytherapy, but still very little objective data is available to help sort out the hype from the legitimate, or the sensical from the ridiculous. Having spent so much time wrestling with these issues, we felt that a second edition of this book would be valuable for the growing number of physicians, patients, and insurers with an interest in brachytherapy.

TOUGH POLITICS

Prostate brachytherapy has always been controversial. There remains almost a visceral dislike of it among many mainstream, otherwise rational radiation oncologists and urologists. The reasons are varied and include residual skepticism borne from inferior results with older retropubic techniques, as well as a natural disdain toward a newer modality viewed as competition for more established procedures. Whatever the reason, it is sometimes unduly difficult to get good quality articles on the topic of brachytherapy accepted for publication in mainstream journals. In this book, we have the luxury of sharing our experiences, impressions, musings, and gripes without concern for "getting past the reviewer."

IMPLANTS AREN'T FOR EVERY PATIENT

While cancer control rates generally look good and morbidity rates are generally relatively low, it has become clear that prostate brachytherapy is not for every patient, something that we've sometimes learned the hard way. In the pages ahead, we provide detailed information about potential complications and what we have learned about who is more likely to experience them. But one of the most frustrating aspects of our experience with brachytherapy has been the difficulty in identifying ahead of time the occasional patient who will develop more serious implant-related problems—and there's no end in sight to this dilemma.

IMPLANTS AREN'T FOR EVERY PHYSICIAN

Performing good prostate brachytherapy requires skill, attention to detail, and tolerance for tedium. Given the current technological limits, there is still a substantial dependence on manual dexterity and familiarity with the physics of brachytherapy—the title of this book was chosen to emphasize this fact. Even as more and more technical information is available to guide newcomers to the field, we still believe that physicians who are too busy with other responsibilities to put a substantial effort into a brachytherapy practice should leave it to someone else.

PERMANENT VERSUS TEMPORARY IMPLANTS

Permanent implants with I-125 or Pd-103 are the predominant form of prostate brachytherapy in the United States. They're favored over temporary, Ir-192 brachytherapy due to encouraging tumor control rates and due to convenience (both for patients *and* physicians). Because of the continued overwhelming preference for permanent implants, we again declined to include temporary implants in this book.

THIS BOOK SHOULD HELP

We witnessed a remarkable reemergence of brachytherapy in the 1990s, and it likely will assume an even bigger role in the future. But we believe a lot of perfecting is still to be done. This text gives us a platform to continue to share our experiences and advice. The descriptions, data, opinions, and ruminations ahead should be helpful to brachytherapists who are just getting started, and to those who have established practices and are looking for ways to improve their techniques. We hope that this second edition helps you to improve your brachytherapy practice.

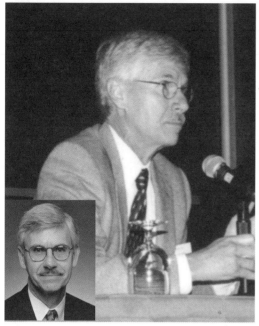

John Blasko

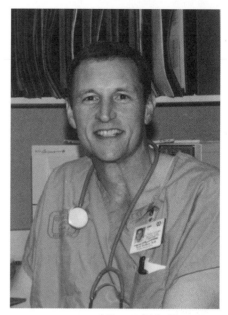

Kent Wallner

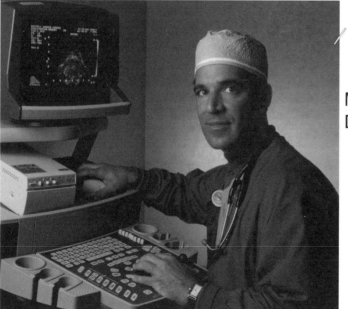

Michael
Dattoli

2

1895–2001

In the four years since we wrote the first edition of this text, we have seen a remarkable shift toward brachytherapy as the treatment of choice for early-stage prostate cancer. While many expected brachytherapy to grow, few expected it to happen so rapidly. Widespread resistance largely melted away as favorable five- to ten-year reports appeared in the late 1990s.(DATTOLI, RAGDE, CRITZ, BLASKO 00, ZELEFSKY, GRADO, BRACHMAN)

THE EARLY DAYS
Prostate brachytherapy, in various forms, has fluctuated in popularity for more than 100 years (**Figure 2-1**). During most of that time, it was more a curiosity than

Century time line

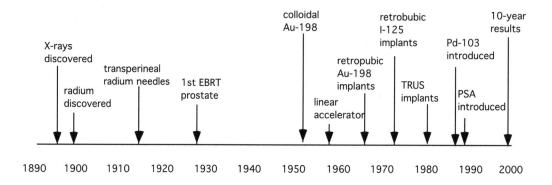

Figure 2-1. Timeline showing major developments in prostate brachytherapy and external beam radiation (EBRT) from 1890 through 2000.

a generally accepted method of treatment. It was never widely accepted by the medical community for a variety of reasons. Barringer, chief of urology at what is now Memorial Sloan-Kettering Cancer Center in New York (MSKCC), was among the first to espouse use of transperineal radium needles for prostate brachytherapy.(BARRINGER) He was impressed with the results, concluding his 1917 JAMA report with:

> *"[B]ecause of the initial success of radium treatment,*
> *I now take the stand that no patient*
> *with prostate cancer should be operated on"*

Since Barringer's time, the evolution of prostate brachytherapy has been punctuated by a few basic ideas, reimplemented in various ways as technology has evolved.

RETROPUBIC IMPLANTS
The first widespread adoption of prostate brachytherapy occurred in the 1970s, when the retropubic method was popularized by Hilaris and Whitmore at MSKCC.(WHITMORE) Early reports appeared favorable, but subsequent reports with longer follow-up were not.(FUKS, SCHELLHAMMER) In retrospect, the introduction of the retropubic method was probably a step backward from Barringer's

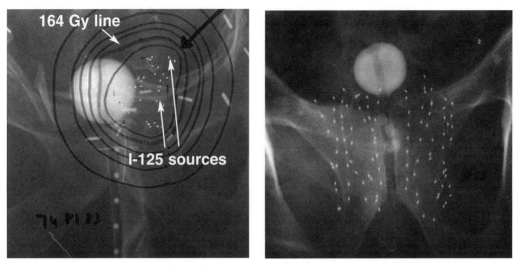

Figure 2-2. On the left is an anterior radiograph of a retropubic implant performed at MSKCC in 1978. You don't need a Ph.D. in physics to recognize that the I-125 sources could not possibly be distributed throughout the prostate. The implant on the right was performed in 1999 with modern, transperineal techniques at the Puget Sound Health Care System VA Hospital. The one on the left is included in long-term reports of retropubic implant results at MSKCC.(FUKS) Unfavorable tumor control rates with poor quality retropubic implants should not have dimmed enthusiasm for modern implant techniques.

transperineal needle placement. The quality of retropubic implants was terrible (**Figure 2-2**), due to technical limitations and lack of dosimetric capabilities.

Although it sounded simple enough to do an implant under direct visualization of the exposed prostate, it was not. The prostate was not well exposed, the operative field was bloody, and without transrectal ultrasound (TRUS) it was impossible to visualize the source location within the prostate—brachytherapists would have had little idea whether placement was properly performed. To compound the technical difficulties, quality assurance was limited—postimplant radiation doses were calculated from plain X rays, without determining their relationship to the prostatic margins (see Chapter 9). Without a system of quality assurance, brachytherapists would not have known how bad a job they were doing with the retropubic method (although they must have had some idea!?).

Prostatectomy: Fool's gold

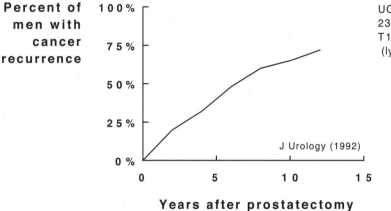

Figure 2-3. First PSA-based tumor control rates with prostatectomy, reported in 1992. The results were dismal, with no plateau on the cancer-free curves. Oncologists began to question whether any patient could be cured surgically.(STEIN)

THE BABY AND THE BATH WATER

Understandably, when unfavorable long-term results for retropubic implants were published, the urologic oncology community went from being enthusiastic to being suspicious of brachytherapy. With introduction of nerve-sparing surgery and widespread availability of linear accelerators, interest in brachytherapy plummeted in the 1980s. Less understandable is the use of unfavorable reports of retropubic implants to vigorously oppose modern prostate brachytherapy. We were often reminded (sometimes with a certain glee) that the results of I-125 prostate brachytherapy, even at its birthplace (MSKCC), were suboptimal. How unimaginative. The retropubic implants of the 1970s were so bad technically, it was obvious to some of us early on that the clinical results would be irrelevant in light of today's transrectal ultrasound, computer technology, and transperineal approach.

It is also commonly remarked that the failures with retropubic implants became evident only with 10- to 15-year follow-up, and that current follow-up with modern techniques is too short to be encouraging. Morons! While long-term follow-up is necessary to assess the curative potential of any modality, the shortcomings of

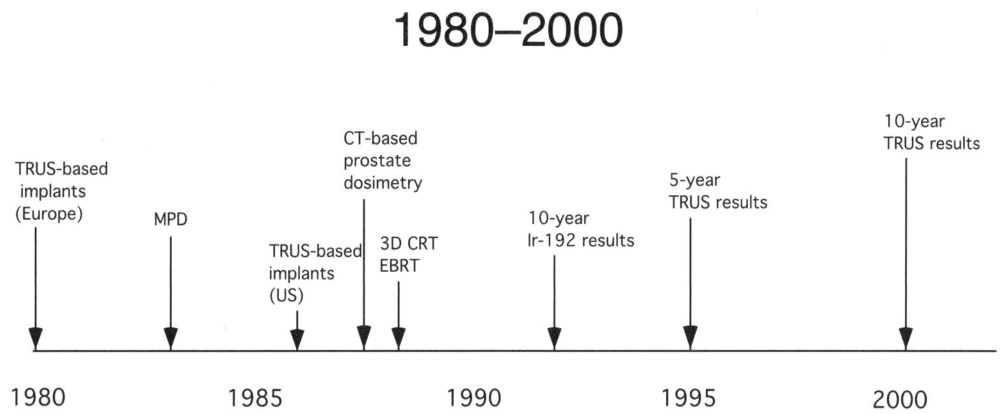

1980–2000

Figure 2-4. Time line showing some of the major developments in prostate brachytherapy from 1980 through 2000.

retropubic implants would have been apparent much earlier if PSA had been available to detect early biochemical evidence of tumor persistence.

(FOOL'S) GOLD STANDARD
Widespread adoption of improved surgical techniques in the 1990s generated renewed enthusiasm for prostatectomy. However, the introduction of PSA-based follow-up showed how ineffective surgery is in eradicating even early stage cancers, forcing a reassessment of the alternatives (**Figure 2-3**).(STEIN, ZIETMAN)

NEW TECHNOLOGIES ARRIVE
The last 15 years witnessed a tremendous surge in prostate brachytherapy (**Figures 2-4 & 2-5**). CT scanners were introduced in the mid-1970s and TRUS in the early 1980s. Computer-based treatment planning became widely available in the late 1970s. By the mid-1980s, these technologies had been combined with the old idea of transperineal implantation, to allow high-quality outpatient prostate brachytherapy.(CHARYULU, HOLM, BLASKO 87, OSIAN)

IR-192 BRACHYTHERAPY
While the rise and fall of retropubic implants was playing out, some brachytherapists took up temporary implants, the most influential and innovative being Nisar Syed, Ajmel Puthawala, and Alvaro Martinez. They treated patients with 30 to 40 Gy external beam radiation plus a temporary Ir-192 boost for an additional 30 to 35 Gy. Source loading was based on CT scan reconstruction of the prostate after the source guides were in place, allowing the radiation dose to be conformed to the

The stats

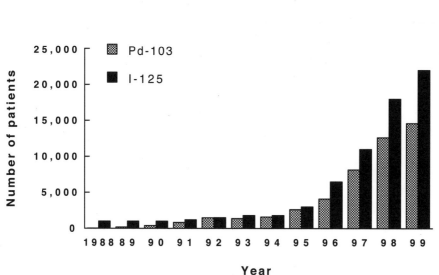

Figure 2-5. Approximate number of implants performed annually in the United States and Canada (courtesy of Theragenics Corporation and Nycomed-Amersham Corporation).

geometry of the prostate. Accordingly, it should be as accurate a system for dose delivery as current TRUS-guided transperineal methods.(SYED)

Despite the pioneering work of Syed and colleagues, the popularity of Ir-192 implants declined substantially in the 1980s. Like retropubic implants, it was eclipsed by the "nerve-sparing" prostatectomy, conformal radiation, and by permanent transperineal implants. Modern high dose rate (HDR) methodology and encouraging five-year results, however, are fueling renewed interest in Ir-192 (**Figure 2-6**).(MARTINEZ, MATE, YOSHIOKA)

WHERE THE CONTROVERSIES WILL GROW
Brachytherapy has some advantages over prostatectomy or external beam radiation, including patient convenience and lower cost. Meanwhile, controversy regarding the ability of brachytherapy to control cancer is decreasing. Where controversy will build over the next few years is how much of an impact brachytherapy has on patients' quality of life (QOL), compared to surgery or external radiation. Mounting evidence shows that brachytherapy has more adverse effect than

HDR versus permanent implants

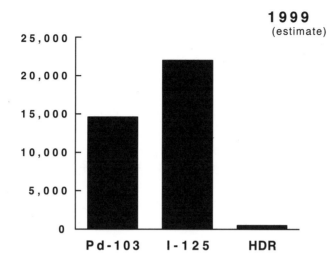

Figure 2-6. Approximate number of permanent implants versus HDR implants in 1999 (HDR stats courtesy of Dr. Philip Devlin).

earlier appreciated. Potency preservation, in particular, may have been too favorably reported.

Several groups are passing the 10-year follow-up mark for transperineal methods, with biochemical-based, cancer-free rates that compare favorably with surgery. But brachytherapy has now entered adolescence—and it will face closer scrutiny by investigators from varied disciplines.

FRINGE PHYSICIANS AND PATIENT ACTIVISM

The wide acceptance of modern prostate brachytherapy was largely due to a handful of physicians determined to proceed despite the admonitions of much of the medical establishment. Drs. Blasko, Ragde, Grimm, and Sylvester were the first prominent advocates in the United States. They were considered for almost 10 years to be out of the mainstream. Now they find themselves center stage before the oncology community.

Resurgent interest in prostate brachytherapy is also largely due to direct patient involvement. In the 1990s patients increasingly began to investigate their treatment options and passing information to other prospective patients through formal (support groups, news articles) and informal (Internet, personal contact) channels. These efforts have had a substantial impact on public awareness of brachytherapy.

Many physicians have grumbled about patients taking the lead in promoting brachytherapy. How ridiculous! If we relied on the entrenched medical establishment to lead the way, we would probably still be in the Dark Ages, treating prostate cancer by bloodletting.

VERY GOOD, BUT NOT PERFECT
As a result of technological developments over the last 10 years, brachytherapy is gaining an increasingly prominent role in the fight against prostate cancer. Much of the prior skepticism has melted away. But with increasing experience, it's clear that brachytherapy is not the runaway best treatment that many believe it is. There *are* some brachytherapy patients who develop implant-related problems that severely impact on their lifestyle. Most of the problems will resolve with time, but doctors and patients should understand that there are pitfalls to this exciting modality. Accordingly, we'll spend much of the next few hundred pages describing the downside as well as the benefits of prostate brachytherapy.

REFERENCES
1. Barringer BS. Radium in the treatment of carcinoma of the bladder and prostate. JAMA 1917; 68:1227-1230.

2. Blasko J C, Ragde H, Schumacher D. Transperineal percutaneous iodine-125 implantation for prostatic carcinoma using transrectal ultrasound and template guidance. Endo/Hypertherm 1987; 3:131-139.

3. Blasko JC, Grimm PD, Sylvester JE, Badiozamani KR, Hoak D, Cavanagh W. Palladium-103 brachytherapy for prostate carcinoma. Int J Rad Oncol Biol Phys 2000; 46:839-850.

4. Brachman DG, Thomas T, Hilbe J, Beyer DC. Failure-free survival following brachytherapy alone or external beam irradiation alone for T1-2 prostate tumors in 2222 patients: results from a single practice. Int J Rad Oncol Biol Phys 2000; 48:111-117.

5. Charyulu KKN. Transperineal interstitial implantation of prostate cancer: A new method. Int J Rad Oncol Biol Phys 1980; 6:1261-1266.

6. Critz FA, Levinson AK, Williams WH, Holladay CT, Griffin VD, Holladay DA. Simultaneous radiotherapy for prostate cancer: 125-prostate implant followed by external-beam radiation. Ca J Sci Am 1998; 4:359-363.

7. Dattoli M, Wallner K, True L, Sorace R, Koval J, et al . Prognostic role of serum prostatic acid phosphatase for 103-Pd-based radiation for prostatic carcinoma. Int J Rad Oncol Biol Phys 1999; 45:853-856.

8. Fuks Z, Leibel SA, Wallner KE, Begg CB, Fair WR, Anderson LL, Hilaris BS, Whitmore WF. The effect of local control on metastatic dissemination in carcinoma of the prostate: Long term results in patients treated with 125-I implantation. Int J Radiat Oncol Biol Phys 1991; 21:337-347.

9. Grado GL, Larson TR, Balch CS, et al . Actuarial disease-free survival after prostate cancer brachytherapy using interactive techniques with biplane ultrasound and fluoroscopic guidance. Int J Radiat Oncol Biol Phys 1998; 42:289-298.

10. Holm HH, Juul N, Pederson JF, Hansen H, Stroyer I. Transperineal 125-Iodine seed implantation in prostatic cancer guided by transrectal ultrasonography. J Urol 1983; 130:283-286.

11. Martinez AA, Kestin LL, Stromberg JS, et al . Interim report of image-guided conformal high-dose-rate brachytherapy for patients with unfavorable prostate cancer: the William Beaumont Phase II dose-escalating trial. Int J Rad Oncol Biol Phys 2000; 47:343-352.

12. Mate TP, Gottesman JE, Hatton J, et al . High dosed-rate after-loading iridium-192 prostate brachytherapy: feasibility report. Int J Rad Oncol Biol Phys 1998; 41:525-533.

13. Osian AD, Anderson LL, Linares LA, Nori D, Hilaris BS. Treatment planning for permanent and temporary percutaneous implants with custom made templates. Int J Rad Oncol Biol Phys 1989; 16:219-223.

14. Ragde H, Elgamal A, Snow P, et al . Ten-year disease free survival after transperineal sonography-guided iodine-125 brachytherapy with or without 45-Gray external beam irradiation in the treatment of patients with clinically localized, low to high Gleason grade prostate carcinoma. Cancer 1998; 83:989-1001.

15. Schellhammer PF, El-Mahdi AM, Wright GL, Kolm P, Ragle R. Prostate-specific antigen to determine progression-free survival after radiation therapy for localized carcinoma of prostate. Urology 1993; 42:13-20.

16. Stein A, deKernion JB, Smith RB, Dorey F, Patel H. Prostate specific antigen levels after radical prostatectomy in patients with organ confined and locally extensive prostate cancer. J Urol 1992; 147:942-946.

17. Syed AM, Puthawala A, Austin P, Cherlow J. Temporary iridium-192 implant in the management of carcinoma of the prostate. Cancer 1992; 69:2515-2524.

18. Whitmore WF, Hilaris B, Grabstald H. Retropubic implantation of Iodine 125 in the treatment of prostatic cancer. J Urol 1972; 108:918-920.

19. Yoshioka Y, Nose T, Yoshida K, et al . High-dose-rate interstitial brachytherapy as a monotherapy for localized prostate cancer: treatment description and preliminary results of a Phase I/II clinical trial. Int J Rad Oncol Biol Phys 2000; 48:675-681.

20. Zelefsky MJ, Hollister T, Raben A, Matthews SM, Wallner KE. Five-year biochemical outcome and toxicity with transperineal CT-planned permanent I-125 prostate implantation for patients with localized prostate cancer. Int J Radiat Oncol Biol Phys 2000; 47:1261-1266.

21. Zietman AL, Edelstein RA, Coen JJ, Babayan RK, Krane RJ. Radical prostatectomy for adenocarcinoma of the prostate: the influence of preoperative and pathologic findings on biochemical disease-free outcome. Urol 1994; 43:828-833.

3

Radiobiology

FEW FACTS, STRETCHED THIN

Radiobiology is a fascinating area of study. Unfortunately, its applicability to clinical decisionmaking is tenuous. Most radiobiologic data is based on theoretical or in vitro experiments. In vivo work has nearly all been derived from transplantable mouse (murine) tumors, which probably behave far differently than spontaneously occurring human tumors (**Table 3-1**).

Nearly all radiobiological data regarding prostate brachytherapy is purely theoretical.(LING 92) While such work is important if we are to make advances beyond what has been learned by clinical trial and error, its practical relevance to current

Table 3-1. Factors that may affect the degree of cell killing, and how much is known about each for human prostate cancers.

Factor	Quantifiable in vivo?
Dose	no*
Dose rate	no*
Damage repair	no
Oxygen enhancement ratio	no
RBE	no
Apoptosis	no
Repopulation	no
Reassortment	no

*even the dose and dose rate can't be quantified precisely, due to rapid fall-off near the sources

medical practice is questionable. The point here is not to belittle such theoretical efforts, but to keep them in perspective.

BRACHYTHERAPY VERSUS EXTERNAL BEAM RADIATION
Brachytherapy and external beam irradiation have three principal differences:

- **dose localization**
- **total dose**
- **dose rate**

All three factors *may* be advantages of brachytherapy over external beam radiation, but data regarding their clinical relevance is scarce.

Dose localization
The rectum is relatively sensitive to radiation, the anterior rectal wall being the principal dose-limiting structure for beam radiation.(LEE, JACKSON) A small rectal area can tolerate a large dose, but as the area irradiated increases so does the risk of complications.(HAN) Even with conformal external radiation, the potential for prostate motion (typically 0.5 cm in the anterior-posterior direction) requires that a relatively large portion of the anterior rectal wall is included in the target volume to avoid underdosing the posterior prostate.

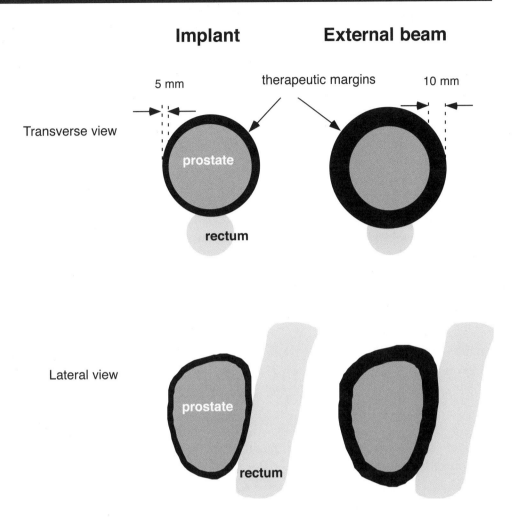

Figure 3-1. Prescription dose in relation to the prostate and rectum for brachytherapy versus beam radiation. Much more rectal surface is included in the high dose region with beam compared to brachytherapy. Lateral view of dose localization to the prostate and rectum with brachytherapy versus beam radiation. With brachytherapy, a smaller portion of the rectum receives the prescription dose, because of rapid dose fall-off and because no allowance need be made for prostate motion.(HAN)

Using brachytherapy, a higher radiation dose can be given to the prostate with less risk of rectal morbidity, probably because of the rapid dose fall-off at the prostatic margins, limiting the rectal surface area that receives the prescription dose or

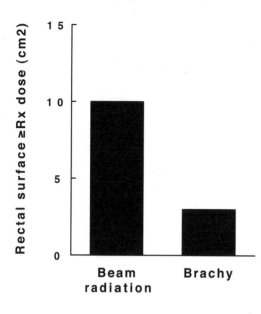

Figure 3-2. Typical anterior rectal wall surface treated to prescription dose or higher with conformal external beam radiation versus brachytherapy.With external beam, approximately twice as much surface receives the prescription dose or higher.(HAN)

higher (**Figure 3-1**). With an implant, approximately 2 to 4 cm^2 rectal surface area receives the prescription dose or higher, in contrast to a typical conformal plan, in which approximately 10 cm^2 of anterior rectal wall receives the prescription dose or higher (**Figure 3-2**).

Bladder tolerance is *not* a dose-limiting concern with prostate brachytherapy or conformal external beam radiation. Because of rapid dose fall-off, no more than 1.0 cm of bladder wall receives the brachytherapy prescription dose. Even with combined brachytherapy plus supplemental beam radiation, bladder irradiation (40 to 50 Gy) is probably of little consequence. Brachytherapy-related urinary morbidity is probably predominantly due to *urethritis*, not cystitis.

Total dose
Total brachytherapy doses are approximately twice those given with external beam radiation (**Figure 3-3**). Total doses of 75 Gy for beam, 144 Gy with I-125, and 124 Gy with Pd-103 are roughly clinically equivalent for patients with pretreatment PSA below 10 ng/ml.(ZELEFSKY 99)

A modification of the TDF tables (time, dose, fractionation) has been made to allow interconvertability between beam radiation and low dose rate brachytherapy.(ORTON) While it reflects current prescription doses, its clinical applicability is unclear.

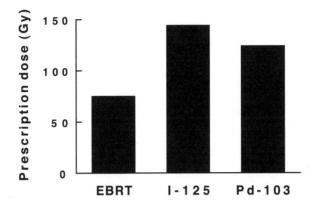

Figure 3-3. Typical external beam prescription dose versus those for I-125 and Pd-103. The brachytherapy dose is approximately twice that delivered with beam radiation.

Dose rate

The most dramatic difference between beam radiation and brachytherapy is in dose rates. The typical initial dose rate of an I-125 or Pd-103 implant is less than 1 percent of the typical 2 to 4 Gy per minute of a linear accelerator (**Figure 3-4**). This marked difference dwarfs the moderate differences in total dose, and may entail substantial differences in radiation damage repair, reassortment, reoxygenation, and redistribution in the cell cycle.

With few exceptions, lower dose rates yield lower cell killing, given the same total dose. As the dose rate gets low enough, its effect diminishes, presumably due to dominance of single hit cell killing. In fact, very little work has been done with dose rates as low as those of I-125/Pd-103 brachytherapy.(LING 95) The comparability of high and low dose rate radiation against human tumors specifically is unknown.

Over what time interval the dose rates should be compared is also unknown. The stated dose rate for any modality is markedly different, depending on the time interval chosen for the denominator. The initial, instantaneous dose rates for beam radiation versus brachytherapy are markedly different, but similar when compared over longer time intervals. For instance, the beam dose rate is typically 10 Gy per week, versus 13 Gy per week for an I-125 implant (**Figure 3-4**). For slow-growing tumors like those of the prostate, dose rates expressed in terms of the longer denominators may be more clinically relevant than those expressed in minutes.

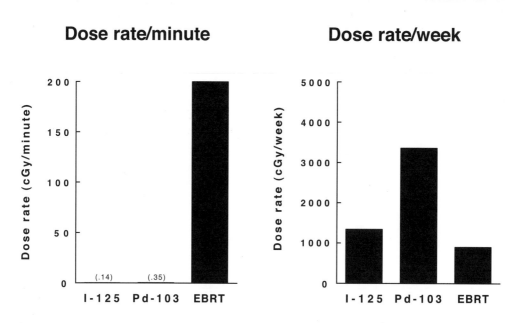

Figure 3-4. The instantaneous dose rate of a linear accelerator is far higher than the dose rate at the periphery of a I-125 or Pd-103 implant (left). However, when compared over a longer time interval, brachytherapy dose rates are similar or greater than that of beam radiation (right). The clinical relevance of how the differences are calculated is not understood.

OXYGEN ENHANCEMENT RATIO (OER)

Sterilizing poorly oxygenated (hypoxic) tumors requires 2.5 to 4.0 times as much radiation as is needed for fully oxygenated tumors. Low dose rate radiation of I-125 or Pd-103 brachytherapy may decrease hypoxia-related radiation resistance.(HALL 74) However, the relationship between the OER and dose rate is complicated, depending on both cell type and the dose rate tested.(LING 85)

While brachytherapy might offer an advantage in eradication of hypoxic tumors, little is known about OER with low dose rate brachytherapy. A wide range of oxygen tensions has been reported in human prostate tumors.(RASEY, MOVSAS 00 & 99) However, judging from the almost uniformly viable appearance of prostate tumors on microscopy, it's unlikely that substantial areas of severe hypoxia exist in most patients' tumors, in contrast to the classic portrayals of histologically evident hypoxic cancer tissue.(HALL 94)

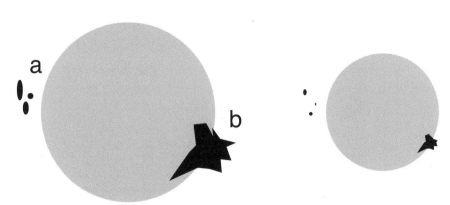

Prehormone   Posthormone

a

b

*Figure 3-5. The physical effect of hormonal therapy in the degree of extraprostatic cancer extension (EPE) depends on which scenario, **a** or **b**, occurs in vivo. If cancer shrinks but remains at a given distance from the prostatic margin, hormonal therapy won't increase the likelihood of eradicating early EPE. However, if the radial extent of cancer decreases (scenario **b**), adjuvant hormonal therapy could increase the likelihood of EPE eradication.*

ADJUVANT HORMONAL THERAPY

There are two rationales for combining androgen deprivation with brachytherapy—physical and biologic. Decreasing the prostate size decreases the volume of rectum, bladder, and small bowel receiving beam radiation.(ZELEFSKY, FORMAN) The same may hold true for brachytherapy rectal wall doses, conceivably decreasing the risk of complications.(WATERMAN) Additional physical advantages to implanting a hormonally downsized prostate include easier access to the anterior prostate in patients for whom pubic arch interference is likely, and a lower number of sources needed.

Perhaps the most clinically important potential advantage of hormonally downsizing the prostate is the possibility that it could facilitate eradication of extraprostatic cancer extension (EPE), if the shrinkage means that EPE retracts back toward the prostatic margin (**Figure 3-5**). However, no studies have been published regarding the effect hormonal therapy has on the magnitude of EPE.

In addition to the potential for physical advantages to hormonal downsizing, hormonal deprivation *may* enhance radiation sensitivity. Adjuvant therapy could

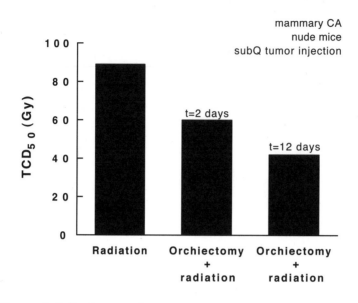

Figure 3-6. Radiation dose required to control 50 percent of androgen-dependent mammary tumors in mice. The hormonal sensitizing effect was greater if more time elapsed between orchiectomy and radiation, possibly due to continued tumor shrinkage with longer antiandrogen effect. (t = time between orchiectomy and radiation)(ZIETMAN)

favorably alter the oxygen milieu of prostate cancer.(RIPPLE) Zietman and colleagues showed that hormonal deprivation increases the radiation sensitivity of androgen-dependent mammary tumors, carried in nude mice.(ZIETMAN) The radiation sensitivity enhancement was most marked if hormonal deprivation was complete more than 48 hours prior to radiation, possibly due to greater volume reduction (**Figure 3-6**). While Zietman and colleagues are to be congratulated for bringing some scientific rigor to the exploration of the biologic effect of hormonal manipulation, the clinical relevance of their experiments in a subcutaneous, transplantable mouse mammary tumor to human prostate cancer is uncertain.

Two large randomized RTOG clinical trials of hormonal ablation combined with radiation have shown a benefit in terms of suppressing overt metastases, but no difference in survival (**Figure 3-7**).(PILEPICH 97 & 95) The most likely explanation is that androgen ablation suppresses the clinical, biochemical, and pathologic evidence of cancer after beam radiation, but does not enhance tumor eradication. This explanation would be consistent with multiple negative surgical trials demonstrating a similar phenomenon with presurgical hormonal ablation.(KLOTZ)

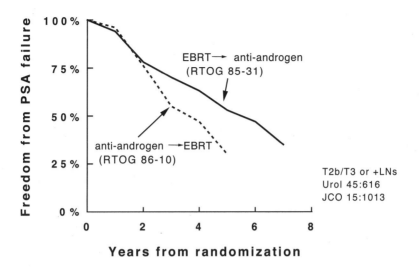

Figure 3-7. Although clinically evident tumor recurrence is delayed with hormonal deprivation, there is still no evidence of a plateau on the disease-free survival curve, whether hormonal ablation preceded (RTOG 86-10) or followed (RTOG 85-31) beam radiation.

Laverdiere and colleagues reported that androgen blockade decreases the likelihood of a positive biopsy after conventional dose external beam radiation.(LAVERDIERE) The effect was most marked if androgen blockade was continued for six months after completion of external radiation (**Figure 3-8**). The findings are compelling but could easily be explained as another example of cancer masking, without a real change in the cure rate. Longer biochemical follow-up should clarify this issue. Unfortunately, the general applicability of Laverdiere's work is hampered by the small patient numbers and incomplete follow-up biopsies.

To date, only one study has shown a clear survival benefit with adjuvant hormonal therapy and external beam radiation.(BOLLA) Patients with clinical stage T3-T4 (any histology) or high grade T2 tumors had a statistically significant improvement in five year overall and disease-free survival. These EORTC findings have been criticized partly because more than 25 percent of the adjuvant patients were still receiving hormonal therapy at the time of the analysis. Additional factors of some concern in the generalizability are the unusually high tumor control rates with or without hormonal therapy, using conventional doses of radiation that have

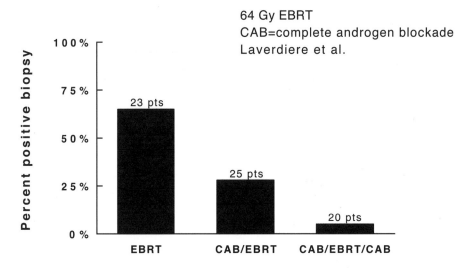

Figure 3-8. Positive biopsy rates after 64 Gy external beam radiation alone, beam radiation preceded by three months androgen blockade, or beam preceded (three months) and followed (six months) by androgen blockade.(LAVERDIERE)

been so ineffective in nearly all studies of patients with more locally advanced cancers.(ZIETMAN 97)

There are still no in vitro, in vivo, or controlled clinical studies regarding the effect of hormonal ablation on brachytherapy radiation sensitivity. Favorable results in uncontrolled studies of brachytherapy patients receiving combined androgen blockade may be explained by better local control with brachytherapy, having nothing to do with adjuvant hormonal therapy.(SYLVESTER) A retrospective, matched-pair analysis of implant patients by Potters and colleagues showed no difference in biochemical freedom from relapse in patients with or without androgen deprivation prior to brachytherapy, regardless of PSA or Gleason score.(POTTERS) The same was reported by Dattoli and colleagues for patients with locally advanced disease.(DATTOLI 99)

APOPTOSIS
Apoptosis is "signal-induced, programmed" cell death, seemingly distinct from mitotic death due to indiscriminate DNA damage. It occurs as a natural involution process in lymphocytes, and to some extent in other tissues. It is probably the mechanism of prostate cell death following androgen deprivation.(MCDONNELL)

The role of apoptosis in radiation-related death of prostate cancer is unclear. It accounts for only a small percent of radiation cell killing in most human cell types, and there is scant evidence that it is important for radiation against prostate cancer.(ALGAN, POLLACK)

HYPERTHERMIA
Hyperthermia is the use of elevated temperature to enhance the cytotoxic effect of radiation. Hyperthermia may act primarily by suppressing sublethal damage repair.(BENHUR, PAULUS) The thermal enhancement ratio varies from 1.0 to 5.0, depending on the temperature and time the hyperthermia is given. Temperatures of 41° to 42°C for 30 to 90 minutes are most practical with the technology currently available.

Hyperthermia generated substantial enthusiasm in the 1980s, when a variety of external and interstitial heating devices were designed for clinical use. Prostate cancer was studied widely, due to accessibility by interstitial heating with radiofrequency antennae. Unfortunately, only locally advanced or recurrent tumors were studied.(PRIONAS) Patients with locally advanced tumors were generally not curable with any local modality available at the time, and the chance of showing a benefit from hyperthermia would have been miniscule.

While there were anecdotal reports of good local response, patients did poorly overall, as would be expected. It is still unclear whether hyperthermia would add to local control.(ALGAN) In the meantime, it has generally fallen out of favor due to technical difficulties achieving homogeneous hyperthermia with available technology.

I-125 VERSUS PD-103
A long-running controversy regards the best isotope for prostate brachytherapy. Theoretical arguments abound, and the ultimate answer may well be that none is clearly superior. But isotope choice *may* be important, and resolving the controversies will require large, well-designed human trials.

Much has been written about the advantages and disadvantages of I-125 versus Pd-103. It has been argued that inferior results with the implants done with I-125 in the 1970s were due to suboptimal radiobiologic properties. Probably not. Retropubic implants were technically poor (see Chapter 2). And the high failure rates likely had little to do with the isotope choice.

In vitro

Low energy photons have a higher linear energy transfer (LET), leading to higher radiobiologic effect (RBE). The higher RBE presumably results from more energy deposition per cell that the photon traverses. The average energy of Pd-103 photons is 21 keV versus 30 keV for I-125, so that Pd-103 would be expected to have a slightly higher LET and RBE.

The RBE of I-125 versus Pd-103 has been compared in only one system—rat embryo cells transfected with Ha-ras oncogene.(LING 95) Using this system, Ling and colleagues reported an I-125 RBE of 1.4, compared to 1.9 for Pd-103. A difference of this magnitude is numerically substantial, and may justify a reduction in total dose by approximately 30 percent. Unfortunately, it has been studied in only one (in vitro) system, and may have little relevance to human prostate tumors.

There are no in vitro studies comparing I-125 to Pd-103 against prostate cancer specifically, due in part to the limited number of cell lines available. There are several rodent models, and only a handful of human models. And the applicability of laboratory-grown immortal murine cancer cell lines to the clinic is highly questionable.

In vivo

Nag and colleagues studied the effect of I-125 versus Pd-103 in transplantable Nb AI-1 prostate tumors in Noble rats.(NAG) At similar doses, tumor growth delay and tumor eradication rates were increased by a factor of 2 or more with Pd-103 versus I-125. The increased tumorcidal effect of Pd-103 was higher than what would be expected by its higher RBE alone, suggesting an enhanced therapeutic ratio.

The results of Nag and colleagues, while intriguing, were based on a limited number of animals (five per group). Large interanimal differences in tumor response to identical treatment require that experiments be repeated multiple times, to give more confidence in the findings. Their findings should also be viewed skeptically because of inconsistencies within the data, especially in that tumor control rates did not increase with increasing dose. Also, their dosimetry was likely far from precise. More in vivo work is needed, using larger numbers of animals and a variety of prostate tumor types, to determine the generalizability of such findings.

Theoretical arguments

Ling has written about the relative efficacy of I-125 and Pd-103, based on theoretical calculations. Based on the biologic effective dose (BED) formula, he calculated that Pd-103 would be more likely to be effective against faster-growing

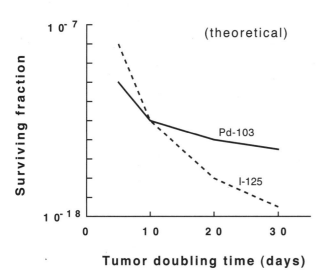

Figure 3-9. Surviving cell fractions following I-125 or Pd-103 versus tumor doubling times. Numbers are theoretical, based on biological equivalent dose calculations.(LING 92) Below is the equation used to determine cell survival levels. The equation contains five variables, the values for which are unknown.

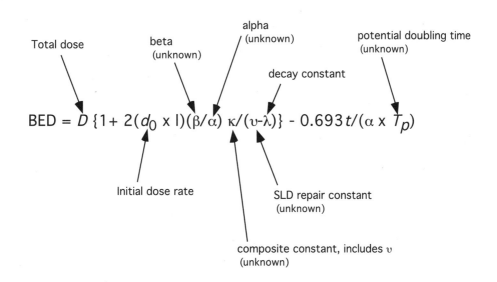

tumors—those with a shorter doubling time (**Figure 3-9**).(LING 92) While interesting and potentially valuable work, its applicability to the clinic is questionable, due to the highly theoretical nature of the data. For instance, a tumor doubling time of less than 10 days is found to be a criteria for better tumor control with Pd-103, while probably all prostate cancers have doubling times far in excess of 10 days.

The core equation used by Ling to calculate the surviving fraction with various isotopes includes five variables of which virtually nothing is known for prostate cancer in humans (**Figure 3-9**). Although the variables would presumably be equivalent for different patients and should essentially "cancel out" in the comparisons between isotopes, use of equations with so little basis in reality should raise skepticism about relevance. This work is of theoretical importance and a good starting point for planning in vitro and in vivo experiments. Basing clinical decisions on it, however, is absurd.

I-125 versus Pd-103: Tpot

Potential tumor doubling time (Tpot) is a balance between the cell proliferation rate and the cell-loss rate. If the proliferation rate increases, or the loss rate decreases, Tpot decreases and tumors grow faster. Tpot can be estimated by the ratio of DNA synthetic phase (S-phase) and the labeling index.(BEGG)

Tpot variability could substantially affect time-related radiation effects. It has been argued that tumors with a more rapid proliferation rate, or shorter Tpot, should be treated with a shorter acting isotope to allow less time for cell repopulation during the radiation interval.(LING 92)

Determination of tumor doubling times is still in its infancy. Results with human tumors in general have been mixed.(BOURHIS) Using an antibromodeoxyuridine monoclonal antibody, the percent of S-phase cells has been correlated with Gleason score.(NEMOTO) Using bromodeoxuridine administered prior to needle biopsy, Scrivner and colleagues showed that the labeling index correlated with Gleason score.(SCRIVNER) In contrast, Haustermans and colleagues found no correlation between Tpot and Gleason score.(HAUSTERMANS)

It is possible that such indexes of tumor growth rates could be used to guide isotope choice. Use of such tests, however, is clouded by tumor heterogeneity, by which different parts of a tumor have different S-phase fractions, just as there is heterogeneity of the Gleason score within a tumor. To date, no clinical reports are available regarding Tpot and radiation response in human prostate cancer.

I-125 versus Pd-103: Clinical

To date, retrospective studies have failed to show a difference in morbidity or tumor-control rates for low-risk patients.(CHA, GELBLUM) In one retrospective study, Yale investigators showed a lower complication rate with Pd-103, but the Pd-103 patients were treated in the later time periods, such that any decrease in

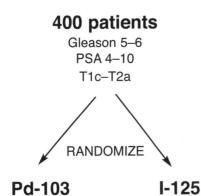

400 patients
Gleason 5–6
PSA 4–10
T1c–T2a

RANDOMIZE

Pd-103   **I-125**

Figure 3-10. Design of an ongoing randomized trial between I-125 and Pd-103 for early stage, low-risk cancers. The study has accrued 300 patients as of July 2001 (WALLNER)

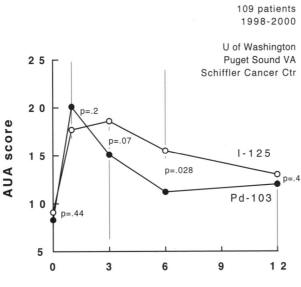

Figure 3-11. Mean AUA scores return to baseline sooner after Pd-103 implantation than after I-125.(WALLNER)

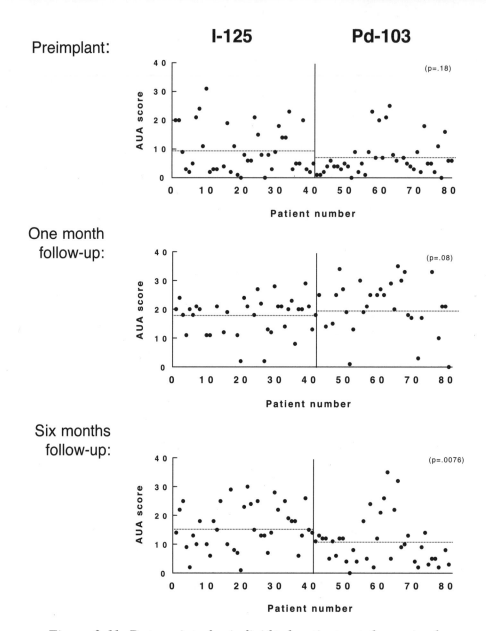

Figure 3-11. Data points for individual patients at the preimplant, one and six months time points. Although the differences between isotopes are statistically different, note the large amount of scatter in the data.

complications may have been due simply to better implantation technique, rather than a true difference in biology.(PESCHEL)

Because of patient-selection criteria related to preconceived notions regarding isotope choice, retrospective studies are unlikely to definitively answer questions regarding the effect of isotope choice on cure rates and morbidity. One ongoing prospective study led by Wallner, Merrick, and colleagues is accruing 400 patients, randomized to I-125 versus Pd-103 (**Figure 3-10**). An early look at the quality-of-life outcomes shows quicker resolution of radiation-related symptoms at six months postimplant, but with substantial scatter in the data (**Figures 3-11 &13-12**). Preliminary data regarding tumor control rates will be available by 2004.

DO WE NEED A RADIATION SENSITIZER?
Much effort has been expended to develop chemical radiation sensitizers (enhancers), but without success. In fact, radiation sensitizers may be of limited value for prostate cancer, given the high negative biopsy rates after brachytherapy.(PRESTIDGE) It appears that local control can be achieved in most cases. The remaining impediment to increased cure rates will be the presence of micrometastases at the time of diagnosis. Better systemic cytotoxic agents would likely be more helpful than a radiation sensitizer.

HUMAN TUMORS—THE GREAT UNKNOWN
Almost nothing is known about radiobiology of brachytherapy against prostate human tumors specifically. Existing in vivo and vitro work has been done primarily with rodent-derived cell lines, with questionable applicability to human prostate cancers. Work with more closely related tumor models might offer some insight as to how best to use the isotopes available, and perhaps how best to combine them with beam radiation. This is an opportunity for the radiation oncology community to revive radiobiology, an area that has been hard hit by cynicism and budgetary constraints.

REFERENCES
1. Algan O, Stobbe CC, Helt AM, Hanks GE. Radiation inactivation of human prostate cancer cells: the role of apoptosis. Radiat Res 1996; 146:267-275.

2. Begg AC, McNally NJ. A method to measure the duration of DNA synthesis and the potential doubling time from a single sample. Cytometry 1997; 6:620-623.

3. BenHur E, Elkind MM, Bronk BV. Thermally enhanced radioresponse of cultured Chinese hamster cells: inhibition of repair of sublethal damage and enhancement of lethal damage. Radiat Res 1974; 58:38-51.

4. Bolla M, Gonzalez D, Warde P, et al . Improved survival in patients with locally advanced prostate cancer treated with radiotherapy and goserelin. NEJM 1997; 337:295-300.

5. Bourhis J, Dendale R, Hill C, Bosq J. Potential doubling time and clinical outcome in head and neck squamous cell carcinoma treated with 70 Gy in 7 weeks. Int J Radiat Oncol Biol Phys 1996; 35:471-476.

6. Cha CM, Potters L, Ashley R, et al . Isotope selection for patients undergoing prostate brachytherapy. Int J Rad Oncol Biol Phys 1999; 45:391-395.

7. Dattoli M, Wallner K, True L, Sorace R, Koval J, et al . Prognostic role of serum prostatic acid phosphatase for 103-Pd-based radiation for prostatic carcinoma. Int J Rad Oncol Biol Phys 1999; 45:853-856.

8. Forman JD, Kumar R, Haas G, Montie J. Neoadjuvant hormonal downsizing of localized carcinoma of the prostate: Effects on the volume of normal tissue irradiation. Ca Invest 1995; 13:8-15.

9. Gelblum DY, Potters L, Ashley R, Waldbaum R, Wang X, Leibel S. Urinary morbidity following ultrasound-guided transperineal prostate seed implantation. Int J Rad Oncol Biol Phys 1999; 45:59-67.

10. Hall EJ. Radiobiology for the radiologist. Philadelphia: J. B. Lippincott, 1994.

11. Hall EJ, Roizin-Towle LA, Colvett RD. RBE and OER determinations for Radium and Californium-252. Radiol 1974; 112:425-430.

12. Han B, Wallner K. Dosimetric and radiographic correlates to prostate brachytherapy-related rectal complications. (submitted) 2002;

13. Han B, Wallner K, Aggarwal S, Armstrong J, Sutlief S. Treatment margins for prostate brachytherapy. Sem in Urol Oncol 2000; 18:137-141.

14. Haustermans KMG, Hofland I, Van Poppel H, et al . Cell kinetic measurements in prostate cancer. Int J Rad Oncol Biol Phys 1997; 37:1067-1070.

15. Jackson A, Skwarchuk MW, Zelefsky MJ, Cowen DM, et al . Late rectal bleeding after conformal radiotherapy of prostate cancer (II): Volume effects and dose-volume histograms. Int J Rad Oncol Biol Phys 2001; 49:685-698.

16. Klotz LH, Goldenberg SL, Jewett M, Barkin J, et al . CUOG randomized trial of neoadjuvant androgen ablation before radical prostatectomy: 36-month post-treatment PSA results. Urol 1999; 53:757-763.

17. Laverdiere J, Gomez JL, Cusan L, Suburu ER. Beneficial effect of combination hormonal therapy administered prior and following external beam radiation therapy in localized prostate cancer. Int J Rad Oncol Biol Phys 1997; 37:247-252.

18. Lee WR, Hanks GE, Hanlon AL, Schultheiss TE, Hunt MA. Lateral rectal shielding reduces late rectal morbidity following high dose three-dimensional conformal radiation therapy for clinically localized prostate cancer: further evidence for a significant dose effect. Int J Rad Oncol Biol Phys 1996; 35:251-257.

19. Ling CC. Permanent implants using Au-198, Pd-103 and I-125: radiobiological considerations based on the linear quadratic model. Int J Radiat Oncol Biol Phys 1992; 23:81-87.

20. Ling CC, Li WX, Anderson LL. The relative biological effectiveness of I-125 and Pd-103. Int J Radiat Oncol Biol Phys 1995; 32:373-378.

21. Ling CC, Spiro IJ, Mitchell J, Stickler R. The variation of OER with dose rate. Int J Radiat Oncol Biol Phys 1985; 11:1367-1373.

22. McDonnell TJ, Troncoso P, Brisbay SM, Logothetis C. Expression of the pro-toooncogene bel-2 in the prostate and its association with emergence of androgen-independent prostate cancer. Ca Res 1992; 52:6940-6944.

23. Movsas B, Chapman JD, Greenberg RE, Hanlon AL, et al . Increasing levels of hypoxia in prostate carcinoma correlate significantly with increasing clinical stage and patient age: an Eppendorf pO2 study. Cancer 2000; 89:2018-2024.

24. Movsas B, Chapman JD, Horwitz EM, et al . Hypoxic regions exist in human prostate carcinoma. Urol 1999; 53:11-18.

25. Nag S, Sweeney PJ, Wienthjes MG. Dose-response study of Iodine-125 and Palladium-103 brachytherapy in a rat prostate tumor (Nb-AI-1). Endocur/Hypertherm 1997; 9:97-104.

26. Nemoto R, Uchida K, Shiimazui T, Hattori K. Immunocytochemical demonstration of S phase cells by anti-bromodeoyuridine monoclonal antibody in humna prostate adenocarcinoma. J Urol 1989; 141:337-340.

27. Orton CG, Webber BM. Time-dose factor (TDF) analysis of dose rate effects in permanent implant dosimetry. Int J Radiat Oncol Biol Phys 1977; 2:55-60.

28. Paulus JA, Tucker RD, Loening SA, Flanagan SW. Thermal ablation of canine prostate using interstitial temperature self-regulating seeds: New treatment for prostate cancer. J Endourol 1997; 11:295-300.

29. Peschel RE, Chen Z, Roberts K, Nath R. Long-term complications with prostate implants: Iodine-125 vs. Palladium-103. Radiat Oncol Invest 1999; 7:278-288.

30. Pilepich MV, Caplan R, Byhardt RW, Lawton CA. Phase III trial of androgen suppression using goserelin in unfavorable-prognosis carcinoma of the prostate treated with definitive radiotherapy: Report of Radiation Therapy Oncology Group Protocol 85-31. J Clin Oncol 1997; 15:1013-1021.

31. Pilepich MV, Sause WT, Shipley WU, Krall JM. Androgen deprivation with radiation therapy compared with radiation therapy alone for locally advanced prostatic carcinoma: A randomized comparative trial of the Radiation Therapy Oncology Group. Urol 1995; 45:616-623.

32. Pollack A, Ashoori F, Sikes C, et al . The early supra-additive apoptotic response of R3327-G prostate tumors to androgen ablation and radiation is not sustained with multiple fractions. Int J Rad Oncol Biol Phys 2000; 46:153-158.

33. Potters L, Torre T, Ashley R, et al . Examining the role of neoadjuvant androgen deprivation in patients undergoing prostate brachytherapy. J Clin Oncol 2000; 18:1187-1192.

34. Prestidge BR, Hoak DC, Grimm PD, Ragde H, Cavanagh W, Blasko JC. Posttreatment biopsy results following interstitial brachytherapy in early-stage prostate cancer. Int J Radiat Oncol Biol Phys 1997; 37:31.

35. Prionas SD, Kapp DS, Goffinet DR, Ben-Yosef R. Thermometry of interstitial hyperthermia given as an adjuvant to brachytherapy for the treatment of carcinoma of the prostate. Int J Radiat Oncol Biol Phys 1993; 28:151-162.

36. Rasey JS, Koh W-J, Evans ML, et al . Quantifying regional hypoxia in human tumors with positron emission tomography of fluoromisonidazole. Int J Rad Oncol Biol Phys 1996; 36:417-428.

37. Ripple M, Henry W, Rago R, Wilding G. Prooxidant-antioxidant shift induced by androgen treatment of humna prostate carcinoma cells. J Natl Ca Inst 1997; 89:40-48.

38. Scrivner DL, Meyer JS, Rujanavech N, Fathman A. Cell kinetics by bromodeoxyuridine labeling and deoxyribonucleic acid ploidy in prostatic carcinoma needle biopsies. J Urol 1991; 146:1034-1039.

39. Sylvester J, Blasko JC, Grimm PD, et al . Neoadjuvant androgen ablation combined with external-beam radiation therapy and permanent interstitial brachytherapy boost in localized prostate cancer. Mol Urol 2000; 3:231-236.

40. Wallner K, Merrick G, True L, Kattan M, Cavanagh W, Simpson C, Butler W. I-125 versus Pd-103 for low risk prostate cancer: Preliminary urinary functional outcomes from a prospective randomized multicenter trial. Journal of Brachytherapy International 2000; 16:151-155.

41. Waterman FM, Dicker AP. Effect of post-implant edema on the rectal dose in prostate brachytherapy. Int J Rad Oncol Biol Phys 1999; 45:571-576.

42. Zelefsky MJ, Leibel SA, Burman CM, Kutcher GJ. Neoadjuvant hormonal therapy improves the therapeutic ratio in patients with bulky prostatic cancer treated with three-dimensional conformal radiation therapy. Int J Radiat Oncol Biol Phys 1994; 29:755-761.

43. Zelefsky MJ, Wallner KE, Ling CC, Raben A, et al . Comparison of the 5-year outcome and morbidity of three-dimensional conformal radiotherapy versus transperineal permanent iodine-125 implantation for earl-stage prostatic cancer. J Clin Oncol 1999; 17:517-522.

44. Zietman AL, Coen JJ, Shipley WU, Willett CG, Efird JT. Radical radiation therapy in the management of prostatic adenocarcinoma: The initial prostate specific antigen value as a predictor of treatment outcome. J Urol 1994; 151:640-645.

45. Zietman AL, Nakfoor BM, Prince EA, Gerweck LE. The effect of androgen deprivation and radiation therapy on an androgen-sensitive murine tumor: An in vitro and in vivo study. Ca J 1997; 3:31-36.

4

TRUS, CT, or MR?

The introduction of transrectal ultrasound (TRUS) was the primary technological breakthrough behind the resurgence of prostate brachytherapy, making it possible to image the prostate for treatment planning and to monitor needle position during the implant procedure. Computerized tomography (CT) played a supporting role in the resurgence of prostate brachytherapy, being the basis for post-implant dosimetry (quality assurance). In the future, both CT and magnetic resonance imaging (MR) may play a larger role.

Preimplant prostate contours, used to determine the number and arrangement of sources, can be derived from TRUS, CT, or MR images. Each modality has its

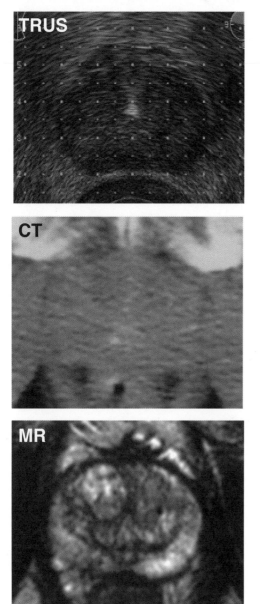

Figure 4-1. Cross section at mid prostate, viewed by TRUS, CT, and MR. TRUS usually gives a sharp image of the prostate contour, while MR gives a better image of internal architecture. CT typically gives the least sharp image of internal architecture and outer contour but shows the spatial relationship between the prostate gland, pubic bones, and rectum.

advantages and disadvantages. Currently, nearly all brachytherapists use TRUS for planning and intraoperative visualization. However, there is substantial interest in substituting MR or CT for TRUS.(HURWITZ, ZAIDER, PICKETT)

The appearance of the prostate and the periprostatic region varies markedly between imaging techniques (**Figure 4-1**). But despite their qualitative differences, the prostate shape and size are fairly consistent between modalities, if interpreted correctly. Until we have a reliable way to image microscopic disease within the prostate, it is the prostatic *margins* that determine how many and in what arrangement the sources should be placed.

Past reports of inconsistent prostate volume determinations with different imaging techniques were more likely due to image misinterpretation than to problems with the modalities per se. Unfortunately, interpretation pitfalls have led to a contradictory body of literature.

TRUS

Quick and easy real-time imaging is the most compelling aspect of TRUS, allowing visualization of needles within the prostate during the procedure. Whether you're doing pre- or intraoperative planning (see chapter 6), the prostate contour and the volume it defines is the primary determinant of the radioactivity needed and how it is placed. The sharp contour of TRUS images minimizes interobserver inconsistencies. In particular, the posterior prostate contour is sharply delineated, helping to avoid excessive rectal doses.

Although real-time TRUS images show a fairly sharp prostatic margin, the images may underestimate the true prostatic size. Several conflicting reports describe the relation between TRUS-based volumes and those determined from the prostatectomy specimen. Rahmouni and colleagues, from Johns Hopkins University (JHU), compared preoperative TRUS and MR prostate volumes with those of the resected gland.(RAHMOUNI) In their hands, the TRUS volume was only 70 percent of that measured at the time of prostatectomy (**Figure 4-2**).

The JHU investigators' finding that TRUS grossly underestimates the prostate volume might be criticized on the grounds that the prostatic volumes were calculated by the elliptical volume formula (.525 x D1 x D2 x D3 [where D1–D3 are the prostatic orthogonal dimensions]) rather than step-section planimetry. However, other investigators have reported that prostate volumes are similar, on average, when determined by step-section planimetry or elliptical volume estimation.(TERRIS) In fact, Stone and colleagues reported that prostate volumes are generally *smaller* with step-section planimetry than with an elliptical volume approximation. If so, underestimation of the prostate volume by step-sectioning could be even more marked than that reported by Rahmouni.(STONE)

Other investigators have found less discrepancy between TRUS volume and the volume of the resected prostate.(BARTSCH) Differences among investigators might be explained by disparity in how TRUS images are interpreted, formulas used to

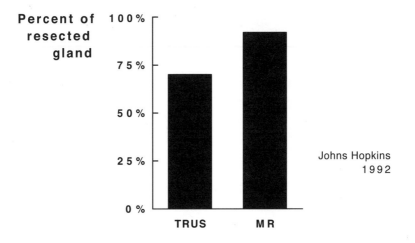

Figure 4-2. Prostate volume measured from prostatectomy specimens versus pre-op TRUS or MR.(RAHMOUNI)

approximate the volume, equipment differences, or how the specimens are processed.

The biggest disadvantage of TRUS is the potential for inter- and intraobserver variability. Average differences of 5% to 25% have been reported when patients are rescanned by the same ultrasonographer on the same day.(BATES, BAZINET) For scans performed in succession by two different observers, a variability of about 10% has been reported.(BATES) The lack of reproducibility is not explained by image interpretation alone, because computer-assisted interpretation does not diminish the inter- or intraobserver variability.(NATHAN) Variability in prostate volume determinations is not explained by differences in ultrasound probe angulation, which leads to only 2 to 4% changes in the volume.(NATHAN) Another potential confounding issue is that prostate volume and shape may change in fully awake versus anesthetized patients. The degree of variability may be less if planimetry, rather that dimension-estimated volumes, is used.(AARNINK)

Reproducibility problems may be partly explained by real, physiologic variations. Prostate volume, measured by TRUS or MR, has been reported to change by approximately 10% from day to day, a variation that is consistent between TRUS and MR; these are likely *real* changes in volume rather than an inconsistent TRUS technique.(AL-RIMAWI)

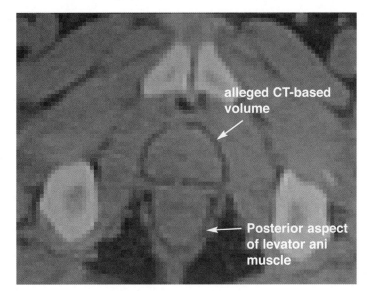

Figure 4-3. Magnification of previously published CT-based prostate margin drawn by Roach and colleagues at UCSF, comparing prostate volumes by CT versus MR.(ROACH) *In this example, the levator muscles are included in the target volume, giving an artificially large CT prostate volume. Excluding nonprostatic tissue, like the levator ani, should lead to a more accurate prostate volume determination. Dr Roach agrees (personal communication).*

We have seen some pretty weird TRUS volume studies from outside institutions, probably due to excessive probe pressure against the prostate (see chapter 6). The effect that reproducibility problems have on clinical outcomes is unknown, but it could be substantial. Falsely low prostate volumes could lead to inadequate dose coverage, and falsely high volumes could lead to complications from overradiation of normal tissues.(NARAYANA)

Despite some early claims to the contrary, TRUS cannot reliably image the presence or extent of intraprostatic cancers.(RIFKIN)

CT
The primary advantages of CT over other techniques are that CT can image sources more clearly and delineate the pubic bones more precisely than the other modalities can. Also, CT is far less operator-dependent that TRUS and requires minimal patient preparation.

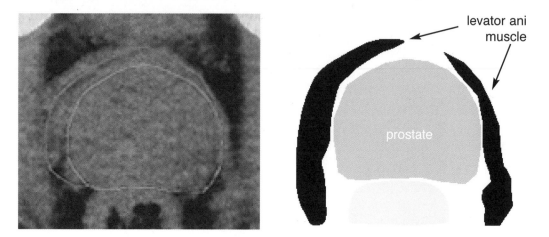

Figure 4-4. In this example of CT interpretation at Fox Chase Cancer Center, the levator ani muscle has been included with the authors' determination of the CT-based lateral prostatic margin, giving a falsely large prostate volume.(KAGAWA) The outer light line is their tracing of the prostate on the left, based on CT. The inner light line is their tracing of the prostate from MR, overlaid on the CT image. On the right is a line drawing of their published image, with K. Wallner's tracing of levator ani muscles and prostate as they appear on the Fox Chase CT image, nearly identical to the Fox Chase MR tracing!

Like TRUS, there are conflicting reports regarding the accuracy of CT prostate volume determination, with most investigators reporting that CT volumes are larger than those determined by TRUS. Roach and colleagues, for example, reported that CT volumes were approximately 30% larger than MR-based volumes.(ROACH) The volumes determined by the UCSF investigators, however, were probably excessive. Judging from the representative case shown in the Roach paper, the levator ani musculature was included within the target volume (**Figure 4-3**). Doing so would erroneously increase the prostatic volume. Similar overinterpretation of the prostate contour was evident in a publication from Fox Chase Cancer Center (**Figure 4-4**). **Figure 4-5** shows a particularly striking example of the separation between the prostate and the levator ani musculature.

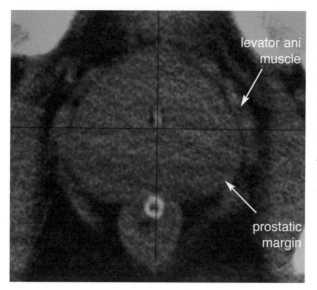

levator ani
muscle

prostatic
margin

Figure 4-5. Unusually clear example of the separation between prostatic margin and levator ani musculature. This degree of clarity is not typical, but it serves to illustrate the potential to overdraw the prostatic volume if the levator ani muscles are included.

To clarify the use of CT versus TRUS for preplanning, CT and TRUS images from ten consecutive, unselected patients from the University of Washington were analyzed by Badiozamani and colleagues.(BADIOZAMANI) Each patient underwent a preimplant TRUS volume study and pelvic CT scan on the same day. To test for consistency between observers, the CT volumes were drawn independently by Badiozamani, Wallner, and Blasko. The CT-based volumes ranged from 31 cc to 48 cc and the TRUS-based volumes ranged from 27 cc to 46 cc. There was close agreement in the determinations between imaging modalities (**Figure 4-6**), includ-

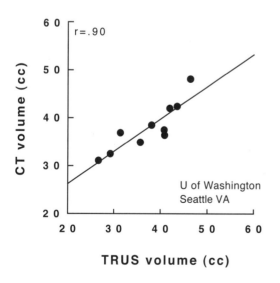

r=.90

U of Washington
Seattle VA

Figure 4-6. Prostate volume measured by TRUS versus CT. If the levator ani muscles are not included in the prostate volume, the volumes are almost identical. (BADIOZA-MANI)

4.7

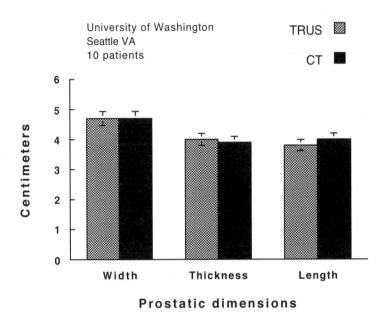

Figure 4-7. Anterior-posterior (thickness), lateral, and cranio-caudal dimensions determined by CT versus TRUS.

ing the anterior-posterior, lateral, and cranio-caudal prostatic dimensions (**Figure 4-7**). The measurements were consistent between observers (**Figure 4-8**). The practical significance of the University of Washington study is that CT and TRUS images can be substituted for each other in preimplant prostate volume determinations, if the CT images are not overinterpreted.

The primary limitation of CT-based implants is the lack of real-time imaging. While intra-op CT scanning would offer some advantages over current TRUS-based methods, intra-op CT scanning is currently not practical due to technical costs and lack of working space in most CT facilities. Portable scanners are commercially available, but to date they have not generated much interest by the prostate brachytherapy community. With wider availability of faster scan reconstruction capability and smaller, portable scanners or CT simulators, real-time intraoperative CT scanning could catch on. It would enable intraoperative CT-based dosimetric analysis, and the opportunity to add supplemental sources as needed to achieve adequate prostatic dose coverage.

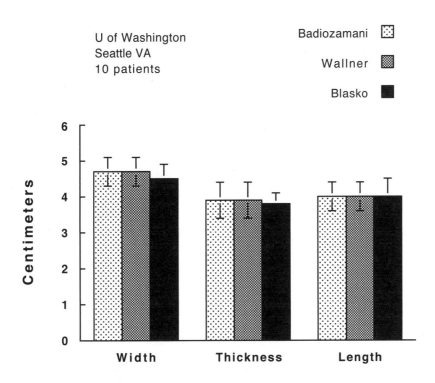

Figure 4-8. In the UW study of CT versus TRUS imaging, interpretation of prostate CT images in each dimension was consistent between the three physician authors.

MR

MR images show a dramatically sharper prostatic margin than CT or TRUS, potentially decreasing the subjectivity in image interpretation and making the planning and evaluation processes more reproducible. MR also shows the most detailed image of the internal architecture of the prostate. But while striking in their degree of detail, the clinical utility of parenchymal imaging is questionable, because nearly all of the prostate should still be treated to prescription dose to sterilize areas of potential microscopic disease.

The primary disadvantage of MR, like that of CT, is that real-time MR is not readily available. However, there is some interest in developing easier access to real-time imaging, and more widespread adoption of MR techniques may occur.(HURWITZ, DUBOIS, AMDUR, MOERLAND, ZAIDER) Another disadvantage of MR, in the current clinical setting, is its price. Patient charges for a diagnostic pelvic MR are two to three times those for a TRUS or CT, extra charges that are difficult to justify in

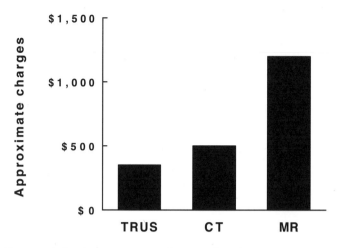

Figure 4-9. Approximate charges for diagnostic TRUS , CT, or MR.

the absence of a large randomized trial showing higher cure rates with MR versus TRUS-based implants (**Figure 4-9**).

DOES IT MATTER?

Controversy continues as to the relative accuracy, reproducibility, and practical merits of the different prostate imaging modalities. That the clinical results with modern transperineal brachytherapy appear favorable, even with widely varying techniques, probably means that the differences described above are of little practical consequence. Good treatment planning and operator skill are likely far more important than the particular imaging equipment used. However, substantial differences in imaging technology or image interpretation could have serious consequences—underestimation of prostate volume could lead to substantial underdose of the prostatic periphery, and overestimation could increase the likelihood of complications.(NARAYANA)

A significant practical reason for clarifying the relative accuracy of the various imaging modalities is the ability to interchange prostate volume information between modalities. If CT, TRUS, and MR images give similar prostate volumes, one set of images can be substituted for the other, making the choice of modality more one of convenience. For instance, CT images are routinely used at the Veterans Administration Puget Sound Health Care System to plan TRUS-based implants. Doing so avoids more labor-intensive TRUS imaging for brachytherapy planning. Additionally, it allows for preplanning of out-of-state patients without having them make a preliminary trip just to have a planning TRUS done to our specifications, because CT scans are rarely subject to technical differences between institutions.

REFERENCES

1. Aarnink RG, De La Rosetter JJ, Debruyne FMJ, Wijkstra H. Reproducibility of prostate volume measurements from transrectal ultrasonography by an automated and a manual technique. Br J Urol 1996; 78:219-223.

2. Al-rimawi M, Griffiths DJ, Boake RC, Mador DR. Transrectal ultrasound versus magnetic resonance imaging in the estimation of prostatic volume. Br J Urol 1994; 74:596-600.

3. Amdur RJ, Gladstone D, Leopold KA, Harris RD. Prostate seed implant quality assessment using MR and CT image fusion. Int J Radiat Oncol Biolo Phys 1999; 43:67-72.

4. Badiozamani KR, Wallner KE, Cavanagh W, Blasko J. Comparability of CT-based and TRUS-based prostate volumes. Int J Rad Oncol Biol Phys 1999; 43:375-378.

5. Bartsch G, Egender G, Hubscher H, Rohr H. Sonometrics of the prostate. J Urol 1982; 127:1119-1121.

6. Bates TS, Reynard JM, Peters TJ, Gingell JC. Determination of prostatic volume with transrectal ultrasound: A study of intra-observer and interobserver variation. J Urol 1996; 155:1299-1300.

7. Bazinet M, Karakiewicz PI, Aprikian A, Trudel C. Reassessment of nonplanimetric transrectal ultrasound prostate volume estimates. Urol 1996; 47:857-862.

8. Dubois FD, Prestidge BR, Hotchkiss LA, Bice WS, Prete JJ. Source localization following permanent transperineal prostate intersititial brachytherapy using magnetic resonance imaging. Int J Radiat Oncol Biol Phys 1997; 39:1037-1041.

9. Hurwitz MD, Cormack R, Tempany CM, et al . Three-dimensional real-time magnetic resonance-guided interstitial prostate brachytherapy optimizes radiation dose distribution resulting in a favorable acute side effect profile in patients with clinically localized prostate cancer. Tech Urol 2000; 6:89-94.

10. Kagawa K, Lee WR, Schultheiss TE, Hunt MA, Shaer AH, Hanks GE. Initial clinical assessment of CT-MRI image fusion software in localization of the prostate for 3D conformal radiation therapy. Int J Radiat Oncol Biol Phys 1997; 38:319-325.

11. Moerland MA, Wijrdeman HK, Beersma R, Bakker CJG. Evaluation of permanent I-125 prostate implants using radiography and magnetic resonance imaging. Int J Radiat Oncol Biol Phys 1997; 37:927-933.

12. Narayana V, Roberson PL, Winfield RJ, McLaughlin PW. Impact of ultrasound and computed tomography prostate volume registration on evaluation of permanent prostate implants. Int J Radiat Oncol Biolo Phys 1997; 39:341-346.

13. Nathan MS, Seenivasagam K, Mei Q, Wickham JEA. Transrectal ultrasonography: why are estimates of prostate volume and dimension so inaccurate? Br J Urol 1996; 77:401-407.

14. Pickett B, Vigneault E, Kurhanewicz J, Verhey L, Roach M. Static field intensity modulation to treat a dominant intra-prostatic lesion to 90 Gy compared to seven field 3-dimensional radiotherapy. Int J Rad Oncol Biol Phys 1999; 43:921-929.

15. Rahmouni A, Yang A, Tempany C, Frenkel T. Accuracy of in-vivo assessment of prostatic volume by MRI and transrectal ultrasonography. J Comp Assist Tomo 1992; 16:935-940.

16. Rifkin MD, Zerhouni EA, Gatsonis CA, Quint LE. Comparison of magnetic resonance imaging and ultrasonography in staging early prostate cancer. NEJM 1990; 323:621-626.

17. Roach M, Faillace-akazawa P, Malfatti C, Holland J. Prostate volumes defined by magnetic resonance imaging and computerized tomographic scans for three-dimensional conformal radiotherapy. Int J Rad Oncol Biol Phys 1996; 35:1011-1018.

18. Stone NN, Stock RG, DeWyngaert JK, Tabert A. Prostate brachytherapy: Improvements in prostate volume measurements and dose distribution using interactive ultrasound guided implantation and three-dimensional dosimetry. Radiat Oncol Invest 1995; 3:185-195.

19. Terris MK, Stamey TA. Determination of prostate volume by transrectal ultrasound. J Urol 1991; 145:984-987.

20. Zaider M, Zelefsky MJ, Lee EK, et al . Treatment planning for prostate implants using magnetic-resonance sprectroscopy imaging. Int J Rad Oncol Biol Phys 2000; 47:1085-1096.

5

Sources

I-125, Pd-103, and Ir-192 are the radioisotopes commonly used for prostate brachytherapy. Radioactive gold (Au-198) has some theoretical appeal, but it is not widely available because of its short half-life and onerous radiation protection requirements secondary to its high energy.(BUTLER, LOENING)

TEMPORARY VERSUS PERMANENT IMPLANTS

Prostate brachytherapy can be done with permanent or temporary source placement. Ir-192 brachytherapy, with ribbons of sources placed inside plastic hollow catheters, is termed *temporary,* because the sources are removed after the dose is delivered.

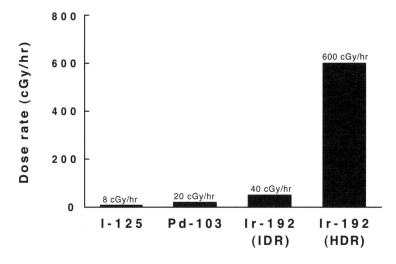

Figure 5-1. Initial dose rate to the prostate periphery with I-125, Pd-103 or Ir-192 implants. (IDR=intermediate dose rate, HDR=high dose rate)

Traditionally, Ir-192 sources were left in place for two to four days, delivering a 20–30 Gy boost to an abbreviated course of external beam radiation (~40 Gy). The boost was delivered at about 50 cGy/hour, an *intermediate* dose rate. Intermediate dose rate temporary implants have been largely replaced by *high dose rate* (HDR) Ir-192 implants, delivering 10–20 Gy in a few minutes.

Dose rates for removable Ir-192 implants are far higher than those for I-125 or Pd-103 permanent implants (**Figure 5-1**), but the clinical implications of the different rates are not clear (see chapter 3). Clinical results, comparable to permanent implants, have been reported for Ir-192 implants.(MATE, MARTINEZ)

Temporary HDR brachytherapy has its practical advantages and disadvantages. The principal advantage is that source insertion time can be modified to adjust for less-than-ideal needle placement, as determined from real-time CT or TRUS.(EDMUNDSON) The option to adjust the loading time is appealing because it allows modification of the implant dosimetry *after* needle placement. With permanent implants, the only way to modify dosimetry after the sources are placed is to take the patient back to the operating room to place more sources. And if too

Table 5.1. Pros and cons of permanent versus temporary implants.

	Pros	Cons
I-125/Pd-103:	Convenient Substantial PSA-based data	Can't alter source loading
Ir-192:	Can alter source loading Re-use sources	Need for supplemental external beam radiation Less convenient

many permanent sources are inadvertently placed, they cannot be removed, short of doing a prostatectomy.

A second advantage of temporary or *remote afterloading* techniques (HDR) is that after the source is removed, no radioactivity remains and no radioprotection precautions are needed. A third advantage of HDR is the ability to reuse sources. Each Ir-192 source typically lasts for three to four months. At $10,000 per source change, reusing them offers a significant savings over I-125 or Pd-103 sources, which cost several thousand dollars per patient. (But a significant cost savings would be seen only in a large patient volume practice, due to the purchase price and maintenance of the HDR machine.)

The biggest disadvantage to temporary implants is the routine use of supplemental external beam radiation. To date, long-term reports of Ir-192 brachytherapy have used it as a boost to 40–45 Gy external beam radiation. In contrast, permanent implants are typically used as sole therapy, avoiding the inconvenience and cost of supplemental beam radiation. There is interest in devising proper dose schemes to use temporary implants as stand-alone therapy, but meaningful tumor cure rate data for HDR alone won't be available until at least 2005.

A second disadvantage of HDR is the need for overnight hospitalization or repeated needle placement on different days, as opposed to the one-time, outpatient I-125 or Pd-103 procedure. Another concern is that giving the entire implant dose (≥ 8 Gy) in a single day may invite complications. A third disadvantage of HDR is the need for radiation shielding of the treatment area, an expensive endeavor for some out-of-hospital patient-care centers. The use of temporary Ir-192 implants has fallen in popularity, relative to permanent implants (see Figure

Half-life

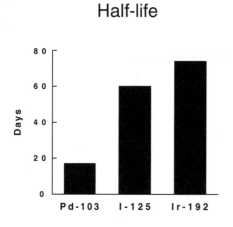

Tissue half-value layer

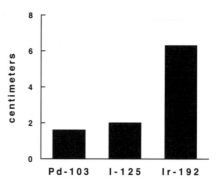

Average photon energy

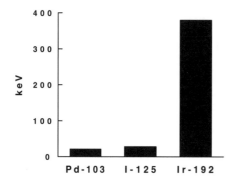

Figure 5-2. Physical characteristics of radionuclides used for prostate brachytherapy.

2-6). While Ir-192-based implants have some appealing aspects, a significant shift back to their use in the near future seems unlikely.

PERMANENT IMPLANTS

I-125 and Pd-103, the commonly used radionuclides for permanent prostatic implants, differ in their half-life and photon energy, factors that may influence their biologic effects (**Figure 5-2**).

Iodine-125

I-125 is produced in a nuclear reactor, from Xe-124. I-125 decays, by electron capture and internal conversion, to Te-125. In the process, it emits photons of 27, 31, and 36 keV, for an average energy of 29 keV. I-125's low average energy of 29 keV

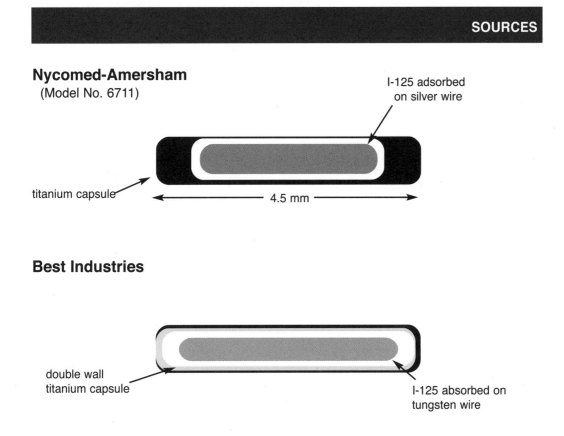

Nycomed-Amersham
(Model No. 6711)

I-125 adsorbed on silver wire

titanium capsule

4.5 mm

Best Industries

double wall
titanium capsule

I-125 absorbed on
tungsten wire

Figure 5-3. Construction of Nycomed-Amersham and Best Industries I-125 sources.

minimizes shielding requirements. The halfvalue layer thickness of lead is only 0.02 mm.

The I-125 is adsorbed on a silver rod, which is encased in a titanium capsule (**Figure 5-3**). It's the inner wire or markers, not the outer titanium capsule, that is radiographically visible (**Figure 5-5**). The outside dimensions of the source are 4.5 x 0.8 mm. I-125 is typically used at a source strength of 0.3 to 0.9 mCi (**Figure 5-6**).

I-125 has been the most widely used radionuclide. Its relatively long half-life of sixty days is a practical advantage in that it can be stored for several weeks prior to use.

Some authors have attributed the inferior results with retropubic implants performed in the 1970s to the choice of I-125 as the isotope. Morons. Poor results in

Theragenics

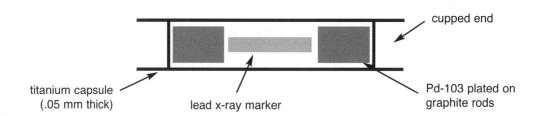

Figure 5-4. Construction of Theragenics Pd-103 source.

retropubic series were almost certainly due to poor source placement, not the source itself (see chapter 2).

Until recently, Nycomed-Amersham was the only company to manufacture I-125 sources. A growing number of companies have introduced alternative I-125 sources.(NATH 93, HEDTJARN)

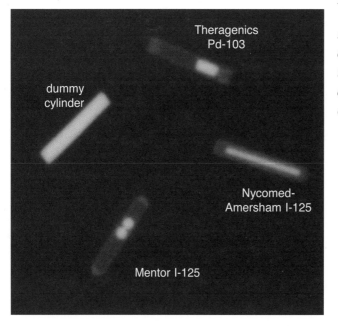

Figure 5-5. Distinct appearance of sources on plain radiographs, due to use of different radiodense markers.

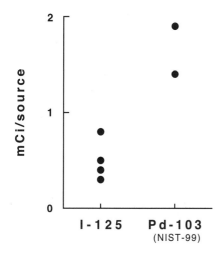

Figure 5-6. Activity ranges commonly used for I-125 and Pd-103. Some brachytherapists advocate use of the lower activity sources for boost implants, combined with supplemental external beam radiation.

Pd-103

Pd-103 is the second most commonly used isotope for permanent implants. It was initially produced in a nuclear reactor, during a process in which Pd-103 absorbs a neutron, but it is currently produced in a cyclotron by bombarding rhodium with protons. It decays by electron capture and internal conversion to Rhodium-103. Photons of 20, 23, 40 and 357 keV are emitted, with an average energy of 21 keV. Pd-103 sources are the same size as I-125 sources (4.5 x 0.8 mm), but they appear differently on radiographs, depending on the manufacturer.(LI, MEIGOONI) For TheraSeed®, the original and still dominant source, Pd-103 is plated on radiolucent graphite rods at each end of the source (**Figures 5-4 & 5-5**). A lead wire is added to the center of the source to make it easily visible on X-ray films.

Pd-103 sources are typically used at 1.3 to 1.8 mCi (NIST-99), with the lower activity sources generally used for boost implants combined with supplemental external beam radiation (**Figure 5-6**).

Pd-103's shorter half-life of seventeen days may be a radiobiologic advantage (**Table 5-2**). Another potential advantage of Pd-103 could be a shorter duration of radiation prostatitis.(WALLNER) The difference in average energy between I-125 and Pd-103 has only minor effects on most treatment planning parameters.(DICKER)

Table 5-2 Pros and cons of I-125 versus Pd-103.

	Pros	**Cons**
I-125	Longer shelf life	Low dose rate(?)
	Less expensive	Longer duration
	Available in strand form	side effects(?)
Pd-103	Radiobiologic advantage(?)	Short shelf life (7 days)
	Shorter duration of side effects(?)	
	Rectal sparing(?)	

The biggest disadvantage of Pd-103 compared to I-125 is its short shelf life—Pd-103 can be held only for about a week before the activity is too low to be practical (too many sources would be required).

AU-198
Au-198, or *radioactive gold*, has been used on a smaller scale since the 1950s. It has a very short half life (2.5 days) and relatively high average energy (600 keV), meaning that its dose rate is substantially higher than even Pd-103, and that there is far more tissue penetration. Radiobiologically, a gold implant is similar to doing HDR, but with permanent sources. The advantage over I-125 or Pd-103 is a lower likelihood of cold spots, and better coverage of periprostatic tissue.

The primary disadvantage of Au-198 is that its half life makes it impractical to ship far from the manufacturing site. Because of its high energy, patients remain hospitalized for about one day afterward to allow the dose rate decline to Nuclear Regulatory Commission (NRC)-mandated levels.

UNITS OF MEASURE
Several changes in source calibration that were made in the late 1990s affected I-125 and Pd-103 in different ways. For Pd-103, there were several alterations in the apparent activity, due to changing the international Cd-109 standardization sources every three years, implementation of an air-kerma strength standard (S_k) and a change in the dose rate constant.(NATH, WILLIAMSON) The cumulative effect of these changes has been summarized in an American Brachytherapy Society article, recommending that the stated prescription dose for a Pd-103 implant be changed from 115 Gy to 125 Gy, with the simultaneous adoption of the NIST-99 air-kerma strength standard for Pd-103 using the new dose rate constants, which are unique for each source manufacturer (**Figure 5-7**).(BEYER)

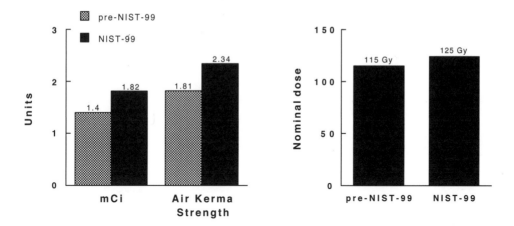

Figure 5-7. Stated mCi and air-kerma strengths and nominal Pd-103 monotherapy doses, before and after adoption of the NIST wide angle free air chamber (WAFAC) calibration.

For I-125, the American Association of Physicists in Medicine (AAPM) Radiation Therapy Committee Task Group No. 43 (TG-43) recommended a switch to air-kerma parameters developed by the Interstitial Collaborative Working Group (ICWG).(NATH 95, YU) The clinical ramifications, apart from the fact that differences among manufacturers could be better accounted for, was a change from a

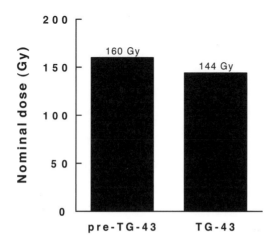

Figure 5-8. Changes in nominal prescription dose for I-125 monotherapy, with adoption of TG-43 dose calculation formalisms.(NATH 95)

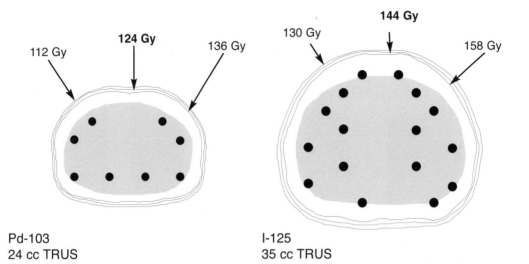

Figure 5-9. Before fretting too much over the change in prescription doses with TG-43 and NIST-99 recommendations, note that the differences in treatment margins are almost imperceptible from 10% to +10% of the ABS-recommended monotherapy doses.(BEYER)

stated prescription dose of 160 Gy to 144 Gy, assuming the TG-43 formalism was simultaneously implemented (**Figure 5-8**).(LUSE, BICE)

The changes in *nominal* doses for Pd-103 and I-125 amount to approximately an 8% increase for Pd-103 and a 10% decrease for I-125. Compared to the substantial variability in treatment margins used by brachytherapists around the world (see Chapter 6), these dose specification changes are probably not of major significance (**Figure 5-9**). This book, includes some inconsistencies between quoted studies, because published data spans the time intervals in which the dosimetry changes have been made. Rather than go back and alter the stated doses, we have tried to specify, when necessary, the period from which the dose calculations were made. When implemented as recommended by the AAPM and ABS, these changes in stated doses, along with dose formalisms, should result in the same long-term success already reported.(BLASKO, DATTOLI, CRITZ, ZELEFSKY) And, yes, additional small adjustments in the NIST-99 calibration standard and associated dose rate constant are being considered but should have minimal clinical significance.

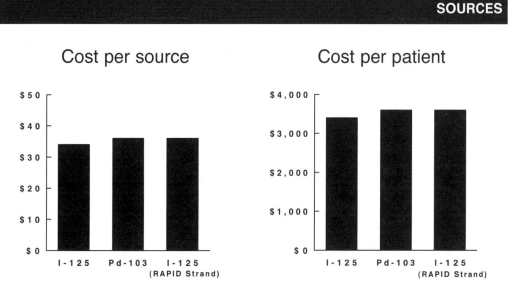

Figure 5-10. Cost of sources, assuming 100 sources to implant a 40 cc prostate gland.

COST

As of 2001, both I-125 and Pd-103 sources cost about $40 to $50 apiece. Using the typical low activity I-125 sources (0.3-0.4 mCi/source), the cost of an implant with either isotope is similar. Because the cost per source is similar regardless of activity, the option to use higher activity sources is a potential cost advantage to I-125, which has a greater range of available sources strengths than Pd-103 has (**Figure 5-6**).(MAGUIRE, WANG) Suture-mounted I-125 (RAPID Strand™) cost about $4 more per source than loose I-125 sources (**Figure 5-10**).

ANISOTROPY

Both I-125 and Pd-103 sources have more dose attenuation at the ends of the sources than at the central plane due to absorption at the thick ends of the metal capsule, and due to some absorption by the silver or aluminum carrier itself (**Figure 5-11**). Decreased dose at the ends of the source could significantly affect the dose distribution of the implant itself, particularly if the sources are uniformly aligned. In practice, sources typically are more randomly oriented. Currently, the actual orientation is not taken into account for implant evaluation, because it would be technically difficult to enter precise orientation data. Instead, commercial planning programs allow for a uniform correction factor, assuming random source rotation from the longitudinal prostatic axis. Calculating the actual anisotropy effect would add a substantial degree of complexity to planning and evaluation of the dose distribution, but it could be automated with the proper software. The clinical relevance of this, however, is likely minimal.

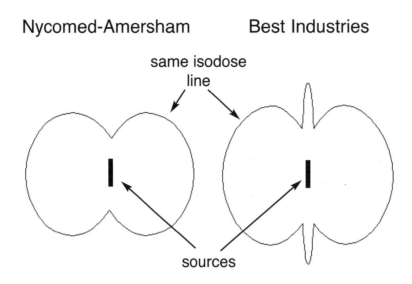

Nycomed-Amersham   Best Industries

Figure 5-11. Effect of source orientation on dose distribution. The isodose lines are constricted at the source ends (anisotropy). Anisotropy could cause substantial underdosage in the longitudinal axis of an implant, when all sources are closely aligned in the longitudinal direction.(MEIGOONI)

SOURCE INSERTION

There are two principle ways to insert sources—preloaded needles and the Mick Applicator®. Each has its pros and cons. Most brachytherapists choose one or the other method, and use it exclusively.(PRESTIDGE)

Mick Applicator®

The Mick Applicator®, manufactured in various models since 1972, has a needle retraction mechanism through which sources are fed from a magazine cartridge (**Figure 5-12**). The primary advantages of the applicator are decreased radiation exposure to personnel, its flexibility to change source spacing at the time of the implant, ease in adding extra sources ad hoc, simplified sterilization procedures and simpler device source loading. Accordingly, the Mick is preferred for intra-operative treatment planning. Limitations of the Mick® Applicator are that it occasionally jams (easy to correct) and that it requires some getting used to. About half of brachytherapists use a Mick® Applicator, and half use preloaded needles.(PRESTIDGE)

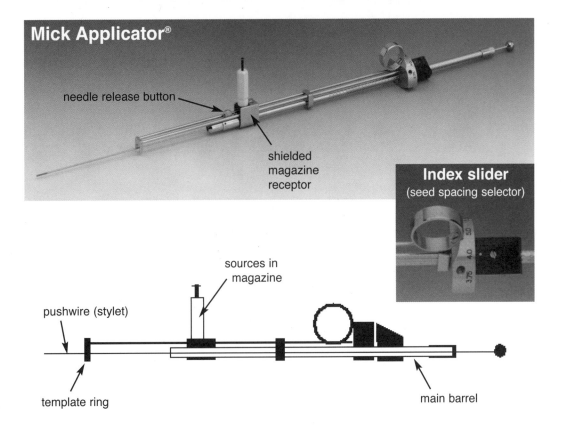

Mick Applicator®

needle release button

shielded
magazine
receptor

Index slider
(seed spacing selector)

50

4.0

3.75

sources in
magazine

pushwire (stylet)

template ring

main barrel

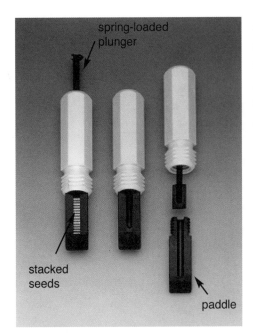

spring-loaded
plunger

stacked
seeds

paddle

*Figure 5-12. Mick Applicator® (top).
Sources are fed into the hollow needle by magazines for 10 to 20
sources (left). The index slider
allows for fine adjustment of source
spacing.*

Mick Applicator® needles

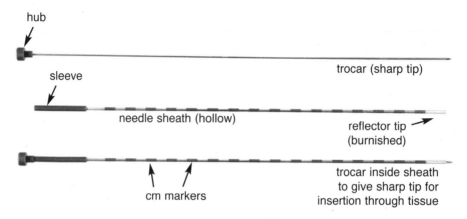

Figure 5-13. Mick Applicator® needles have a trocar that is placed inside the sheath to provide a sharp tip for insertion, and then removed prior to attaching the applicator to insert sources through the hollow sheath.

pushrod out   pushrod in

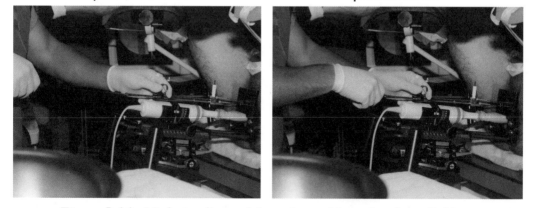

Figure 5-14. Mick Applicator® in action, with pushrod out (left) or in (right). Moving the pushrod in drives a source from the magazine, out the tip of the hollow sheath.

Preloaded needles

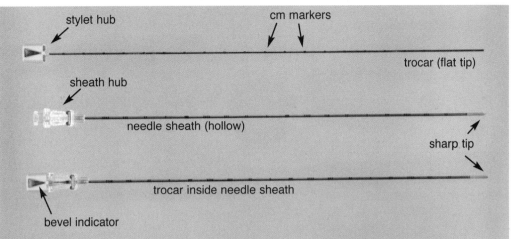

Figure 5-15. Preloaded needles have an inner stylet and hollow sheath. The sources and spacers are loaded prior to starting the procedure (below). After insertion, the needle is withdrawn over the stylet, leaving the sources in place. Centimeter markers on the stylet indicate how many sources are in the needle, depending on how many cm of stylet protrude out the sheath. The bevel indicator shows which way the bevel tip points, which is the direction the needles tend to deviate as they pass through tissue. The sheath hub is funnel shaped to facilitate source preloading.

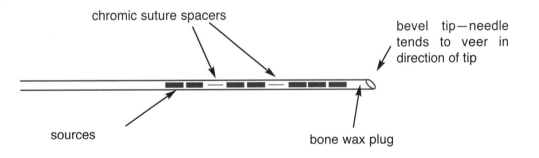

Preloaded needles: the sequence of events

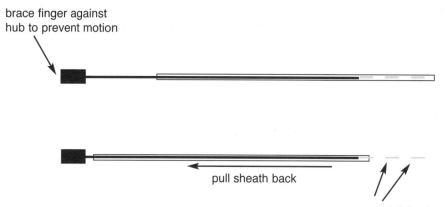

brace finger against
hub to prevent motion

pull sheath back

sources left in place

*Figure 5-16. Schematic of preloaded needles. After insertion, the
sheath is withdrawn over the stylet, leaving the sources in place.*

needle with sources loaded, advanced into patient

sheath drawn back, with free sources now in place

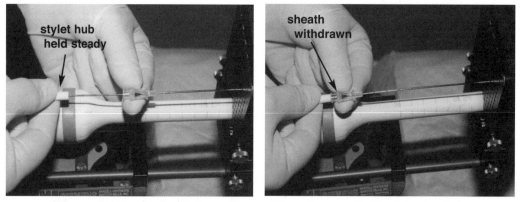

stylet hub
held steady

sheath
withdrawn

*Figure 5-17. Preloaded needles, with stylet out (left) or in (right).
Pulling the sheath back leaves the free sources in place in the
patient.*

Preloaded needles

Preloaded needles, manufactured in 18-gauge, are loaded with sources before starting the case. To provide gaps where needed, absorbable spacers (No. 3 chromic gut suture material) of appropriate multiples of 5.5 mm are placed between the sources (**Figure 5-15**). Devices are available to help with the tedious task of preloading sources into the needles (**Figures 5-18 and 5-19**).

One advantages of preloaded needles is that they are easier to learn to use, with less operator dependence on proper source spacing. Disadvantages are that they are time-consuming and tedious to set up, offer less intraoperative source placement flexibility, and increase radiation exposure to the staff.

Choosing a method

The choice between preloaded needles versus the Mick® Applicator has substantial practical implications—give it serious thought before you buy (**Table 5-3**). In addition to the points mentioned above, there can be significant cost differences between the two methods, depending on the number of cases you do (**Figure 5-20**). The Mick has higher start-up costs, but avoids personnel time to load needles. It becomes especially cost-saving if a limited number of needles are used per patient.

SUTURE-MOUNTED SOURCES

Suture-mounted I-125 sources (RAPID Strand™, Nycomed-Amersham) are mounted in #1 Vicryl™ (polyglactin 910). The suture is stiffened and sterilized with ethylene oxide gas prior to being shipped inside a plastic spacing jig, packed inside a stainless steel shielding tube (**Figure 5-21**). Suture-mounted sources are more likely to maintain their position, and should not migrate if one or two sources of the suture are protruding partly out of the prostate. Theoretically, they could allow for wider periprostatic coverage, but their true clinical benefit is unclear. While proper placement at one centimeter intervals is assured with RAPID Strand™, one centimeter spacing may not be the best way to achieve coverage in certain parts of the prostate. If you need intraoperative flexibility in source placement, you'll probably use RAPID Strand™ for most of the sources, and end up placing some sources with a Mick® Applicator.

The primary disadvantage of suture-mounted sources has been their tendency to stick inside the needles. Plugging the needle tips with heated Anusol™ provides lubrication and helps prevent needle jamming problems. There is clearly an "art" to proper use of RAPID Strand™.(BUTLER) If you're thinking about using them, it

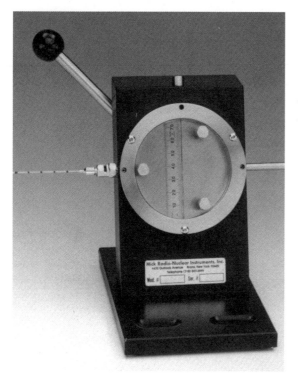

Figure 5-18. Seed loading device (Seed Hopper™) from Mick Radio-Nuclear Instruments Inc. The Seed Hopper™ facilitates loading, provides shielding, and allows visual verification of proper loading.

Mick Radio-Nuclear   Radiation Therapy Products

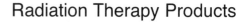
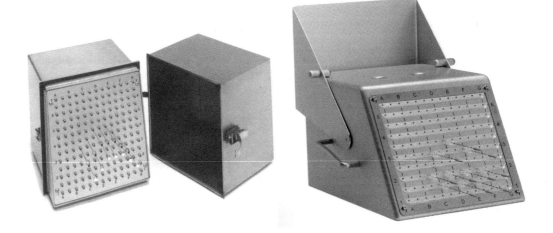

Figure 5-19. Hot boxes used to hold needles from time of loading to time of insertion. Numbers and letters on the margins of the box correspond to those on the TRUS template.

Start-up costs

Per case costs

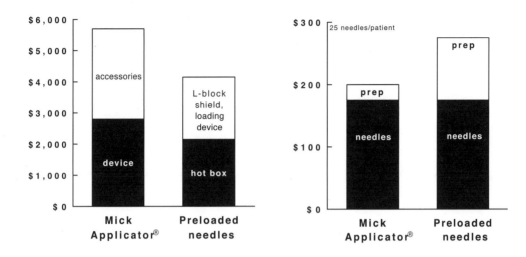

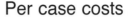

Figure 5-20. Start-up and per case costs for Mick Applicator® versus preloaded needles. Start-up costs are greater for the Mick, but per case costs are greater for pre-loaded needles. The overall cost advantage depends on case volume—the more implants you do, the greater the cost advantage to using the Mick Applicator®.

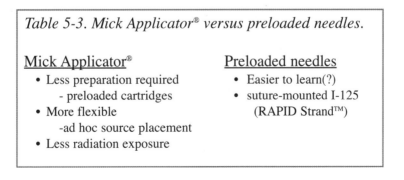

Table 5-3. Mick Applicator® versus preloaded needles.

Mick Applicator®
- Less preparation required
  - preloaded cartridges
- More flexible
  - ad hoc source placement
- Less radiation exposure

Preloaded needles
- Easier to learn(?)
- suture-mounted I-125
  (RAPID Strand™)

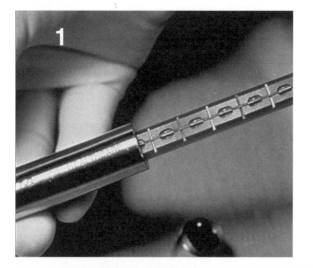

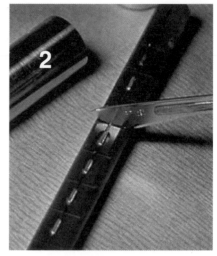

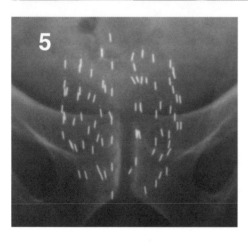

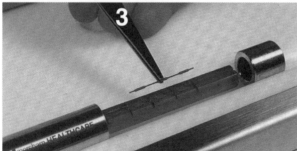

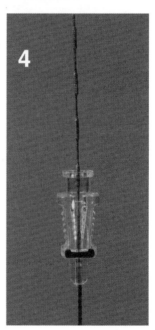

Figure 5-21. Suture-mounted I-125 sources (RAPID Strand™ Nycomed-Amersham) are shipped inside a plastic spacing jig, which is inside a stainless steel shielding tube. The strand should be cut between the sources with a razor-sharp blade, and then picked up with tweezers, grasping only the portion that holds a source. (Photos courtesy of Nycomed-Amersham and Dr. Peter Grimm)

would be wise to first spend some time observing a skilled brachytherapist with substantial experience.

SO MANY WAYS...

There are already a variety of source placement techniques and equipment to carry them out. More manufacturers are getting involved, offering a larger variety of equipment. Some of the new ideas are simply technology-run-amok, making a quick and efficient procedure less so, and with no better final result. Nonetheless, there's still plenty of room for improvement to make the procedure more efficient and less prone to operator error.

REFERENCES

1. Beyer D, Nath R, Butler W, et al . American Brachytherapy Society recommendations for clinical implementation of NIST-1999 standards for Pd-103 brachytherapy. Int J Rad Oncol Biol Phys 2000; 47:273-275.

2. Bice WS, Prestidge BR, Prete JJ, Dubois DF. Clinical impact of implementing the recommendations of AAPM Task Group 43 on permanent prostate brachytherapy using I-125. Int J Rad Oncol Biol Phys 1998; 40:1237-1241.

3. Blasko JC, Grimm PD, Sylvester JE, Badiozamani KR, Hoak D, Cavanagh W. Palladium-103 brachytherapy for prostate carcinoma. Int J Rad Oncol Biol Phys 2000; 46:839-850.

4. Butler EB, Scardino PT, Teh BS, et al . The Baylor College of Medicine experience with gold seed implantation. Sem Surg Oncol 1997; 13:406-418.

5. Butler WM, Merrick GS. I-125 Rapid Strand™ loading technique. Radiat Oncol Invest 1996; 4:48-49.

6. Critz FA, Williams WH, Benton JB, Levinson AK, Holladay CT, Holladay DA. Prostate specific anitgen bounce after radioactive seed implantation followed by external beam radiation for prostate cancer. J Urol 2000; 163:1085-1089.

7. Dattoli M, Wallner K, True L, Sorace R, Koval J, et al . Prognostic role of serum prostatic acid phosphatase for 103-Pd-based radiation for prostatic carcinoma. Int J Rad Oncol Biol Phys 1999; 45:853-856.

8. Dicker AP, Lin C-C, Leeper DB, Waterman FM. Isotope selection for permanent prostate implants? An evaluation of 103-Pd versus 125- based on radiobiological effectiveness and dosimetry. Sem in Urol Oncol 2000; 18:152-159.

9. Edmundson GK, Yan D, Martinez AA. Intraoperative optimization of needle placement and dwell times for conformal prostate brachytherapy. Int J Rad Oncol Biol Phys 1995; 33:1257-1263.

10. Hedtjarn H, Carlsson GA, Williamson JF. Monte Carlo-aided dosimetry of the Symmetra model 125.S06 125-I, interstitial brachytherapy seed. Med Phys 2000; 27:1076-1085.

11. Li Z, Palta JR, Fan JJ. Monte Carlo calculations and experimental measurements of dosimetry parameters of a new 103-Pd source. Med Phys 2000; 27:1108-1112.

12. Loening SA. Gold seed implantation in prostate brachytherapy. Sem Surg Oncol 1997; 13:419-424.

13. Luse RW, Blasko J, Grimm P. A method for implementing the American Association of Physicists in Medicine Task Group-43 dosimetry recommendations for I-125 transperineal prostate seed implants on commercial treatment planning systems. Int J Rad Oncol Biol Phys 1997; 37:737-741.

14. Maguire PD, Waterman FM, Dicker AP. Can the cost of permanent prostate implants be reduced? An argument for peripheral loading with higher strength seeds. Tech Urol 2000; 6:85-88.

15. Martinez AA, Kestin LL, Stromberg JS, et al . Interim report of image-guided conformal high-dose-rate brachytherapy for patients with unfavorable prostate cancer: the William Beaumont Phase II dose-escalating trial. Int J Rad Oncol Biol Phys 2000; 47:343-352.

16. Mate TP, Gottesman JE, Hatton J, et al . High dosed-rate after-loading iridium-192 prostate brachytherapy: feasibility report. Int J Rad Oncol Biol Phys 1998; 41:525-533.

17. Meigooni AS, Sowards K, Soldano M. Dosimetric characteristics of the InterSource-103 palladium brachytherapy source. Med Phys 2000; 27:1093-1100.

18. Nath R, Anderson LL, Luxton G, Weaver KA, Williamson JF, Meigooni AS. Dosimetry of interstitial brachytherapy sources: Recommendations of the AAPM Radiation Therapy Committee Task Group No. 43. Med Phys 1995; 22:209-234.

19. Nath R, Melillo A. Dosimetric characteristics of a double wall 125-I source for interstitial brachytherapy. Med Phys 1993; 20:1475-1483.

20. Prestidge BR, Prete JJ, Buchholz TA, Friedland JL, Stock RG, Grimm PD, Bice WS. A survey of current clinical practice of permanent prostate brachytherapy in the United States. Int J Rad Oncol Biol Phys 1998; 40:461-465.

21. Wallner K, Merrick G, True L, Kattan M, Cavanagh W, Simpson C, Butler W. I-125 versus Pd-103 for low risk prostate cancer: Preliminary urinary functional outcomes from a prospective randomized multicenter trial. Journal of Brachytherapy International 2000; 16:151-155.

22. Wang H, Wallner K, Sutlief S, Blasko J, Russell K, Ellis W. Transperineal brachytherapy in patients with large prostate glands. Int J Cancer 2000; 90:199-205.

23. Williamson JF, Coursey BM, DeWerd LA, et al . Recommendations of the American Association of Physicists in Medicine on 103-Pd interstitial source calibration and dosimetry: Implications for dose specification and prescription. Med Phys 2000; 27:634-642.

24. Yu Y, Anderson LL, Li Z, Mellenberg DE, Nath R, Schell MC, Wu A, Blasko JC. Permanent prostate seed implant brachytherapy: Report of the American Association of Physicists in Medicine Task Group No. 64. Med Phys 1999; 26:2054-2076.

25. Zelefsky MJ, Hollister T, Raben A, Matthews SM, Wallner KE. Five-year biochemical outcome and toxicity with transperineal CT-planned permanent I-125 prostate implantation for patients with localized prostate cancer. Int J Rad Oncol Biol Phys 2000; 47:1261-1266.

6

Design

Treatment planning, or preimplant dosimetry, refers to the determination of how many sources will be used and where they will be placed. Planning has traditionally been performed a week or more ahead of the implant procedure, but there is growing interest in intraoperative planning. Whether you choose to do your planning ahead of time or not, the same principles apply.

Despite a rapidly growing body of favorable clinical reports, prostate brachytherapy treatment planning remains a mysterious endeavor, based more on gut instinct than on a critical look at the relationship between planning parameters and outcomes. Although the stated prescription doses are fairly uniform, there is still sub-

Minimal probe pressure   Excessive probe pressure

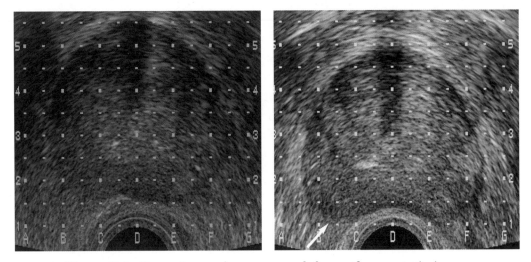

Figure 6-1. Excessive probe pressure deforms the prostatic image. These two mid prostatic images of the same patient were taken with minimal (left) or substantial (right) probe pressure, causing artifactual drooping of the posterior-lateral margins (arrow). Note that increased probe pressure also moves the prostate lower on the grid.

stantial variability from one implant team to another in the way the doses are instituted, primarily due to inconsistencies in the use of treatment margins and to marked dose inhomogeneity. The best way to avoid problems in your own practice is to understand the differences that exist and the potential pitfalls in transferring nominal doses from one implant team to another.

PLANNING IMAGES
Implants are planned from images of the prostate, taken at 5 mm intervals from the prostatic base through the apex. The patient should be in the lithotomy position, similar to that for the implant procedure itself. It's best to come as close as reasonably possible to the position the patient will be for the implant procedure. It's also important that the prostate is not deformed by excessive probe pressure (**Figure 6-1**) and that it remains centered on the grid with the posterior margin aligned along a grid row (**Figure 6-2**).

The most proximal image is considered the *zero plane* or *0.0 plane*. It is located by visualizing the most proximal image or *base*, usually including a portion of the seminal vesicles (**Figure 6-3**). Sagittal imaging can be used to check that your 0.0

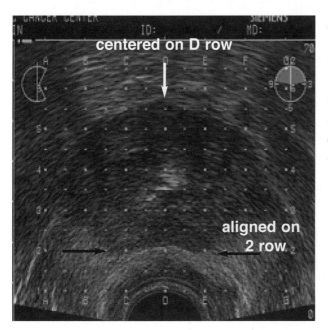

Figure 6-2. You're less likely to make mistakes going from the plan to the operating room if the prostate is consistently centered on the grid, with the back of the gland aligned along the same row for each case.

plane cuts through the top of the prostate. Images and source positions are typically specified by their distance from the zero plane. Going caudally, transverse planes are numbered by their distance (in cm) from the 0 plane (i.e., the *1.0 plane* is 1.0 cm caudal to the 0.0 plane). The most caudal image, or *apex*, typically is indistinct on transverse imaging but can be readily verified on sagittal imaging (**Figure 6-3**).

TARGET DEFINITIONS
ICRU 50 treatment planning definitions were written for external beam treatment planning, but are generally applicable to brachytherapy.(ICRU, HAN) The *gross target volume* (GTV) is the prostate itself, as visualized on the TRUS images. The *clinical target volume* (CTV) is designed to cover the prostate plus periprostatic regions of potential microscopic tumor spread. For external beam planning, the *planning target volume* (PTV) includes a margin around the CTV to allow for variability in patient setup and prostatic motion. For prostate brachytherapy, the PTV is not as relevant, since the prostatic position on the template should not change. But the GTV and CTV treatment planning parameters can be applied equally well to prostate brachytherapy as to external beam radiation. The *treatment margin (TM)*, is the perpendicular distance between the GTV and the prescription isodose (**Figure 6-4**). The *treated volume* (TV) is that enclosed by the prescription isodose.

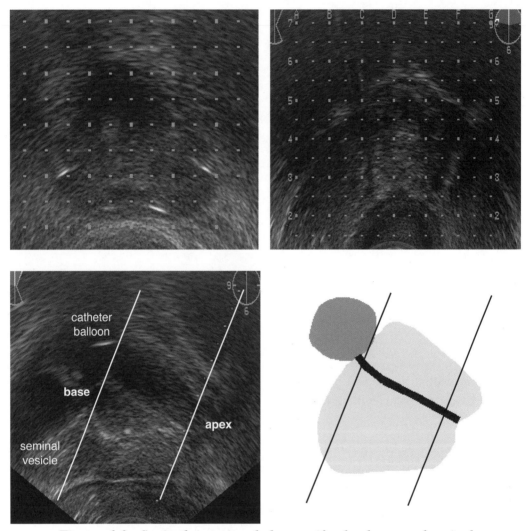

Figure 6-3. Sagittal imaging helps verify the base and apical planes. The transverse images (top) of the base and apex are typically less distinct than those of the midprostate. The sagittal view (bottom images) helps confirm the base and apical planes, in part because the continuous prostatic contour can be visually extrapolated from midportions of the prostate. (white lines show transverse imaging planes).

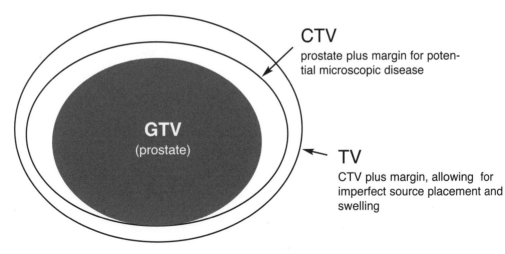

Figure 6-4. Schematic of GTV, CTV, and TV.(ICRU, HAN)

It's important to realize how crucial these treatment planning concepts are in determining how much tissue is treated and what dose is actually delivered to the prostate, rectum, and urethra. In contrast to external beam radiation, brachytherapy delivers doses far higher than the prescription dose, due to high dose regions near the implanted sources and the use of treatment margins.

To start the treatment planning process, the prostatic margin (GTV) is identified on the TRUS images and transferred into a planning program. Admittedly, identi-

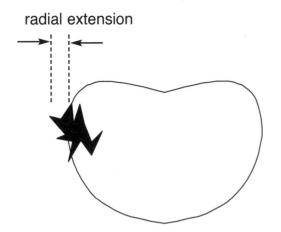

radial extension

Figure 6-5. Schematic of EPE, measured radially, from the urethra to the prostatic margin. The degree of radial extracapsular cancer extension is limited to within 3 mm in nearly all patients (see chapter 11).

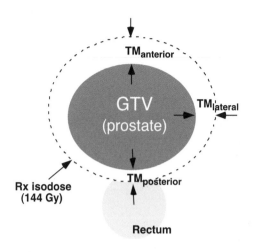

Figure 6-6. Treated margin (TM) measurement points used by Han and colleagues.(HAN)

fying the prostate margins is a bit of an *art*, because the margins appear fuzzy, especially at the apex, where the prostatic tissue blends into the nearly isodense pelvic floor musculature. When in doubt, we err on the side of being generous with margin identification. A policy of generosity seems safe, since the visualized margins are typically sharp posteriorly, near the rectum—the most dose-limiting structure.

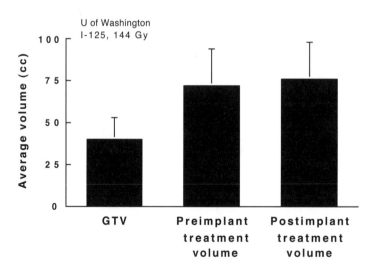

Figure 6-7. GTV, preimplant TVs, and postimplant TVs. Note that the TVs were nearly twice as large as the GTVs.

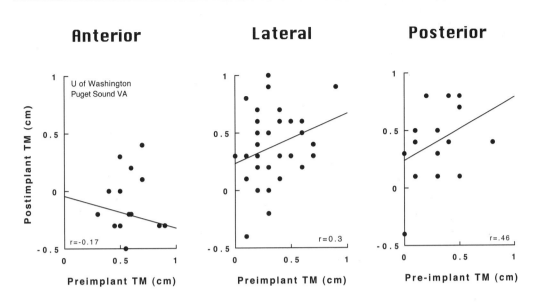

Figure 6-8. Preimplant TMs versus postimplant TMs (right and left lateral margins are grouped together).

MARGIN SIZE

While modern TRUS equipment has made the identification of the GTV fairly simple, there is surprisingly little data regarding the optimum treatment planning margins to add to the GTV. In practice, "a few mm" have typically been added, but the optimal magnitude of the TM has not been rigorously studied. The problem with the arbitrariness of the magnitude of the margins is that the actual dose to the prostate may be far different than the prescription dose, depending on how large a TM is used. Fortunately, recent studies regarding the extent of EPE and the effect of implant-related edema on postimplant TMs are bringing us closer to a more rational choice of treatment margins.(HAN, MERRICK 02)

Extraprostatic cancer extension (EPE)

Ideally, brachytherapy delivers a tumorcidal dose to the prostate, with a sufficient margin to encompass the likely extent of extracapsular disease extension (ECE) (**Figure 6-5**). According to prostatectomy specimen studies, EPE is nearly always limited to within 3 mm (radially) of the prostatic edge, so that a 3 mm TM should suffice.(DAVIS 99, SOHAYDA)

Preimplant versus postimplant TMs

In the absence of source placement errors or implant-related prostate swelling, a planning TM of 3 mm should be sufficient to achieve a postimplant margin of 3

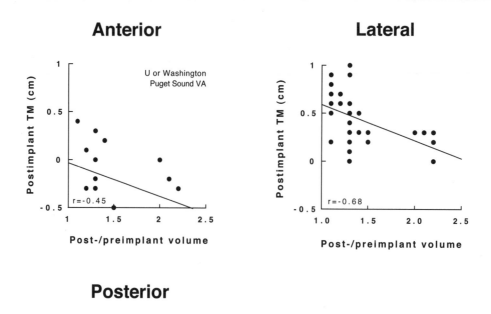

Posterior

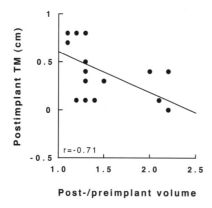

Figure 6-9. Postimplant TMs versus the ratio of the postimplant to preimplant prostate volume.

mm. But in order to achieve adequate margins on the *post*implant prostate, some allowance must be made for source placement error and implant-related swelling that continues over much of the active life of the isotopes.(WILLINS 98, WATERMAN 98)

In a landmark effort to determine what preimplant TMs are likely to achieve an adequate periprostatic cancericidal dose, Han and colleagues correlated preimplant with postimplant TMs (day 0).(HAN) The distances between the GTV and treated margin were determined by measuring the distance between the ultrasound-defined prostatic margin and the prescription isodose, perpendicular to the prosta-

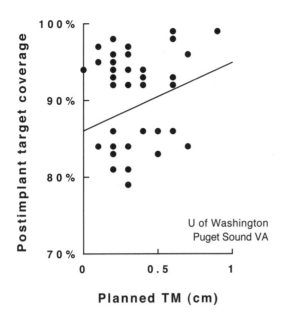

Figure 6-10. Target coverage versus lateral preimplant TMs. Larger TMs were associated with greater postimplant prostatic coverage, but the correlation was loose due to variable implant-related prostatic swelling.

tic margin (**Figure 6-6**). Each patient's preimplant TMs were then compared to his corresponding post-implant TMs. Postimplant parameters were taken from postimplant CT scans, interpreted by a single, experienced investigator (KW).

There were several disconcerting findings in this first systematic look at the treatment planning parameters by an experienced implant group with a long track record of high tumor control rates. First, the preimplant TVs were nearly twice as large as the GTVs. This huge increase from the GTV to the TV shows how big an impact the use of planning margins can have on the tissue volume irradiated (**Figure 6-7**). The postimplant TVs were similar to the planned TVs, evidence that the plans were accurately implemented. Second, the planning TMs varied substantially between patients, due to lack of a consistent policy regarding their magnitude. The good news was that the actual postimplant TMs were generally similar to their corresponding planned TMs, albeit with substantial scatter in the data (**Figure 6-8**). The exceptions were primarily anteriorly, where the postimplant TMs were substantially smaller than those planned due to larger edema-related increases in the anterior-posterior prostatic dimension. (BADIOZAMANI)

The loose correlation between pre- and postimplant treatment margins is explained by the variable, implant-related prostatic dimensional changes. As expected,

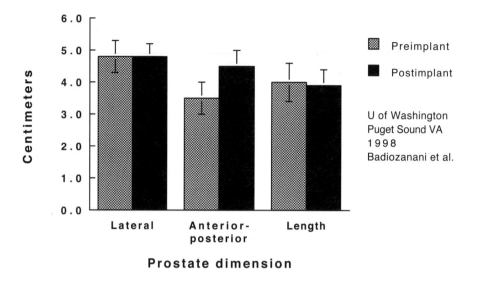

Figure 6-11. Prostatic dimensions before and after implant procedure. (AP=anterior-posterior dimension)

patients with a greater implant-related volume increase tended to have smaller postimplant treatment margins (**Figure 6-9**). And as you would guess, the postimplant prostate coverage (V100, see chapter 9) was higher when larger planning TMs were used, but the correlation was loose due to the unpredictable and highly variable degree of implant-related swelling (**Figure 6-10**).

Despite the loose correlation between the preimplant planning margins and the postimplant margins, in most patients, a minimum 2–3 mm postimplant margin was achieved. Additionally, the prostate typically shrinks back to its original size within 30 days following the implant procedure, so that the functional TM should increase somewhat.(WATERMAN 98, WILLINS 98) While the arbitrary use of TMs has led to surprisingly favorable tumor control rates, a more uniform treatment planning policy seems desirable, if only to make the treatment planning process more consistent between institutions.

ANTICIPATING SWELLING
The major impediment to closer matching between pre- and postimplant treatment margins is the inconsistency of implant-related prostate swelling. The prostate volume increases by approximately 25% by the completion of the implant procedure, but with a large degree of variability between patients.

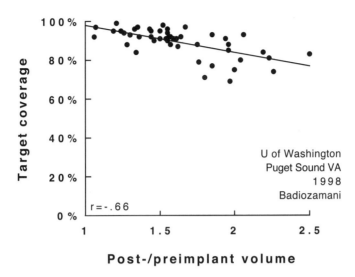

Figure 6-12. Fraction of post-implant target coverage versus degree of procedure-related swelling.

One solution to implant-related volume changes and their impact on the post-implant TMs actually achieved would be to anticipate the degree of swelling for a given patient when planning his implant, i.e., customizing the planned TMs. Nice idea, but predicting swelling in the individual patient has proven impossible so far, being unrelated to the number of needles, radioisotope, or the number of sources.(WATERMAN 98)

In the hope of being able to customize each patient's planning TMs to accommodate his expected degree of implant-related swelling, Badiozamani and colleagues compared implant-related volume changes with pre-implant clinical parameters, including preimplant volume, hormonal ablation, and preimplant external beam radiation in 50 patients.(BADIOZAMANI) On average, the postimplant prostate volume increased by a factor of 1.7 compared to the preimplant volume. In most patients, the greatest size increase was in the anterior-posterior dimension. Changes in the lateral and craniocaudal (length) dimensions were smaller and inconsistent (**Figure 6-11**). And as expected, the degree of postimplant target coverage was less in patients with greater volume increase (**Figure 6-12**). The absolute volume change was similar in patients with small versus large pre-implant prostate volume, but the proportional increase was less in patients with a larger prostate volume (**Figure 6-13**). Because patients with a small pre-implant prostate had proportionately greater volume increase, their postimplant target cov-

6.11

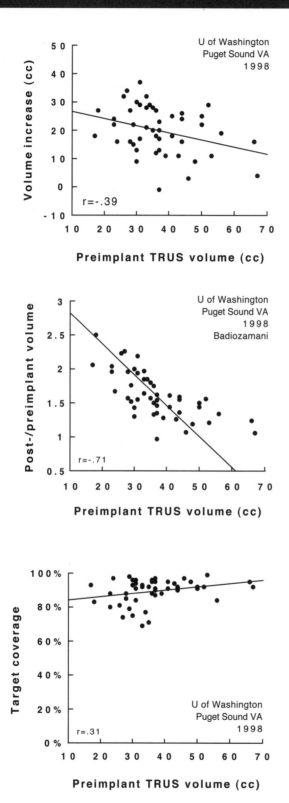

Figure 6-13. Absolute (top panel) and proportional (lower panel) prostate volume increase versus preimplant TRUS volume. Fraction of postimplant target covered by prescription dose versus preimplant volume (lower panel).

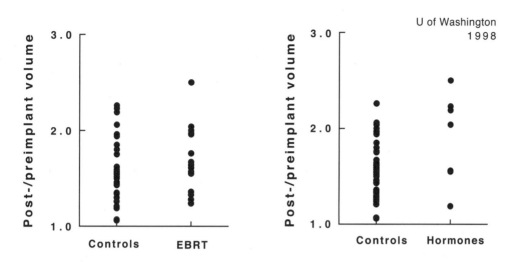

Figure 6-14. Degree of implant-related swelling versus use of pre-implant supplemental external radiation (left) or hormonal deprivation (right).

erage was generally *lower*, contrary to popular belief. Preimplant hormonal therapy or supplemental external beam radiation had no consistent effect on postimplant volume changes (**Figure 6-14**).

In a broad sense, Badiozamani's findings suggest that TMs should be larger for patients with smaller prostate volumes, and should not be influenced by prior hormonal manipulation or external beam radiation. However, no single parameter can accurately predict the degree of swelling for an individual patient. A practical solution to the unpredictability of implant-related prostate volume changes remains to be determined. Similar findings have been more recently reported from the University of California, San Francisco.(SPEIGHT)

PROSTATIC REGIONS
So far, we've considered how implant-related prostatic swelling affects the postimplant treatment margins. Another factor to consider in the choice of preimplant margins is prostatic cancer regionalization. Cancers occur more frequently in the posterior-lateral regions, where EPE is also more common.(ROSEN, MCNEAL)

It seems logical to use larger treatment margins where EPE is greatest—posterior-laterally and at the base (**Figure 6-15**).(SOHAYDA) In prostatectomy studies from Cleveland Clinic, there were *no* instances of EPE at the anterior portion of the prostate, so that anterior TMs probably should be minimized (Sohayda, personal communication).

Seminal vesicles

With a typical implant, only the most proximal portion of the seminal vesicle, the region between the bladder and the prostatic base, receives a cancericidal dose (**Figure 6-16**). It's not practical to implant portions of the seminal vesicles that extend cephalad to the base of the prostate, because they move when pushed by a needle tip, and sources deposited in or near the more distal portions of the seminal vesicles tissue tend to bunch up or migrate. Stock and colleagues calculated that seminal vesicle tissue above the top of the prostate typically receives less than 50% of the prescription dose.(STOCK) Biopsies are generally done of the more cephalad portion of the vesicles, so that finding cancer in such biopsies means that external beam radiation would be needed to achieve cancercidal doses.

Extensive seminal vesicle invasion, reaching above the prostate to the commonly biopsied regions of the vesicles, is not treated with brachytherapy and may be synonymous with metastatic disease. However, early cases of vesicle invasion, typically limited to the confluence of the vesicles with the vas deferens, would likely be covered with a cancercidal brachytherapy dose.(DAVIS 01) In drawing the CTV it is, in fact, difficult to separate the seminal vesicles from the posterior prostate and we routinely include the periprostatic seminal vesicle within the TV (**Figure 6-17**). Sources *do* fix properly in the region of the confluence of the seminal vesicles and the ejaculatory ducts, the site of early seminal vesicular cancerous invasion.(VILLERS) Accordingly, *early* seminal vesicle invasion is highly treatable with brachytherapy, and such patients may still be highly curable with an implant alone.

Base

In the report by Sohyada and colleagues, radial EPE measurements were largest at the prostatic base, where it seems logical to use larger margins due to a concern for greater EPE, and because the prostatic margins are less sharply defined on TRUS images. The use of more generous margins at the base does not appear to lead to a higher likelihood of adverse rectal or sexual effects, partly because the rectum tends to be further from the prostate at that point.

Midprostate

Perhaps smaller TMs can be used at the midprostate, because it is sharply visualized and because the rectum appears to limit the geographic posterior EPE extent. The authors tend to use greater TMs posterior *laterally*, where the EPE is greater and where excessive rectal doses are unlikely to occur.

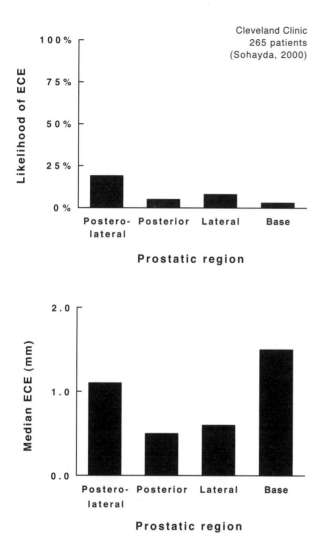

Cleveland Clinic
265 patients
(Sohayda, 2000)

Figure 6-15. The likelihood (top panel) and radial extent (bottom panel) of EPE vary by the region of the prostate. In this series by Sohayda and colleagues at the Cleveland Clinic, EPE was most common at the posterior-lateral margins, and of greatest radial extent at the base. The apex was not analyzed separately, due to lack of a well-defined capsule in that region.

Apex

Surgical resection margins are frequently positive at the prostatic apex, in part because tumor can track outside the prostate where the neurovascular bundles pierce the capsule posteriorly.(STAMEY) Because of the risk of tumor extension through the apical region, the apex is drawn generously on the planning images. Extraprostatic sources usually "fix" well in the region of the apex, imbedded in the pelvic floor musculature.

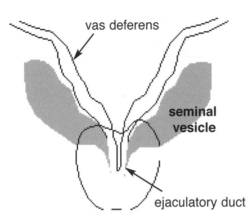

Figure 6-16. Position of of seminal vesicles in relation to vas deferens and prostate. The portion of the vesicles most prox- imal to the prostate are indistinguishable on TRUS from the prostate itself (see Figure 6-17).

Generous apical treatment margins do not appear to lead to an excessive risk of urinary incontinence, but could contribute to overradiation of the penile bulb, which may adversely affect sexual function (see chapter 16). Overirradiation of the prostatic apex may also lead to stricture formation (see chapter 15).

URETHRAL DOSES
Probably the hardest-learned lesson from the early TRUS experience was that of urethral tolerance. In their initial experience, Blasko and colleagues used a homo-

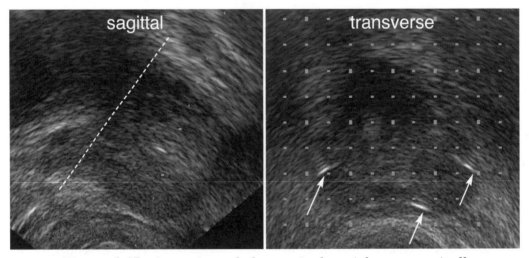

Figure 6-17. A portion of the seminal vesicles are typically included with the prostatic base, so that brachytherapy may erad- icate early vesicle invasion. In this case, sources (arrows) are vis- ible in seminal vesicle tissue near the prostate.

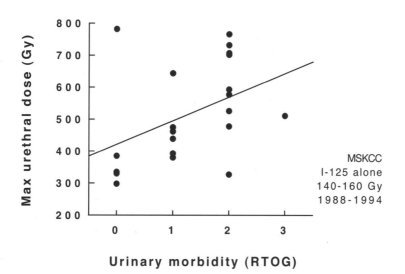

Figure 6-18. RTOG urinary morbidity versus the Maximal urethral dose. There was a suggestion of higher morbidity in patients with a higher maximal dose, but with a lot of scatter in the data.

geneous source loading pattern, assuming urethral tolerance to be nearly infinite. It was not until a substantial incidence of superficial urethral necrosis was seen that a concerted effort was made to switch to peripheral loading (see chapter 15). In 1995, Wallner and colleagues showed that excessive urethral doses were associated with increased urinary morbidity, and recommended that maximal urethral doses be kept below 250% of the prescription dose (**Figure 6-18**).(WALLNER 95) Other measures of urethral doses were no better at predicting morbidity than was the maximal dose. At this time, there is no apparent clinical benefit to more sophisticated dosimetric parameters.(BUTLER)

The correlation between urethral doses and urinary morbidity, first described by Wallner and colleagues, has not been reproduced by others, probably because more recent investigators have consistently used peripheral loading patterns without the central dose extremes of homogeneous loading patterns. Correlations between urethral dose and morbidity will be much less demonstrable in the setting of smaller urethral dose ranges. When doing your treatment planning, a rule of thumb is to keep the urethral dose between 150% and 250% of the prescription dose, a goal that is easily met using modified peripheral source placement patterns.(MERRICK 00) On the other extreme, make sure to keep the urethral dose comfortably *above* the prescription dose, perhaps a minimum of 150% of prescription, to allow for the possibility of some source misplacement and for implant-related prostatic swelling that might actually bring the central dose below cancericidal levels.(WATERMAN 98, LEIBOVICH)

Assuming that urethral doses *are* important in minimizing morbidity, some brachytherapists advocate identifying the urethra on the planning images, to help avoid placing sources too near it, but most brachytherapists don't bother. We assume that it is midline and keep sources 1 cm or more from the midprostate, because the midpoint typically estimates the urethral dose accurately.(WATERMAN 00) If a patient turns out at the time of implant to have a markedly asymmetric urethra, some needle adjustments can be made intraoperatively—typically simply moving one or more needles several mm away from wherever the urethra is. This sort of intraoperative adjustment should have no significant effect on the overall prostate coverage.

Rectum
Although rectal complications are typically of most concern to the radiation oncologist, their low incidence in most series has made it almost impossible to make meaningful guidelines regarding maximal safe rectal doses. Even in the early experience at MSKCC, where the rectal complication rate was relatively high, Wallner and colleagues were unable to establish clear guidelines to minimize rectal morbidity. While some rectal complications have been clearly related to errant source placement, most cases were not (see chapter 14). We typically accept a posterior treatment margin of 3–5 mm. As such, a small portion of the anterior rectal wall usually receives the prescription dose or higher. As long as you're careful not to exceed that, or place sources behind the back edge of the prostate, the chance of serious complications appears to be small (see chapter 15).

TOTAL ACTIVITY
Before the widespread availability of desktop computers and TRUS-based pre-planning, the total activity needed to treat the prostate was determined from standardized tables, based on past experience. The prostatic volume was estimated using three orthogonal dimensions and the total activity was spaced at approximately 1 cm intervals throughout the prostate.(ANDERSON 76, ANDERSON 91)

Dosimetry for permanent implants is now computerized, and can be more closely tailored to an individual patient's prostate. Instead of relying on standard tables, sources are placed at the prostate periphery, typically at 1.0 cm spacing. After a preliminary source placement on the computer screen, the target coverage is cal-

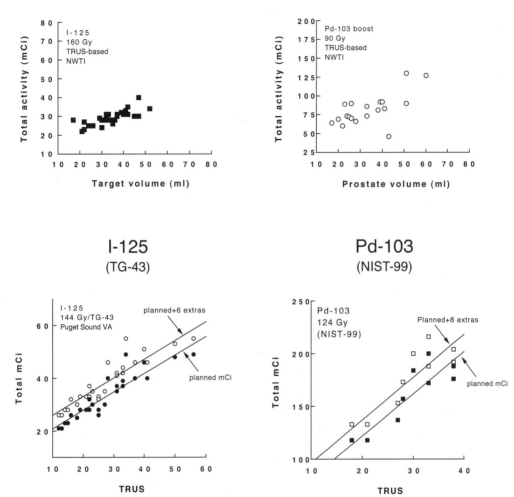

Figure 6-19. Examples of total activity used for I-125 or Pd-103. The scatter and slope of the relationship between prostate volume and total activity will vary, depending on the treatment margins used in the planning process and the degree of peripheral versus homogeneous source placement. The upper panels are from the pre-TG-43/pre-NIST-99 days, and the lower panels are more recent.

culated and sources are added or deleted to achieve the desired coverage of the entire target periphery.

The total activity needed for an implant increases as the prostate volume increases (**Figure 6-19**). However, the correlation is imperfect because the actual activity for a given target volume will depend on the shape of a particular prostate, how much effort is made to minimize the rectal and urethral dose, and how generous the treatment margins are. Adopting the total activity tables of another brachytherapy team should be undertaken with caution.

SOURCE STRENGTH

A wide variety of source strengths have been used for prostate brachytherapy, with no clinical evidence of any effect on outcomes. I-125 sources typically vary in strength from 0.2 to 0.9 mCi and Pd-103 sources vary from 1.4 to 2.0 mCi (NIST-99). Using higher activity sources reduces the number required.(MAGUIRE) However, it has been argued that use of high activity sources could lead to a higher complication rate or less adequate target coverage.

Cumes and colleagues analyzed fourteen I-125 patients, concluding that higher activity sources were more likely to lead to complications.(CUMES) They recommended that individual I-125 source strength be limited to 0.4 mCi or less. Their data, however, comes from patients implanted at Stanford with the retropubic method following recurrence of cancer after external beam radiation or prior retropubic implant. Only seven patients had high activity sources. Drawing *any* conclusion based on such skimpy data exceeds the limits of common sense.

Contrary to the Stanford experience, a detailed analysis of I-125 patients at MSKCC showed no relationship between source strength and urinary or rectal morbidity (**Figure 6-20**). The MSKCC experience is more convincing than that of Stanford because it is based on many more patients, without previous treatment, and implanted in a fairly uniform fashion. The lack of a relationship between source strength and morbidity should not be surprising—radiation-related complications result from the dose delivered, not the individual source strength.

It is possible that higher source strength would lead to higher "hot spots" in the immediate vicinity of the sources and increase the likelihood of complications, but there is no clinical data to support such an argument. At MSKCC, I-125 source strengths of 0.5-1.0 mCi have routinely been used since 1988 and the complication rate, since 1992, has been low.(WALLNER) Rectal and urethral complications in

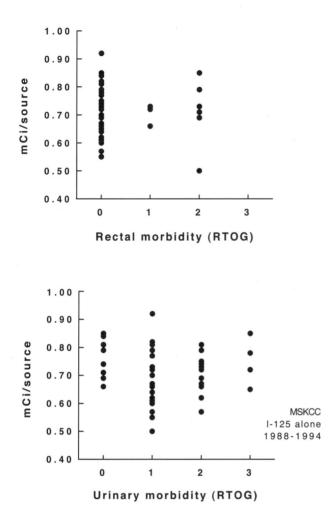

Figure 6-20. There was no relationship between source strength and the degree of rectal or ure-thral morbidity following I-125 implantation at MSKCC (140-160 Gy). (RTOG 1=rectal bleeding or minimal urinary symptoms, RTOG 2=rectal ulceration or the need for alpha blockers to relieve urinary symptoms). (WALLNER)

the early experience were almost surely related to suboptimal source placement, rather than to individual source strength.

One argument for using lower strength sources is that there may be less likelihood of underdosing if a few sources are incorrectly placed. With a greater number of lower activity sources the potential for error is spread out over a greater number of sources, so that misplacement of a few is of less consequence, an argument for which there is some merit.

Homogeneous loading

Peripheral loading

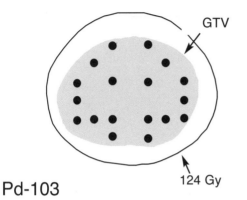
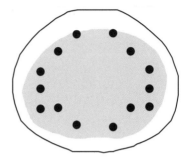

Pd-103

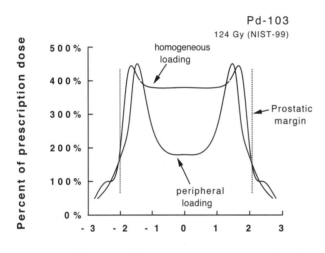

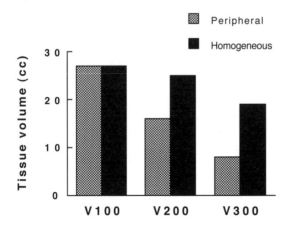

*Figure 6-21.
Homogenous versus
peripheral loading pat-
terns for Pd-103 (124
Gy). The homogeneous
pattern (top left)
achieves the intended 5
mm TM using 108 1.9
mCi sources, but with
central doses about four
times the prescription
dose (left). By removing
26 sources from the cen-
ter of the prostate, the
central doses are
decreased to about twice
the prescription dose,
with very little effect on
the treatment margin.
The most striking differ-
ence between the two
placement patterns is the
larger high dose regions
within the prostate
(V200 and V300).*

Homogeneous loading

Peripheral loading

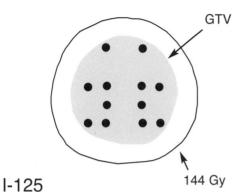

GTV

I-125

144 Gy

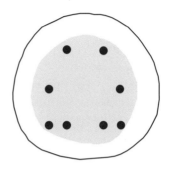

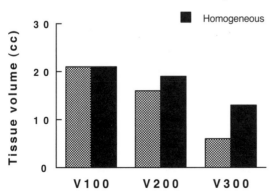

I-125
144 Gy (NIST-99)

homogeneous
loading

Percent of prescription dose

500%

400%

300%

Prostatic
margin

200%

peripheral
loading

100%

0%

-3   -2   -1   0   1   2   3

Distance from prostate center (cm)

Peripheral

Homogeneous

Tissue volume (cc)

30

20

10

0

V100   V200   V300

*Figure 6-22.
Homogenous versus
peripheral loading pat-
terns using I-125 (144
Gy) for a 21 cc prostate.
The homogeneous pat-
tern (top left) achieves
the intended 5 mm treat-
ment margin, but with
central doses about triple
the prescription dose
(left). By removing 10
central sources, the periurethral doses are
decreased to about twice
the prescription dose,
with very little effect on
the treatment margin.
The peripheral loading
pattern minimizes the
V200 and V300 volumes,
as seen on the graph
(lower left).*

SOURCE SPACING

There is no evidence that any particular lateral or longitudinal spacing is advantageous. Ultrasound templates are constructed with 5.0 mm spacing between needles. Some brachytherapists prefer to maintain a minimum 5.0 mm end-to-end spacing between sources, but there is no evidence that end-to-end placement has any detrimental effect. It's where the *isodoses* are, not the sources per se!

TARGETING THE TUMOR

Prostatic carcinoma is multifocal in 50% to 80% of cases, so that the entire prostate should be treated to the prescription dose.(MCNEAL) It has been suggested that more activity be placed where tumor is known to exist and there is a certain degree of common sense to doing so. Advances in radiographic imaging could facilitate a legitimate targeting of high risk areas within the prostate, but we're not there yet.(ZAIDER)

It is not practical to prescribe a higher dose to one portion of the prostate. Instead, the prostatic margin near the tumor-bearing area can be drawn more generously on the planning images. In practice, brachytherapists commonly place several extra sources "ad hoc" in known tumor-bearing areas at the time of the procedure. This practice is generally safe, but it's probably best to keep extra sources away from the urethra and rectum.

HOMOGENEOUS VERSUS PERIPHERAL LOADING

Sources can be distributed in a regular pattern throughout the prostate or kept toward the periphery. While a homogeneous pattern is conceptually appealing, it leads to excessive urethral doses, easily exceeding 400% of the prescription dose and leading to increased urinary morbidity.(WALLNER)

Limiting sources to the periphery, the prostatic margins can be treated adequately, without excessive central doses (**Figures 6-21 & 22**).(NARAYANA) *Pure* peripheral loading is not practical because with larger prostates, especially, the central portion of the gland may be underdosed if *all* sources were at the periphery. In fact, the current norm is neither pure peripheral nor pure homogenous loading, but a *modified peripheral loading.*(MERRICK 00) With modified peripheral loading the central dose is usually kept below 200% of the prescription dose, minimizing the likelihood of urinary morbidity (see Figures 6-24 and 6-25).

EXTRAPROSTATIC SOURCES

One of most contentious source placement issues is the use of extraprostatic sources. There has long been a perception that extraprostatic sources were likely to migrate, either to the retroperitoneum or in the vasculature (see Figure 8-29).

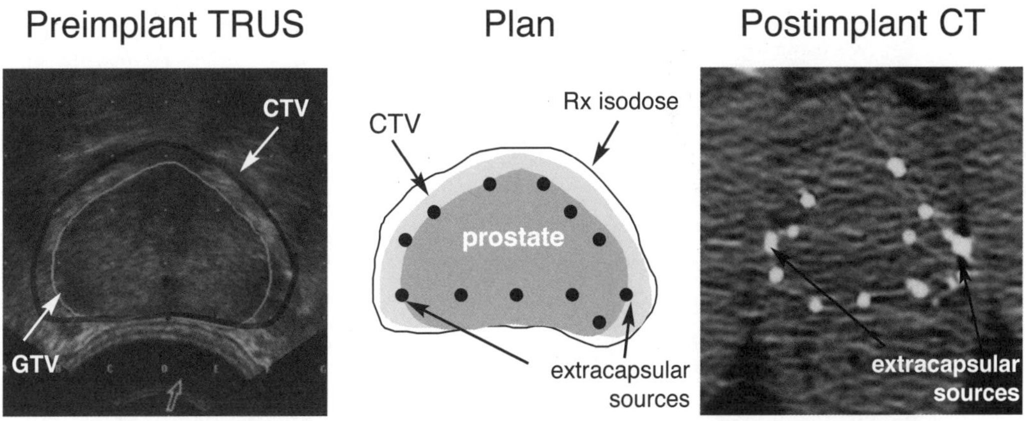

Preimplant TRUS   Plan   Postimplant CT

Figure 6-23. Extracapsular source placement. M. Dattoli has long been an advocate of placing sources 1–5 mm outside of the prostatic capsule.

Accordingly, many brachytherapists refrain from placing sources outside of the prostate. In fact, extraprostatic sources generally do not migrate, a phenomenon that has been well documented.(MERRICK 00, WILLINS 98) Apparently, sources are well imbedded in the periprostatic tissue, whether it is the pelvic floor musculature near the apex, or the periprostatic connective tissue and muscle.

The rationale for placing sources outside is that the extraprostatic coverage can be extended, keeping urethral doses within acceptable limits. A brief perusal of pre-plans in Figures 6-24 and 6-25 shows that the prescription isodose is typically 4–5 mm outside of the most peripheral sources of the implant, so that achieving a 5 mm treatment margin around the prostate will require sources very near the edge of the prostate. Davis and colleagues showed that maximal EPE may be treatable without the use of extraprostatic sources, but many brachytherapists use them routinely (**Figure 6-23**).(DAVIS 00).

SOURCE PLACEMENT MADE EASY
Okay, okay. Take a break. Yes, there is a bewildering maze of treatment planning minutiae with a lot of yet-to-be-resolved issues. But in routine practice, at least as we know it now, treatment planning is actually a quick and easy procedure. With computer-based planning, source placement can be quickly optimized to minimize the central dose, while achieving the prescription dose at the prostatic periphery. And while one could spend endless hours agonizing over a millimeter or two here or there, such agonizing isn't really called for, since we don't know precisely where the treatment margins *should* be.

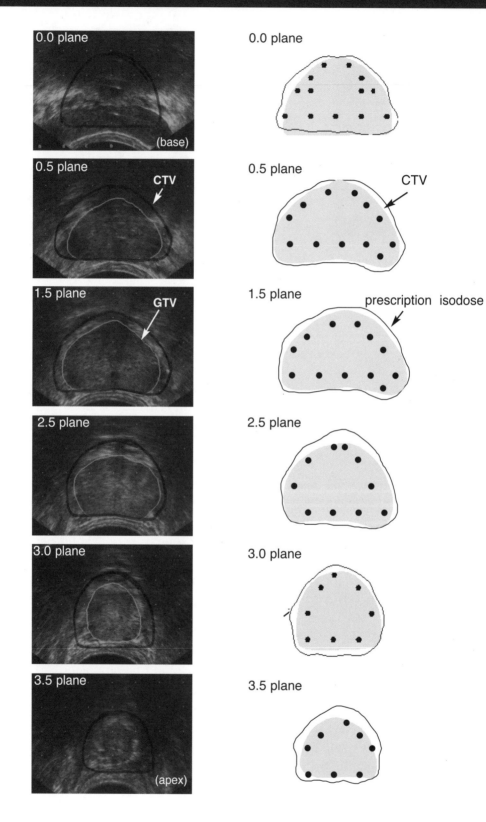

6.26

Figure 6-24 (opposite page). Preimplant TRUS images and plan for 120 Gy Pd-103 implant by M. Dattoli. Note that the clinical target volume (CTV) extends considerably beyond the margin of the prostate (GTV) anteriorly and laterally. This added margin is most striking at the base and apex.

While there are not hard and fast rules for source placement, some general rules of thumb can help keep things simple. First, keep the right and left sides of the prostate symmetric. Second, avoid placing sources near the urethra. Third, when possible, avoid needles with less than three sources, to minimize the number of needles required.

Sources should be placed first around the periphery, at 1.0 cm spacing and keeping within 2–5 mm from the prostatic margin. Sources at the periphery alone often will not give adequate coverage of the entire volume. Additional sources are then placed more centrally and/or peripherally until adequate target coverage is achieved, with acceptable central doses.

Although there are commercially available automatic seed placement programs, with modern treatment planning systems the process can be completed by trial and error within a few minutes by an experienced dosimetrist, adding or moving sources until adequate peripheral coverage is achieved (**Figures 6-24 & 6-25**).

As a guide to the kind of treatment planning used in some favorable, high-profile series, Figures 6-24 and 6-25 show typical plans used by M. Dattoli and J. Blasko. But yours don't need look the same. Remember, even following the guidelines described in the preceding pages, there's plenty of room to be creative with your own plans! As a further guide to how others do it, Merrick and colleagues published a detailed accounting of their own treatment planning technique.(MERRICK 00)

EXTRAS

For better or worse, it's common practice to add extra sources at the time of implant, beyond what is called for in the computer-generated plan. Extra sources are typically added to areas where biopsies are known to be positive, or to regions where source placement appear suboptimal, based on intraoperative TRUS or fluoroscopy images. Adding sources ad hoc is a somewhat risky practice that could lead to excessive urethral or rectal doses. If you choose to do so, it is prudent to

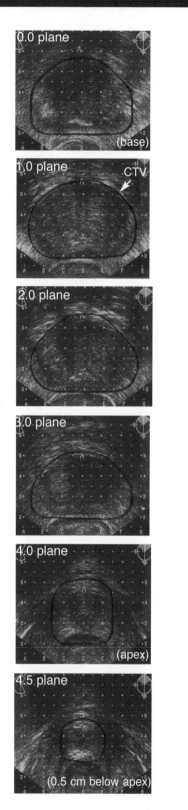

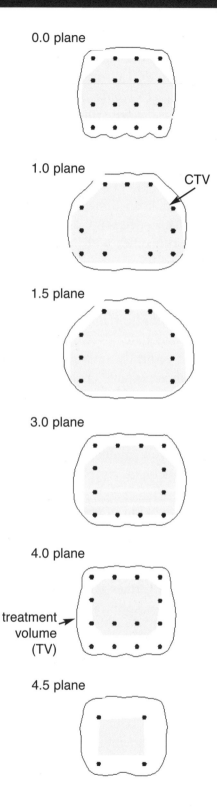

6.28

Figure 6-24 (opposite page). Pre-implant TRUS images and plan for 144 Gy I-125 implant by J. Blasko. Note that JB draws tighter CTV, but makes up for it with larger treatment margins on the plan, with a more generous CTV-to-TM distance, so that the ultimate treatment margin is similar to that of M. Dattoli in Figure 6.23. Like Dattoli, Blasko uses a more generous CTV at the prostatic base and apex (4.0 and 4.5 planes).

keep extras lateral, to minimize additional radiation to the urethra and the rectum.

If you're going to add extras, keep in mind that the typical six to eight extras amount to 5–10% of the total sources, modestly increasing the high dose volumes (**Figures 6-26 & 6-27**). But as long as the extras are kept lateral, rectal and ure-thral doses should be acceptable.

It should be noted that this somewhat haphazard use of extra sources is one of the *voodoo factors* of prostate brachytherapy, being an arbitrary and inconsistent alter-ation of what is supposed to be a precise treatment plan. But it's been a routine pol-icy followed by brachytherapists, achieving high tumor control rates with accept-able morbidity (the authors of this book all do it!).

The days of arbitrary extras are probably numbered. There is considerable interest in the development of intraoperative, postimplant dosimetry. Real-time evaluation would make the use of additional sources to boost inadequately implanted regions a more rational endeavor.

HORMONAL DOWNSIZING
Androgen deprivation typically reduces the prostate volume by approximately 25% to 50%.(SHEARER, ZELEFSKY, FORMAN) When pretreatment androgen depriva-tion is used, dosimetry should be based on the reduced prostate volume. Sufficient time should be given to allow near maximal shrinkage before obtaining the plan-ning images, with most of the shrinkage occurring in the first two months of andro-gen deprivation (**Figure 6-28**).

PREPLANNING VERSUS INTRAOPERATIVE PLANNING
Stone, Stock, and DeWyngaart have reported extensively on TRUS-based implants, without use of pre-planning images. The prostate size is estimated from preimplant office TRUS, and the approximate number of sources needed is deter-mined from a nomogram. At the time of the procedure, two-thirds of the activity

Extra sources: Pd-103

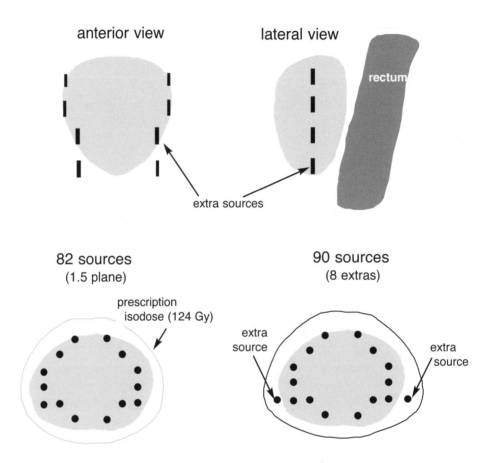

82 sources
(1.5 plane)

90 sources
(8 extras)

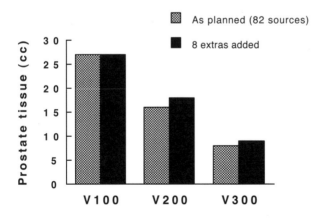

Figure 6-26. Typical placement of eight extra Pd-103 sources, arbitrarily putting four more on each side of the prostate (top panel). The extras amount to 10% of the planned total activity. Note that the effect on the prescription isodose is slight (middle panels), as is the effect on the high dose volumes within the prostate (left).

6.30

Extra sources: I-125

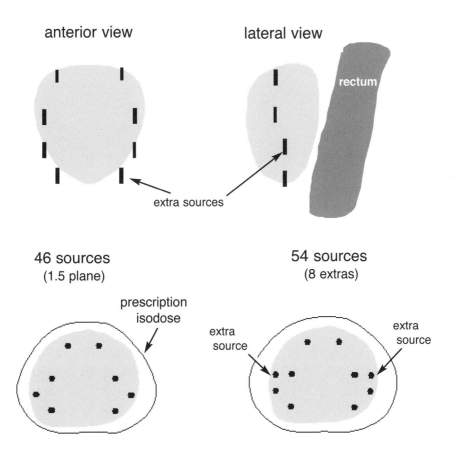

anterior view

lateral view

rectum

extra sources

46 sources
(1.5 plane)

54 sources
(8 extras)

prescription
isodose

extra
source

extra
source

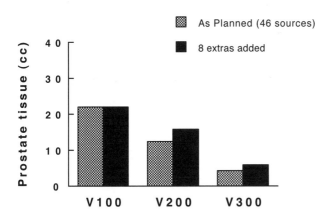

As Planned (46 sources)

8 extras added

Figure 6-27. Typical placement of eight extra I-125 sources, arbitrarily putting four more on each side of the prostate (top panel). The extras amount to 17% of the planned total activity. Even with this substantial addition to the total, note that the effect on the prescription isodose is still small (middle panels), as is the effect on the high dose volumes within the prostate (left).

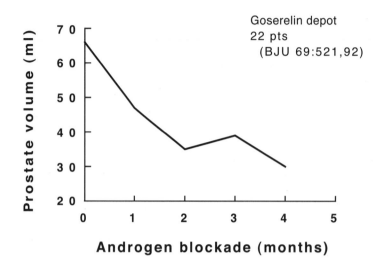

Figure 6-28. Prostate volume reduction after initiating androgen blockade. The volume reduction slows at two months, although the time course varies substantially from patient to patient.(SHEARER)

is placed at the prostatic periphery, and the remainder in the interior of the gland. Satisfactory dosimetry is achievable with their method.(STONE) Now, faster treatment-planning systems allow true intraoperative planning based on intraoperative image capture, and many people are getting into the act.(MESSING, ZELEFSKY 00, GEWANTER, BEYER)

Intraoperative planning has its pros and cons (**Table 6-1**). Probably the most touted advantage is better matching of the planning images with what is actually used, circumventing the potential problem of a discrepancy between the planning versus the intraoperative images some weeks later. While this could be a legitimate advantage, in experienced hands we find that such discrepancies are minimal and likely inconsequential. Reports of improved results with one technique over the other likely reflect inadequate brachytherapy skills, rather than a true advantage to one over the other.

Probably the most appealing aspect of preplanning is the increased time available to evaluate the plan, deciding on minor changes at your leisure. While the time to evaluate may be an advantage, in experienced hands it's probably not a major one.

Table 6-1. Preop versus intraop planning

	Intra-operative	Pre-operative
Pros	Better tailored to image(?)	Less OR time
		Easier seed management
		More time to evaluate plans
Cons	Increase OR time	Need meticulous preimplant TRUS study
	-20-30 minutes+	
	Need extra seeds	
	-10-20+	

From a purely practical standpoint, intra-operative planning has some substantial disadvantages. It can increase operating time by 20–30 minutes or more, and requires a greater degree of physics support intraoperatively. Additionally, it requires extra sources on hand, in case the intraoperative plan calls for more seeds than were anticipated from the preimplant volume. The bottom line—there are many ways to do transperineal implants, and good results are more dependent on the skill and experience of the brachytherapy team than on the particular planning method.

SUPPLEMENTAL EXTERNAL BEAM RADIATION

The use of supplemental beam radiation with prostate brachytherapy has been widely practiced since the days of low dose rate Ir-192 (see chapter 11). There are many possible combinations of brachytherapy and supplemental radiation—the sequencing, radionuclides, and doses can all be varied. While there is no lack of

Table 6-2. Implant boost treatment schemes used by various groups.

Investigator	1st modality	EBRT dose	Isotope	Imp dose	Time between
Blasko	EBRT	45 Gy	Pd-103	90 Gy	2-6 wks
Wallner (1997)	EBRT	50 Gy	Pd-103	60 Gy	2-4 wks
Wallner (1999)	EBRT	20 Gy	Pd-103	105 Gy	1-5 days
Dattoli	EBRT	41 Gy	Pd-103	80 Gy	2-6 wks
	EBRT	20 Gy			0-1 week
Critz	Implant	45 Gy	I-125	80 Gy	3-6 wks
Stone/Stock	Implant	60 Gy	Pd-103	80-90 Gy	8 wks

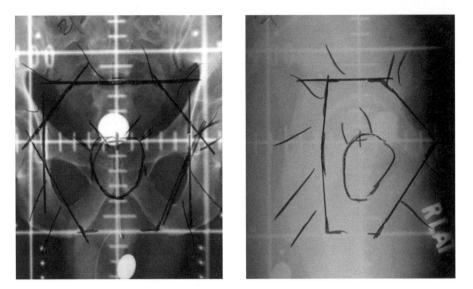

Figure 6-29. Typical anterior and lateral fields used for supplemental external beam radiation. No studies have been done regarding the optimal treatment margins to use in the setting of brachytherapy plus beam radiation.

opinions as to how modalities should be combined, little data is available to support one scheme versus another.

Sequencing
Theoretical arguments can be made for using either radiation sequencing scheme. In the absence of solid data that one is better than the other, preimplant and postimplant supplemental external radiation are both widely used, with what appears to be an acceptable risk of serious complications in experienced hands (**Table 6-2**).(CRITZ, BLASKO, DATTOLI)

Beam radiation is typically given first, followed by brachytherapy, one rationale being that external radiation may shrink the prostate and facilitate coverage by the implant. This rationale is probably flawed in that it's unlikely that the prostate shrinks detectably during several weeks of external radiation.

There is some concern that doing the implant first could lead to a higher incidence of rectal complications, in part because patients still are receiving some implant radiation while the beam radiation is being delivered. In one European report, patients who were implanted first had a very high incidence of rectal complications.(IVERSEN) However, in addition to doing the implant first, the investigators gave large fractions of beam radiation (2.5 Gy per day to the whole pelvis) and a *full* dose I-125 implant. Delivering full doses with both radiation modalities was more likely the cause of frequent rectal complications, rather than their sequencing.

Time between modalities
The time interval between implant and external radiation varies from two to eight weeks in published studies, but there is currently no published data regarding clinical outcomes versus the time interval (**Table 6-2**). Studies of the effect of overall treatment time with external beam alone for prostate cancer have been mixed.(AMDUR, LAI) Shorter times between beam radiation and brachytherapy for cervical carcinoma result in better tumor control rates, an impetus to consider shorter intervals between brachytherapy and supplemental external radiation for prostatic cancer.(LANCIANO) Considering the very low likelihood of serious rectal complications with *any* of the time intervals used, it seems reasonable to decrease the interval to two weeks or less. In fact, K. Wallner and M. Dattoli have arbitrarily decreased the interval to zero to five days, with no obvious increase in morbidity (data not yet published).

Field sizes
Limited external beam radiation fields are the norm, considering the negative RTOG study regarding radiation of pelvic lymph nodes.(ASBELL) Fields typically are designed to cover the prostate and base of the seminal vesicles, with about a 2 cm margin anteriorly and laterally, and a 1 cm margin posteriorly (**Figures 6-29 & 6-30**).

Doses
A wide variety of implant and beam radiation dose combinations could be used (**Table 6-2**). When combined with beam radiation, implant doses are generally dropped to about 50% to 80% of monotherapy doses, ranging from 90–120 Gy with I-125 and 60–113 Gy with Pd-103 (**Figure 6-30**). Caution should be used when extrapolating combined brachytherapy and beam doses between institutions, due to potential differences in treatment margins.

External beam doses of 40–60 Gy are typically used, extrapolating from combined radiation modality treatment of cancer of cervix, head & neck, and sarcomas. Doses for *all* sites have been arrived at empirically.

In an effort to arrive at a more rational dosing policy, a randomized trial is being conducted at the Puget Sound Veterans Affairs Hospital, the University of

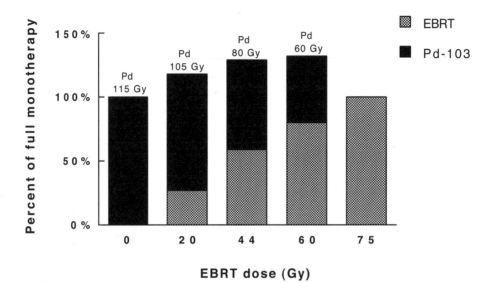

Figure 6-30. Total doses, expressed as percent of monotherapy dose, with various combinations of beam radiation and brachytherapy, estimated by assuming that equivalent full monotherapy doses for Pd-103 and beam radiation are 115 Gy and 75 Gy, respectively.

Washington, and the Schiffler Cancer Center in Wheeling, West Virginia. Patients with intermediate-risk cancer (PSA 10–20 and/or Gleason 7–10) are randomized to 20 versus 44 Gy, with a Pd-103 implant (**Figure 6-31**). Initial results should be available by 2004.

Radionuclides
The optimal isotope choice for use with beam radiation is not clearly established. The majority of favorable, published series have used Pd-103, but there are also encouraging reports of I-125 combined with supplemental external radiation. (CRITZ) Randomized trials are needed.

THE ART OF PROSTATE BRACHYTHERAPY
This chapter, more than any other, points out the inconsistencies between brachytherapists in performing prostate implants. *Art* is a euphemism for the striking lack of scientific evidence regarding the optimal way to design an implant. Much of the variability is due to personal bias rather than legitimate data. But there are probably a lot of ways to get an effective implant—just because the methodology is not standardized doesn't mean that prostate brachytherapy doesn't work.

High versus low dose supplemental beam radiation

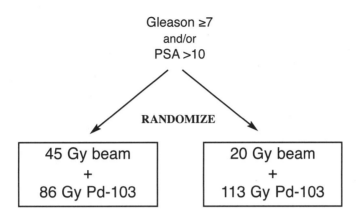

Figure 6-31. Ongoing trial randomizing intermediate risk patients to 44 Gy versus 20 Gy supplemental external beam radiation.

Remember, despite the multitude of uncertainties in brachytherapy treatment planning and the widely varying treatment schemes, the clinical results appear favorable in most hands. Nevertheless, it's important to understand the nuances of implant design in order to maximize cure rates and minimize the likelihood of complications.

REFERENCES
1. Amdur RJ, Parsons JT, Fitzgerald LT, Million RR. The effect of overall treatment time on local control in patients with adenocarcinoma of the prostate treated with radiation therapy. Int J Radiat Oncol Biol Phys 1990; 19:1377-1382.

2. Anderson LL. Spacing nomograph for interstitial implants of I-125 seeds. Med Phys 1976; 3:48-51.

3. Anderson LL. Brachytherapy planning and evaluation. Endo/Hyper Oncol 1991; 7:139-146.

4. Asbell SO, Krall JM, Pilepich MV, Baerwald H. Elective pelvic irradiation in stage A2, B carcinoma of the prostate: Analysis of RTOG 77-06. Int J Radiat Oncol Biol Phys 1988; 15:1307-1316.

5. Badiozamani K, Wallner K, Sutlief S, Ellis W, Blasko J, Russell K. Anticipating prostatic volume changes due to prostate brachytherapy. Radiat Oncol Invest 1999; 7:360-364.

6. Beyer DC, Shapiro RH, Puente F. Real-time optimized intraoperative dosimetry for prostate brachytherapy: A pilot study. Int J Radiat Oncol Biolo Phys 2000; 48:1583-1589.

7. Blasko JC, Grimm PD, Sylvester JE, Badiozamani KR, Hoak D, Cavanagh W. Palladium-103 brachytherapy for prostate carcinoma. Int J Rad Oncol Biol Phys 2000; 46:839-850.

8. Butler WM, Merrick GS, Dorsey AT, Hagedorn BM. Comparison of dose length, area, and volume histograms as quantifiers of urethral dose in prostate brachytherapy. Int J Radiat Oncol Biolo Phys 2000; 48:1575-1582.

9. Critz FA, Williams WH, Levinson AK, Benton JB, Holladay CT, Schnell FJ. Simultaneous irradiation for prostate cancer: intermediate results with modern techniques. J Urol 2000; 164:738-743.

10. Cumes DM, Goffinet DR, Martinez A, Stamey TA. Complications of 125-Iodine implantation and pelvic lymphadenectomy for prostatic cancer with special reference to patients who had failed external beam therapy as their initial mode of therapy. J Urol 1981; 126:620-622.

11. Dattoli M, Wallner K, True L, Sorace R, Koval J, et al . Prognostic role of serum prostatic acid phosphatase for 103-Pd-based radiation for prostatic carcinoma. Int J Rad Oncol Biol Phys 1999; 45:853-856.

12. Davis BJ, Haddock MG, Wilson TM, et al . Treatment of extraprostatic cancer in clinically organ-confined prostate cancer by permanent intersititial brachytherapy: Is extraprostatic seed placement necessary? Tech Urol 2000; 6:70-77.

13. Davis BJ, Pisansky TM, Wilson TM, Rothenberg HJ, Pacelli A, Hillman DW, Sargent DJ, Bostwick DG. The radial distance of extraprostatic extension of prostate carcinoma: implications for prostate brachytherapy. Cancer 1999; 85:2630-2637.

14. Forman JD, Kumar R, Haas G, Montie J. Neoadjuvant hormonal downsizing of localized carcinoma of the prostate: Effects on the volume of normal tissue irradiation. Ca Invest 1995; 13:8-15.

15. Gewanter RM, Wuu C, Laguna JL, Katz AE, Ennis RD. Intraoperative preplanning for transperineal ultrasound-guided permanent prostate brachytherapy. Int J Rad Oncol Biol Phys 2000; 48:377-380.

16. Han B, Wallner K, Aggarwal S, Armstrong J, Sutlief S. Treatment margins for prostate brachytherapy. Sem in Urol Oncol 2000; 18:137-141.

17. ICRU . Prescribing, recording, and reporting photon beam therapy. ICRU Report 50 1993; 1-8.

18. Iversen P, Nielsen L, Bak M, Rasmussen F, Juul N, Torp-Pederson S, Laursen F, Holm HH, von der Maase H. Ultrasonically guided 125Iodine seed implantation with external radiation in management of localized prostatic carcinoma. Urol 1989; 34:181-186.

19. Lai PP, Pilipich MV, Krall JM, Asbell SO. The effect of overall treatment time on the outcome of definitive radiotherapy for localized prostate carcinoma: the Radiation Therapy Oncology Group 75-06 and 77-06 experience. Int J Radiat Oncol Biol Phys 1991; 21:925-933.

20. Lanciano RM, Pajak TF, Martz K, Hanks GE. The influence of treatment time on outcome for squamous cell cancer of the uterine cervix treated with radiation: a patterns-of-care study. Int J Rad Oncol Biol Phys 1993; 25:391-397.

21. Leibovich BC, Blute ML, Bostwick DG, Wilson TM, et al . Proximity of prostate cancer to the urethra: Implications for minimally invasive ablative therapies. Urol 2000; 56:726-729.

22. Maguire PD, Waterman FM, Dicker AP. Can the cost of permanent prostate implants be reduced? An argument for peripheral loading with higher strength seeds. Tech Urol 2000; 6:85-88.

23. McNeal JE, Price HM, Redwine EA, Freiha FS, Stamey TA. Stage A Versus Stage B Adenocarcinoma of the Prostate: Morphological Comparison and Biological Significance. J Urol 1988; 139:61-65.

24. Merrick GS, Butler WM. Modified uniform seed loading for prostate brachytherapy: rationale, design, and evaluation. Tech Urol 2000; 6:78-84.

25. Merrick GS, Butler WM, Dorsey AT, et al . Influence of prophylactic dexamethasone on edema following prostate brachytherapy. Tech Urol 2000; 6:117-122.

26. Merrick GS, Butler WM, Dorsey AT, Lief JH, Benson ML. Seed fixity in the prostate/periprostatic region following brachytherapy. Int J Rad Oncol Biol Phys 2000; 46:215-220.

27. Merrick GS, Butler WM, Wallner KE, Burden LR, Dougherty JE. Extracapsular dose distribution following permanent prostate brachytherapy. (submitted) 2002;

28. Messing EM, Zhang JBY, Rubens DJ, et al . Intraoperative optimized inverse planning for prostate brachytherapy: early experience. Int J Rad Oncol Biol Phys 1999; 44:801-808.

29. Narayana V, Roberson PL, Winfield RJ, Kessler ML. Optimal placement of radioisotopes for permanent prostate implants. Radiol 1996; 199:457-460.

30. Prestidge BR, Bice WS, Kiefer EJ, Prete JJ. Timing of computed tomography-based postimplant assessment following permanent transperineal prostate brachytherapy. Int J Radiat Oncol Biolo Phys 1998; 40:1111-1115.

31. Rosen MA, Goldstone L, Lapin S, Wheeler T, Scardino PT. Frequency and location of extracapsular extension and positive surgical margins in radical prostatectomy specimens. J Urol 1992; 148:331-337.

32. Shearer RJ, Davies JH, Gelister JSK, Dearnaley DP. Hormonal cytoreduction and radiotherapy for carcinoma of the prostate. Br J Urol 1992; 69:521-524.

33. Sohayda C, Kupelian PA, Levin JS, Klein EA. Extent of extracapsular extension in localized prostate cancer. Urol 2000; 55:382-386.

34. Speight JL, Shinohara K, Pickett B, Weinberg VK, Hsu ICJ, Roach M. Prostate volume change after radioactive seed implantation: possible benefit of improved dose volume histogram with perioperative steroid. Int J Radiat Oncol Biolo Phys 2000; 48:1461-1467.

35. Stamey TA, Villers AA, McNeal JE, Link PC, Freiha FS. Positive surgical margins at radical prostatectomy: importance of the apical dissection. J Urol 1990; 143:1166-1173.

36. Stock RG, Lo Y, Gaildon M, Stone NN. Does prostate brachytherapy treat the seminal vesicles: A dose-volume histogram analysis of seminal vesicles in patients undergoing combined Pd-103 prostate implantation and external beam irradiation. Int J Rad Oncol Biol Phys 1999; 45:385-389.

37. Stone NN, Stock RG, DeWyngaert JK, Tabert A. Prostate brachytherapy: Improvements in prostate volume measurements and dose distribution using interactive ultrasound guided implantation and three-dimensional dosimetry. Radiat Oncol Invest 1995; 3:185-195.

38. Wallner KE, Roy J, Harrison L. Dosimetry guidelines to minimize urethral and rectal morbidity following transperineal I-125 prostate brachytherapy. Int J Radiat Oncol Biol Phys 1995; 32:465-471.

39. Waterman FM, Dicker AP. Determination of the urethral dose in prostate brachytherapy when the urethra cannot be visualized in the postimplant CT scan. Med Phys 2000; 27:448-451.

40. Waterman FM, Yue N, Corn BW, Dicker AP. Edema associated with I-125 or Pd-103 prostate brachytherapy and its impact on post-implant dosimetry: an analysis based on serial CT acquistion. Int J Rad Oncol Biol Phys 1998; 41:1069-1077.

41. Willins J, Wallner K. CT-based dosimetry for transperineal I-125 prostate brachytherapy. Int J Rad Oncol Biol Phys 1997; 39:347-353.

42. Willins J, Wallner KE. Time-dependent changes in CT-based dosimetry of I-125 prostate brachytherapy. Radiat Oncol Invest 1998; 6:157-160.

43. Yue N, Chen Z, Peschel R, Dicker AP, Waterman FM, Nath R. Optimum timing for image-based evaluation of 125-I and 103-Pd prostate seed implants. Int J Rad Oncol Biol Phys 1999; 45:1063-1072.

44. Yue N, Dicker AP, Corn BW, Nath R, Waterman FM. A dynamic model for the estimation of optimum timing of computed tomography scan for dose evaluation of 125-I or 103-Pd seed implant of prostate. Int J Rad Oncol Biol Phys 1999; 43:447-454.

45. Zaider M, Zelefsky MJ, Lee EK, et al . Treatment planning for prostate implants using magnetic-resonance sprectroscopy imaging. Int J Rad Oncol Biol Phys 2000; 47:1085-1096.

46. Zelefsky MJ, Leibel SA, Burman CM, Kutcher GJ. Neoadjuvant hormonal therapy improves the therapeutic ratio in patients with bulky prostatic cancer treated with three-dimensional conformal radiation therapy. Int J Radiat Oncol Biol Phys 1994; 29:755-761.

47. Zelefsky MJ, Yamada Y, Cohen G, et al . Postimplantation dosimetric analysis of permanent transperineal prostate implantation: improved dose distributions with an intraoperative computer-optimized conformal planning technique. Int J Rad Oncol Biol Phys 2000; 48:601-608.

7

Patient Preparation

Proper patient preparation should facilitate the implant procedure and decrease the risk of postoperative morbidity. There is a wide variety of preparatory practices, with little data to support one policy over another. The following is a summary of various policies, all of which seem acceptable. Some are more practical than others.

BOWEL PREPARATION
The rectum should be clear of feces to facilitate proper TRUS imaging. Lower GI clearing may also decrease the risk of infection should the rectum inadvertently be pierced. A variety of enemas, diets, and laxative cocktails can be used, all with a

Table 7-1. Lower GI clearing protocols.

	Diet	Enema	Laxative
Blasko	low fiber (24 hr) NPO after midnight	night before & AM of implant	none
Dattoli	NPO after midnight (liquid breakfast for evening cases)	night before (2) & AM (2) of implant	none
Wallner	Liquid breakfast	AM of implant	none

80 to 90% likelihood of success (**Table 7-1**).(POUND) Some regimens are more onerous than others. Given the lack of any apparent difference, it seems wise to use the least expensive, least uncomfortable, and most convenient regimen. We have abandoned the use of laxatives, as they too often lead to intraoperative diarrheal disasters. An early morning enema is usually sufficient. If feces obscures the TRUS image, intra-operative rectal lavage with a large bore tube is a practical (but unpleasant) solution.

INFECTION CONTROL
In the late 1800s, postoperative infection rates fell from nearly 100% to less than 5%, primarily due to adoption of hand-washing and clothing changes. Since that time, a large number of additional antiseptic (tissue) and disinfectant (inanimate objects) maneuvers have been introduced, without much further reduction in the infection rate. Prostate brachytherapy offers a good sampling of the inane infection-control practices of modern medicine.

Shaving
Several investigators have reported a *higher* likelihood of infection if the skin is shaved prior to general surgery, probably resulting from microscopic skin breaks.(SEROPIAN, BIRD) Considering that no case of perineal skin or subcutaneous infection after transperineal prostate brachytherapy has ever been reported, and that shaving may actually *increase* the likelihood of infection, it's a practice that should be avoided.

Cleansing
Whether or not the skin is shaved, it should be cleansed with an antiseptic. There is no substantial difference between commonly used skin cleansers regarding their

*Table 7-2. Clinical data supporting the use of prophylactic antibi-
otics with transperineal prostate brachytherapy.*

antimicrobial effect.(RITTER) Alcohol (70%) is as effective as any other cleanser, but may cause skin irritation. Free iodine (tincture) is no longer used, due to its tendency to cause skin irritation. Iodine complexed with povodine (10% povodine-iodine solution, Betadine™) is less likely to irritate the skin—it works as well as tincture of iodine and reactions to it are rare.

Antibiotics
In general, prophylactic antibiotics are prescribed far more frequently than is supported by the medical literature.(DURACK) Data to support their use for transperineal implantation are scarce. Two randomized trials have shown that prophylactic antibiotics can decrease the incidence of bacteriuria or bacteremia following transrectal biopsy.(RUEBUSH, CRAWFORD) However, no significant decrease in clinically recognized sepsis or urinary infection was shown. Apparently, patients with postsurgical bacteriuria or bacteremia nearly always clear bacteria with natural defenses.

Amazingly, the inconclusive data regarding prophylactic antibiotics for trans*rectal* biopsy have been extrapolated to trans*perineal* brachytherapy, such that antibiotics are routinely given. Extrapolation of inconclusive transrectal biopsy data to transperineal implantation is especially questionable, because transrectal biopsies are done through a contaminated rectal mucosa, whereas transperineal procedures should be clean, if not sterile (depending on whether the rectum is violated).

No randomized trials have tested the benefit of routine antibiotics for transperineal biopsy or implantation (**Table 7-2**). In a nonrandomized retrospective trial, Packer

*Table 7-3. Febrile episodes following transperineal implantation at MSKCC, with or without prophylactic antibiotics.(*WALLNER *96)*

	Patients	Febrile episodes
No antibiotics	114	2 (2%)
no catheter	95	2 (2%)
catheter	19	0 (0%)
Antibiotics	17	0
no catheter	16	0
catheter	1	0

and colleagues found no benefit to antibiotic use in patients with a documented negative urine culture prior to transperineal biopsy.(PACKER)

Implants without antibiotics
Of 131 patients who underwent I-125 implants by K. Wallner at Memorial Sloan-Kettering Cancer Center (MSKCC) from 1987 through 1995, none of 17 patients who received prophylactic antibiotics had a postoperative febrile episode. Of 114 patients who did not receive prophylactic antibiotics, 19 required Foley catheter drainage one day or longer for postimplant urinary retention and two patients (2%) developed a postimplant febrile episode within two weeks of surgery (**Table 7-3**). One patient was treated empirically (outpatient) with trimethoprim/sulfamethoxazole (TMP/SMX) and defervesced. The second patient had a 10-year history of chronic lymphocytic leukemia (CLL) and was probably immunocompromised from chlorambucil therapy. He developed E. Coli sepsis twenty-four hours after the procedure, requiring inpatient antibiotic therapy.(WALLNER 96)

Apart from patients with a history of immunosuppression, the MSKCC data argues against routine antibiotics in favor of a wait-and-see approach, with antibiotics given to those unusual patients who develop postimplant infectious signs. Cutting back on routine prophylactic antibiotics may help minimize emergence of drug-resistant bacterial strains and would save money (**Table 7-4**). More recent investigators have also been unable to find a legitimate reason to continue routine use of prophylactic antibiotics.(DICKER)

When antibiotics might be justified
Some more compelling circumstances for routine antibiotic prophylaxis include rheumatic heart disease, prosthetic devices, or immune compromise. (DAJANI) A

Table 7-4. Acceptable antibiotic regimens (actual charges to the patient could be two to three fold higher than those listed)

	Antibiotic(s)	Dose	Timing	Cost ($US)
Blasko	levofloxacin	500 mg IV	immediately prior	$48
	ciprofloxacin	250 mg	bid x 3 days	$25
Dattoli	levofloxacin	500 mg IV	immediately prior	$48
	ciprofloxacin	500 mg	bid x 7 days	$55
Wallner	none			$0

previous history of prostatitis is probably *not* an indication for antibiotics.(HUGHES)

Preoperative urine culture
The likelihood of asymptomatic urinary infection is so low that it is difficult to justify routine cultures in asymptomatic patients.

Timing
If prophylactic antibiotics are used, they should be given immediately (within one hour) preoperatively, so that they are present at the time of the procedure. They should be effective against the most likely contaminants—presumably E. Coli and Enterococcus faecalis.

BLOOD WORK AND CHEST XRAYS
Considering the minimally invasive nature of transperineal brachytherapy and the apparent rarity of intraoperative complications, routine preoperative complete blood counts (CBC) or blood clotting tests (PT/PTT) are probably unnecessary in otherwise healthy patients. Similarly, routine electrolytes, liver function tests, or pre-op chest Xrays, in otherwise healthy patients without specific indications, are probably unnecessary.(SCHEIN)

ANTICOAGULANTS
Traditionally, aspirin and nonsteroidal anti-inflammatory agents (NSAID) are stopped one week prior to the implant procedure, and coumadin should be stopped three days prior.(KEARON) These policies are probably overly cautious considering the rarity of bleeding complications with needle biopsies, even when patients have recently taken NSAIDs.(HERGET)

DVT PROPHYLAXIS

Patients are in the lithotomy position for approximately one to two hours for the implant procedure, but an increased risk of deep venous thrombosis (DVT) or symptomatic thromboembolism has never been reported. Presumably the risk is very low, and prophylactic measures are not routinely used in these typically otherwise healthy patients. However, prophylactic heparin (6,000 units SubQ immediately prior to the procedure) may be warranted in patients with past history of thrombosis, or other predisposing condition.

OBESE PATIENTS

Obese patients are generally more likely to experience adverse postoperative events, including thromboembolism and heart failure. No excess risk of complications has been reported specifically for transperineal implantation of morbidly obese patients, but prophylaxis against DVT may be warranted.

STERILE BARRIERS

Like prophylactic antibiotics, sterile barriers are used far more than warranted by objective data. It seems sensical that liberal use of sterile gowns or drapes would decrease the likelihood of infectious complications, but this has never been shown. Disposable sterile barriers are unnecessary and wasteful, but often mandated by zealous infection control committees. Considering that transperineal implantation is a minimally invasive procedure, and that the skin is cleansed immediately preoperatively, use of gowns is probably unnecessary.

Sterile leg and pelvic drapes are another common, but highly questionable, anti-infection practice. Drapes can actually *increase* the infection rate by trapping bacteria on the warm, moist surface under the barrier.(LEWIS, ALEXANDER) The routine use of sterile drapes might be justified as a way to define and preserve a sterile field, but should not be necessary in experienced hands.

Face masks have never been shown to decrease the risk of perioperative infection for any surgical procedure. In a large, randomized Swedish trial, masks did not decrease the infectious rate for open operations.(TUNEVALL)

ANESTHESIA

Spinal (epidural), general, or local anesthesia can be used. Of 262 orthopedic patients randomized to general or spinal anesthesia at Cornell University Medical College, there was no safety advantage from either a cardiac or cognitive standpoint.(WILLIAMS-RUSSO) The primary advantage of general anesthesia is quick induction. Patients may recover bladder function more quickly with general ver-

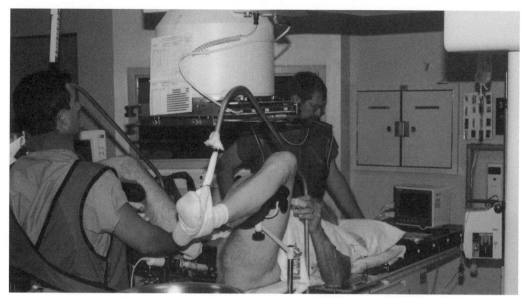

Figure 7-1. Patient is fully awake for an implant procedure in the simulator suite in the Veterans Affairs Puget Sound Health Care System.

sus spinal anesthesia, and spinal anesthesia may prevent perineal discomfort in the immediate postoperative period.

Local anesthesia

Faced with rapidly increasing patient demand and limited operating room time, local anesthesia has been used exclusively for prostate brachytherapy at the Puget Sound VA.(WALLNER 99) The patient is brought into the simulator suite in the radiation oncology department, an IV line is started, and a urinary catheter is inserted. He is then placed in the lithotomy position, using stirrups attached to the simulator table (**Figure 7-1**). A 5 cm patch of perineal skin and subcutaneous tissue is anesthetized by local infiltration of 10 cc of 1% lidocaine, using a 25 gauge 1.5-inch needle (**Figure 7-2, left**). All parenteral lidocaine is given in a 0.5% solution with epinephrine (1:100,000). Immediately following injection into the subcutaneous tissues, the pelvic floor and prostate apex are anesthetized by injecting 15 cc lidocaine solution with approximately eight passes of a 25-gauge 1.5-inch needle.

The transrectal ultrasound (TRUS) probe is then inserted and positioned to reproduce the planning images and a 3.5- or 6.0-inch, 22-gauge spinal needle is inserted into the peripheral planned needle tracks, monitored by TRUS. When the tips of

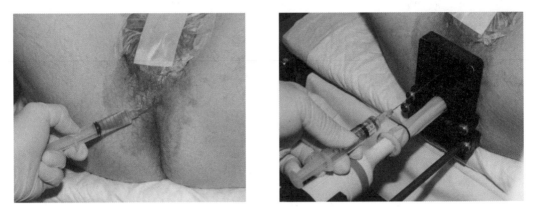

Figure 7-2. Injection of lidocaine into perineal subcutaneous, pelvic floor musculature, and periapical prostatic region (left) and more proximal prostatic tissue (right). The deeper injections can be done with a 6-inch 22-gauge spinal needle, through the TRUS template to monitor position within the prostate.

the needles reach the prostatic base, about 1.0 cc of lidocaine solution is injected in the intraprostatic track, as the needle is slowly withdrawn, for a total volume of 5 to 15 cc (**Figure 7-2, right**). At this point in the procedure, the total dose of lidocaine injected is approximately 100 to 400 mg (**Figure 7-3**). Not all tracks are necessarily injected, depending on the total number and how patients tolerate the injections. A limited number of central tracks are also injected.

When using a Mick® Applicator, a maximum of about six needles are in the patient at any one time. During the implant procedure, an additional 1 cc lidocaine solution is injected into one or more needle tracks if the patient experiences substantial discomfort. The total dose of lidocaine is generally limited to 300 mg. An anesthesiologist is not present for the implant procedure. Lidocaine injections are generally done by a registered nurse.

At the completion of the source placement, the TRUS probe is removed and plain orthogonal pelvic radiographs taken with the catheter in place. Patients are discharged home about two hours after completing the implant.

Patients tolerate brachytherapy under local anesthesia surprisingly well. Their heart rate and diastolic blood pressure usually show minimal changes, consistent with mild discomfort (**Figures 7-4**). Serum lidocaine levels are typically below or

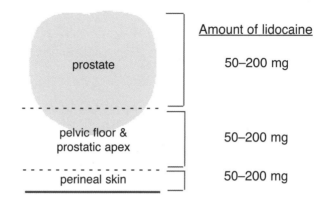

Figure 7-3. Approximate amounts of lidocaine injected into various areas. Other strategies, like injecting into the neurovascular bundles, may be helpful.(NASH)

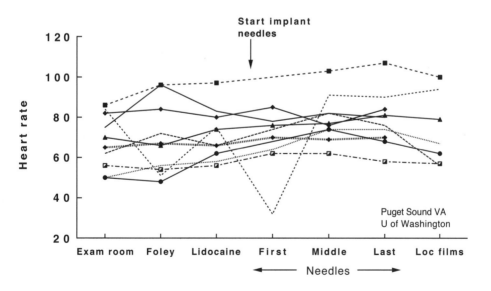

Figure 7-4. Patients' pulse during Foley catheter insertion, lidocaine injections, and the implant procedure.

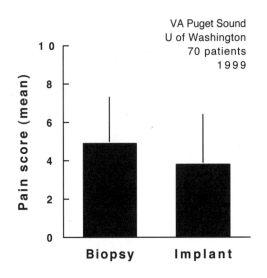

Figure 7-5. Median patient-reported pain scores related to their prostate biopsy versus implant procedure.

at the low range of therapeutic. Postimplant CT-defined target coverage has ranged from 80% to 95%, well within published criteria for technical adequacy.(WILLINS)

As of December 2000, more than 200 patients have received implants under local anesthesia at the Seattle VA; no patient has received an implant under general or spinal anesthesia since June 1999. In all but one case, the implant was completed as planned at the first try, with no deviation in needle or source number due to patient intolerance. However, there was a substantial learning curve, and the procedure has become easier with increasing experience. To evaluate comfort level, patients were interviewed by telephone and asked to rate their pain with the prostate biopsy versus their prostate implant on a scale of 0 to 10.

Of 58 patients interviewed at a median of six months since an implant, the median biopsy pain score was 4.5 and the median implant pain score was 3.0 (**Figure 7-5**). There was no correlation between the two scores (**Figure 7-6**). There is no relationship between the number of needles or the prostate size and the implant pain score (**Figure 7-7**). Five of the 58 patients interviewed by Smathers and colleagues (9%) stated that they would have preferred to have the procedure under general anesthesia (**Figure 7-8**).(SMATHERS)

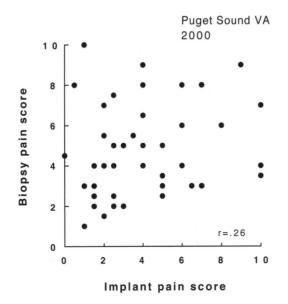

Figure 7-6. There was no relationship between patients' biopsy versus implant pain scores.

The fact that patients typically rate their implant procedure-related pain somewhat *less* than that of their prostate biopsy, a very common procedure that is rarely done under anesthesia, should allay any ethical concerns about decreasing the use of general anesthesia. While a small percentage of patients stated in retrospect that they would have preferred general over local anesthesia, it is also common for patients to express relief over not needing general or spinal anesthesia. Local anesthesia may entail more discomfort with the procedure itself than would be experienced with spinal or general anesthesia, but it offers patients the advantages of a lower risk for postanesthesia dysphoria, and a more rapid return to normal function, and avoids the possibility of postspinal headaches.

In addition to a high degree of patient satisfaction, performing implants under local anesthesia allows for phenomenal logistical and cost advantages. Moving the procedure from an operating room or cystoscopy suite avoids the scheduling difficulties of a busy operating room, and slashes operating and recovery room costs.

That's not to say that performing implants with local anesthesia is without its problems. There's no question that patients are more likely to move, requiring some

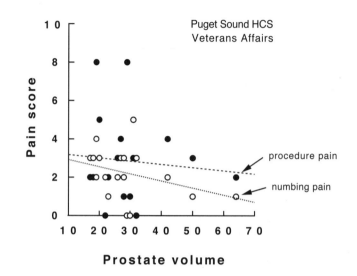

Figure 7-7. Implant pain scores versus TRUS-based prostate volume. Patients with larger prostate volumes tolerate the procedure as well as patients with smaller ones. Numbing pain refers to the infiltration of lidocaine throughout the prostate. Procedure pain refers to placement of the sources.(HOFFMAN)

adjustments in positioning of the TRUS probe. But with an easily adjustable TRUS stand, this has not been a big problem.

While pleased with the overall level of patient acceptance at the Seattle VA, we're still trying to make it better. Nitrous oxide ("laughing gas") facilities have recently been installed in the simulator suite (for the patients, not the staff!). Nonpharmacologic relaxation techniques and/or intravenous midazolam are being given to more anxious patients.

PROPHYLACTIC CORTICOSTEROIDS
Approximately 2% to 10% of patients develop postimplant urinary retention, requiring temporary catheter drainage (see chapter 12). Prophylactically corticosteroids might decrease the likelihood of post-operative urinary retention, the rationale being to prevent postimplant tissue swelling. Corticosteroids are routinely given by M. Dattoli (**Table 7-6**), but they are not currently widely prescribed.

Although the concept is appealing, in a preliminary trial, corticosteroids did not alter implant-related prostatic size changes appreciably, and there is no data that

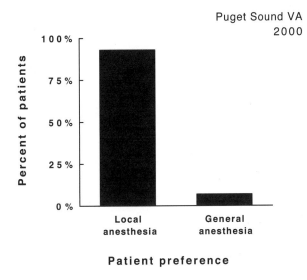

Puget Sound VA
2000

Figure 7-8. If given the choice, patients typically prefer the convenience of local anesthesia.

corticosteroids decrease the likelihood of postoperative prostate swelling or urinary obstruction.(MERRICK 00) Randomized, controlled trials are warranted.

HOSPITALIZATION
The vast majority of implants are performed on an outpatient basis, with consistently low perioperative complications.(HAN, BENOIT) Without data to the contrary, it is hard to justify routine overnight hospitalization. Patients occasionally request to be hospitalized, in case they develop a postoperative problem. Such hospitalization, in the absence of extenuating circumstances, should be discouraged. For the vast majority of patients, it's expensive and unnecessary. Additionally, hospitalization might increase the likelihood of hospital-derived infection with drug-resistant organisms.

An alternative to the cost of overnight hospitalization that still provides the patient an extra sense of security is "23-hour hospitalization," whereby patients are observed overnight but spared the full charge of an overnight hospitalization. M. Dattoli uses 23-hour hospitalization routinely. The urinary catheter is removed at 4:00 AM to allow a voiding trial before discharge.

INFORMING PATIENTS
What and how much to tell patients beforehand is largely a matter of personal practice. We have learned a few things the hard way. Patients commonly get the impression from the news media or overly zealous brachytherapists that side

Table 7-5. Dexamethasone schedule used by M. Dattoli.

- 10 mg IV intra-operative
- 4 mg IV at 8 PM
- 4 mg IV at 6 AM
- discharge with 1-2 week taper schedule

effects with brachytherapy are minimal. When considered in comparison to radical prostatectomy, that is likely true. But there is still some risk of acute urinary retention, and a very high likelihood of longer-term (but temporary) radiation-related prostatitis. It's prudent to make sure that patients are warned in some detail about these probabilities (**Table 7-6**).

The possibility of postoperative fever and bleeding should be mentioned. Patients should be warned that they have a 5% to 10% likelihood of requiring a catheter to relieve urinary retention in the first few weeks following the procedure, and that a small percentage of patients require a catheterization for much longer. Patients should expect to have burning with urination, frequent daytime urination, a significant degree of urinary urgency, and perhaps a very slow stream, especially during the night. The potential use of alpha blockers to alleviate radiation-related urinary symptoms for three months or longer should be mentioned.

Patients should be told that they are likely to experience frequent bowel movements, loose stools, and some rectal urgency for several months after implantation. Rectal symptoms usually resolve within six to twelve months of the procedure, usually earlier than the urinary symptoms.(MERRICK 00) We tell patients that the risk of permanent urinary incontinence or serious rectal bleeding or ulceration has been very low in most reported series.

Considering that many patients choose brachytherapy because of their hope to maintain potency, it's a good idea to warn sexually active patients that they are likely to experience pain with orgasm for several months, and that they are likely to have less ejaculate volume.(MERRICK 01) They should also be warned that a small percent of patients are impotent immediately after the procedure, with some chance that they will improve with time. Although there's no evidence that sexual abstinence is necessary, it seems prudent to use a condom for one month follow-

Table 7-6. Informed patients — a general list of thing that patients should be told about beforehand.

- substantial urinary burning immediately afterward, subsiding over next 24 hours and then returning for 6–12 months
- abnormal bowel function for at least a couple of days
- intermittent gross hematuria for several days, and sometimes later
- 5–10% chance of needing a urinary catheter, for one day or longer
- 0.5%–3% risk of urinary incontinence
- 2–10% risk of intermittent, painless rectal bleeding (spontaneous healing)
- 0.1–1% risk of colostomy

ing Pd-103 implantation and four months after I-125, until the risk of passing a radioactive source is minimized.

Most important, patients should be reminded to call sooner rather than later if they experience symptoms in excess or different from what they have been told. It's much better, for instance, to juggle a patient's alpha-blocker dose over a few weeks, rather than to hear first about his increasing urinary obstruction from the emergency room staff at 4:00 AM.

REFERENCES

1. Alexander JW, Aerni S, Plettner JP. Development of a safe and effective one-minute preoperative skin preparation. Arch Surg 1985; 120:1357-1361.

2. Benoit RM, Naslund MJ, Cohen JK. Complications after prostate brachytherapy in the Medicare population. Urol 2000; 55:91-96.

3. Bird BJ, Chrisp DB, Scrimgeour G. Extensive pre-operative shaving: a costly exercise. N Z Med J 1984; 97:727-729.

4. Crawford ED, Haynes AL, Story MW, Borden TA. Prevention of urinary tract infection and sepsis following transrectal prostatic biopsy. J Urol 1982; 127:449-451.

5. Dajani AS, Taubert KA, Wilson W, Bolger AF. Prevention of bacterial endocarditis: Recommendations by the American Heart Association. JAMA 1997; 277:1794-1801.

6. Dicker AP, Figura AT, Waterman FM, et al . Is there a role for antibiotic pro-phylaxis in transperineal intersitial permanent prostate brachytherapy? Tech Urol 2000; 6:104-108.

7. Durack DT. Prevention of infective endocarditis. NEJM 1995; 332:38-44.

8. Han BH, Demel KC, Wallner KE, Young L. Patient reported short-term com-plications after prostate brachytherapy. J Urol 2001; (in press):

9. Herget EJ, Saliken JC, Donnely BJ, Gray RR, Wiseman D, Brunet G. Transrectal ultrasound-guided biopsy of the prostate: Relation between ASA use and bleeding complications. Can Assoc Radiolol 1999; 50:173-176.

10. Hoffman C, Wallner K, Simpson C, Arthurs S, Sutlief S. A reappraisal of local anesthesia for prostate brachytherapy. (submitted) 2002;

11. Hughes S, Wallner K, Miller G, Miller S, True L. Pre-existing histologic evi-dence of prostatitis is unrelated to post-implant urinary morbidity. (submitted) 2001;

12. Kearon C, Hirsh J. Management of anticoagulation before and after elective surgery. NEJM 1997; 336:1506-1511.

13. Lewis DA, Leaper DJ, Speller DCE. Prevention of bacterial colonization at operation: comparison of iodine-impregnated ("Ioban") drapes with conventional methods. J Hosp Inf 1984; 5:431-437.

14. Merrick GS, Butler WM, Dorsey AT, et al . Influence of prophylactic dexam-ethasone on edema following prostate brachytherapy. Tech Urol 2000; 6:117-122.

15. Merrick GS, Butler WM, Dorsey AT, Galbreath RW, Blatt H, Lief JH. Rectal function following prostate brachytherapy. Int J Radiat Oncol Biolo Phys 2000; 48:667-674.

16. Merrick GS, Wallner KE, Butler WM, Lief JH, Sutlief S. Sexual function after prostate brachytherapy. (submitted) 2002;

17. Nash PA, Bruce JE, Indudhara R, Shinohara K. Transrectal ultrasound guided prostatic nerve blockade eases systematic needle biopsy of the prostate. J Urol 1996; 155:607-609.

18. Packer MG, Russo P, Fair WR. Prophylactic antibiotics and foley catheter use in transperineal needle biopsy of the prostate. J Urol 1984; 131:687-689.

19. Pound DC. Flexible sigmoidoscopy: Techniques and utilization. Baltimore: Williams & Wilkins, 1990.

20. Ritter MA, French MLV, Eitzen HE. The antimicrobial effectiveness of operative-site preparative agents: a microbiological and clinical study. J Bone Joint Surg 1980; 62A:826.

21. Ruebush TK, McConville JH, Calia FM. A double-blind study of timethoprim-sulfamethoxazole prophylaxis in patients having transrectal needle biopsy of the prostate. J Urol 1979; 122:492-494.

22. Schein OD, Katz J, Bass EB, Tielsch JM, et al . The value of routine preoperative testing before cataract surgery. NEJM 2000; 342:168-175.

23. Seropian R, Reynolds BM. Wound infections after preoperative depilatory versus razor preparation. AM J Surg 1997; 121:251-254.

24. Smathers S, Wallner K, Simpson C, Roof J. Patient perception of local anesthesia for prostate brachytherapy. Sem in Urol Oncol 2000; 18:142-146.

25. Tunevall TG. Postoperative wound infections and surgical face masks: A controlled study. World J Surg 1991; 15:383-388.

26. Wallner KE, Roy J, Harrison L. Low risk of perioperative infection without prophylactic antibiotics for transperineal prostate brachytherapy. Int J Radiat Oncol Biol Phys 1996; 36:681-683.

27. Wallner KE, Simpson C, Roof J, Arthurs S, Korssjoen T, Sutlief S. Local anesthesia for prostate brachytherapy. Int J Rad Oncol Biol Phys 1999; 45:401-406.

28. Williams-Russo P, Sharrock NE, Mattis S, Szatrowski TP. Cognitive effects after epidural vs general anesthesia in older adults. JAMA 1995; 274:44-50.

29. Willins J, Wallner K. CT-based dosimetry for transperineal I-125 prostate brachytherapy. Int J Rad Oncol Biol Phys 1997; 39:347-353.

8

Technique

One of the more remarkable things about prostate brachytherapy is the variety of ways to do a good implant. A good result is not as much dependent on which technique you use, but rather how careful and proficient you are with the methods you choose. In this chapter, we'll walk through the implant procedure from start to finish, describing a variety of methods for each step. Take your pick. If you're new to brachytherapy, don't assume that what's here is best for you—do your own reading and then visit with other brachytherapists to decide which techniques best fit your practice setting. If you're a seasoned brachytherapist already set in your ways, consider trying some of the technical variations described here.

Lithotomy   Extended lithotomy

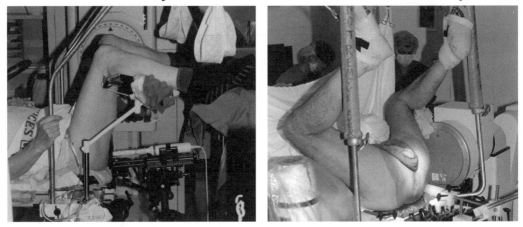

Figure 8-1. Patient positioning. Keep the pelvis square. More extended lithotomy (right) helps avoid pubic arch interference, but be careful to orient the probe such that the prostate lines up on the grid as it did for the planning images (see Figure 8-16).

Often, there are more efficient or downright better ways than what you're accustomed to, partly because the equipment keeps getting better.

PATIENT POSITIONING
After induction of anesthesia, place the patient in the lithotomy position (**Figure 8-1**). Try to reproduce the positioning of the planning scan, realizing that there will always be minor differences. The legs should be symmetrically rotated and extended at the hips and at the knees to avoid rotating the pelvis on the head-to-toe axis. Step back when you think you're done setting up and make sure the patient is as squarely lined up as possible, in the middle of the table. The perineum should be at the very end of the table to allow room to maneuver the ultrasound probe.

The extended lithotomy position helps to avoid pubic arch interference by tilting the pelvis back, moving the pubic bones away from the anterior portion of the prostate. This can be achieved by adjusting the leg stirrups or by pulling the patient's pelvis toward the end of the table, without changing the position of the stirrups. Some brachytherapists place patients in the extended position at the time of initial setup, while others start with the femurs at 90 degrees to the floor, and move to the extended lithotomy position only if pubic arch interference calls for it.

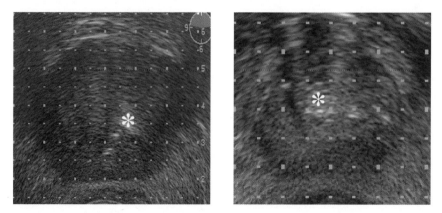

Figure 8-2. Some patients have a remarkably asymmetric urethra (*). The patient on the left has aerated intraurethral gel. The patient on the right has a catheter in place.

A good set of stirrups can really make your life easier. The rigid boots, which are easy to adjust and minimize the likelihood that a patient's legs shift position, are probably best.

URETHRAL VISUALIZATION
There's no shortage of opinions as to how (or even *if*) the urethra should be visualized. Most brachytherapists use some technique to visualize the urethra during the procedure, primarily to make sure that sources are not placed inside it. The biggest problem with intraurethral sources is that they'll be expelled and they won't contribute to the dose as planned. Admittedly, most patients' urethras are midline, and simply avoiding source placement in the prostate midline is enough to keep out of the urethra. But some patients have a markedly asymmetric urethra and its visualization really helps (**Figure 8-2**).

A catheter is the simplest, most reliable way to visualize the urethra and bladder neck. Their downside is that they produce a large ultrasound void (**Figure 8-3**). There is some concern that having a catheter in place during the procedure will lead to urethral tears if the urethral lining gets caught between an advancing needle tip and the catheter. This doesn't seem to be the case, since many brachytherapists use a catheter routinely and persistent postimplant gross urethral bleeding is unusual. Concern has also been raised that a catheter might deform the prostate, altering the source placement. Unlikely—the prostate is a very firm gland, and a flexible catheter shouldn't change its shape.

transverse view

saggital view

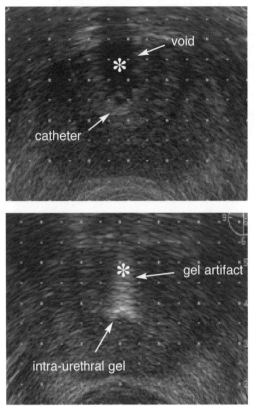
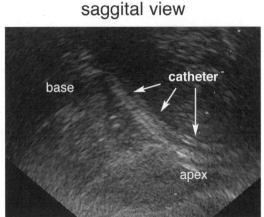

Figure 8-3. Top panels show transverse and sagittal TRUS images with a Foley catheter in place and an ultrasound void behind it (*). The left panel shows a transverse image with aerated intraurethral gel, with substantial artifact behind it (*).

An advantage of a catheter is that the balloon marks the prostatic base on fluoroscopy, so long as the balloon is snug against it (**Figure 8-4**). Place some traction on the catheter, to make sure that the balloon is pulled against the prostate.

As an alternative to keeping a catheter in during the procedure, M. Dattoli uses one prior to starting the implant, placing 50 cc of 100% Renografin™ into the bladder, and taking a lateral fluoroscopic view. The image is held on the second fluoroscopy screen throughout the implant procedure, to serve as a reference as to where the urethra is. After the reference image is taken the catheter is removed for the remainder of the implant procedure (**Figure 8-5**). Dye is left in the bladder during the procedure to help visualize the interface between bladder and prostate on lateral or anterior fluoroscopy.

Another popular urethral visualization technique is installation of aerated gel (**Figure 8-3**). Sterile water soluble lubricating jelly or ultrasound gel is passed back and forth between two syringes until it turns milky white. It is then instilled

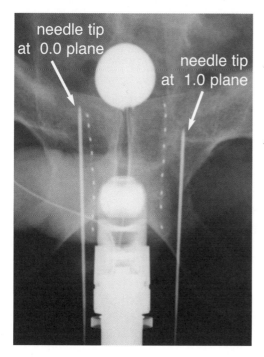

Figure 8-4. The catheter balloon is a simple marker of the prostatic base. Positioning the needle tip at the lower edge of the balloon on fluoroscopy is one way to double check that you're at the 0.0 plane.

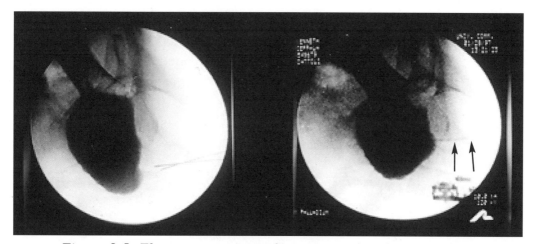

Figure 8-5. Fluoroscopy screen during procedure by M. Dattoli. On the right is preprocedure view with urinary catheter in place (arrows) and 50 ml Renografin™ in the bladder. The right-sided image is kept during the procedure, to help identify the urethra. The left-sided screen is used during the procedure to help monitor needle and source placement. (Note posterior crossing stabilization needles on the left screen.)

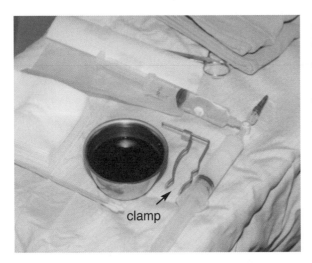

Figure 8-6. Gel is aerated by repeatedly passing it between syringes through a stopcock. Once instilled, a penile clamp is applied to keep the gel from leaking out.

through the urethra using a 20 cc syringe with a luer lock tip with a catheter tip. A penile clamp keeps it from leaking out (**Figure 8-6**).(SYLVESTER) During the procedure, the gel will often not be visible on some TRUS slices, but can be milked into view by pressing on the anterior pelvic wall.

Scrotum
The scrotum should be kept away from the perineum. It can be held up to the abdominal wall with tape or a rolled up, wet cloth towel (**Figure 8-7**). Using towel clips to fasten the scrotal skin against the anterior abdominal wall adds unnecessary trauma to the procedure.

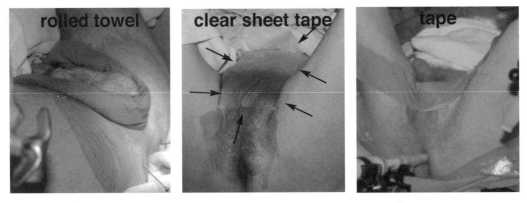

Figure 8-7. Scrotal solutions. A rolled surgical towel or tape are usually sufficient to keep the testicles out of the perineal field.

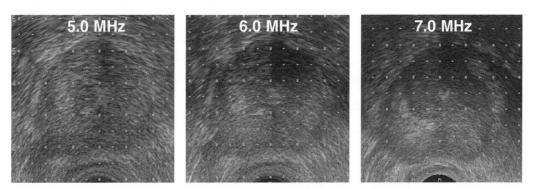

Figure 8-8. Various TRUS frequencies—6.0 MHz typically gives the best overall tissue contrast, but the differences aren't huge.

TRUS probe

Current TRUS probes are remarkably durable and easy to set up. Frequencies of 5.0, 6.0 and 7.0 MHz are standard. Higher frequencies give better tissue visualization closer to the probe. A 6.0 MHz tip generally provides the best overall resolution (**Figure 8-8**).

Probe covers

The probe should be covered generously with lubricant. Water-soluble gel seems to be as good as specially-designated "ultrasound gel." Most brachytherapists use at least one probe cover, primarily to keep the probe clean. A variety of covers can be used, with no obvious advantage of one over the other (**Figure 8-9**). The more

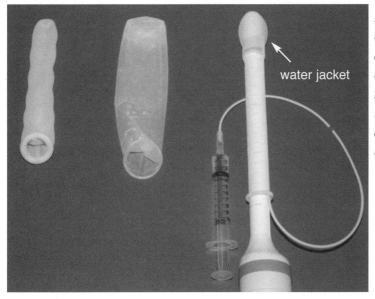

water jacket

Figure 8-9. A variety of probe covers are available. We're not convinced that they make much difference in image quality, despite wide differences in price.

Apex
(transverse view)

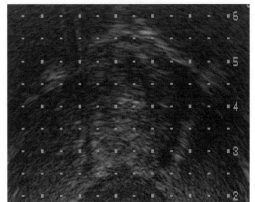

Sagittal view

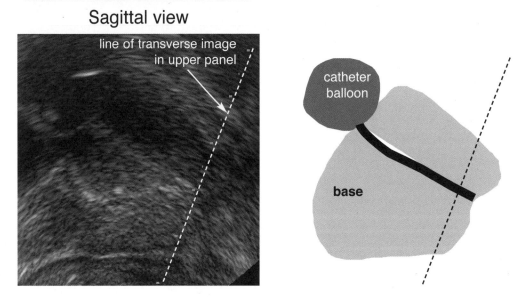

line of transverse image
in upper panel

catheter
balloon

base

Figure 8-10. The transverse image on the left shows poor visualization of the prostatic apex because it blends in with the tissue-equivalent pelvic floor. The sagittal view (lower left) offers a clearer view of the apical margins, in part because the continuous prostatic contour can be visually extrapolated from more proximal portions of the prostate.

sophisticated covers include a water bag that can be filled from a syringe reservoir, allegedly improving coupling between the probe and the rectal wall. An outer condom can be used, but may interfere with image quality. Use ample lubricant between inner and outer condoms.

While implants can be done well with transverse imaging alone, sagittal imaging helps visualize the prostatic base and apex and verify proper needle location and depth (**Figure 8-10**). Biplane probes, capable of transverse and sagittal imaging, are now considered standard for prostate brachytherapy. There's a wide variability

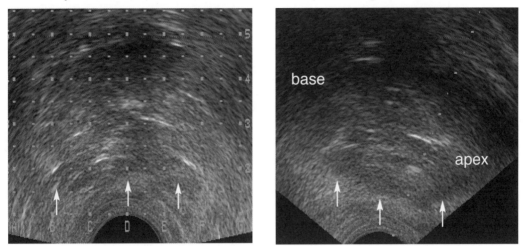

midprostate, transverse   sagittal view

Figure 8-11. Transverse and sagittal images with sources in place. The posterior rectal wall (arrows) commonly becomes obscured toward the end of the case, and it can usually be better seen on sagittal imaging (right).

in the degree to which sagittal imaging is used. It's not absolutely essential, but it's good to have it available.

Some brachytherapists use sagittal imaging in lieu of fluoroscopy to check that sources are not pulled distally with the receding needle tip. Sagittal imaging is especially valuable toward the end of a case, when source artifact can obscure the prostate-rectum interface on transverse view (**Figure 8-11**).

Stepping unit and stabilizer
The TRUS probe is supported on a *stepping unit*, allowing it to be moved caudal or cephalad at 0.5 cm intervals. The unit should hold the probe steady, without obstructing access to the perineum (**Figure 8-12**). Set the carriage in the middle of its range before inserting the probe, to allow maximal range of useful motion.

A stable, but easily adjustable stepping unit (and stand) can make the difference between a pleasant versus a frustrating implant experience. Even under anesthesia patients commonly move. Sometimes you'll have to make adjustments intraoperatively for pubic arch interference. A variety of units are available, and your choice could be the most important equipment decision you'll make. Ask for advice from experienced colleagues *before* you buy ($10,000–$16,000).

Barzell-Whitmore   Radiation Therapy Products

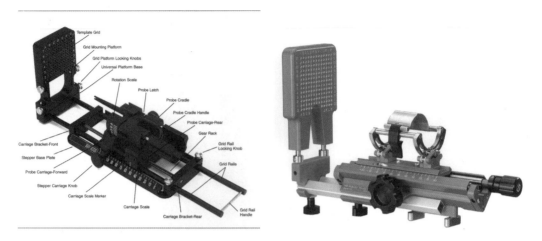

Figure 8-12. A variety of stepping units allow movement of the TRUS probe at 5 mm increments.

The stepping unit is supported by a *stabilizing stand*, either table-mounted or floor-mounted (**Figures 8-13**). The principle advantage of a table-mounted stand is that it moves with the table if the table position is changed during the case. Table-mounted stands are typically lighter and more portable.

PROBE POSITIONING
To begin imaging the prostate, place the probe tip against the anus, and press gently until the sphincter gives way. The probe should advance easily and the prostate will come into view. Make gross probe adjustments by moving the stand itself. Make small changes with the fine adjusters on the stepping unit/stand. If the image is not clear, move the probe in and out to clear gas from the interface between the probe and the anterior rectal wall (**Figure 8-14**). If unsuccessful, completely withdraw and reinsert the probe. If gas or fecal artifact persists, an intraoperative enema using a 30 French red rubber catheter attached to a large syringe will usually clear the offending material.

RECREATE THE PREPLANNING IMAGES
Before placing needles, make sure that the imaging planes match those for the planning images. The images often do not match *exactly*, due in part to daily changes in the prostate shape and volume, or to technical factors. But they should be very close. Use common sense. Don't get too crazy about a couple of millime-

Barzell-Whitmore

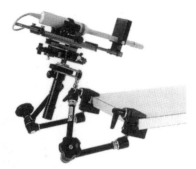

Barzell-Whitmore

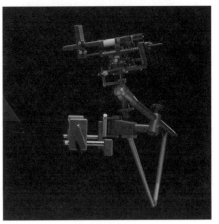

Radiation Therapy Products

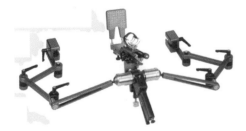

Amerteck

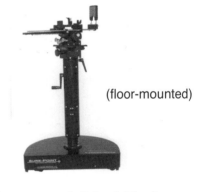

(floor-mounted)

Accuseed (Med-Tec)

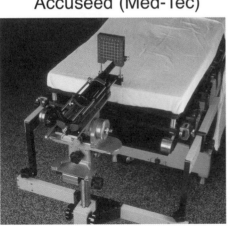

Accuseed (Med-Tec)

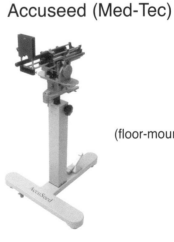

(floor-mounted)

Figure 8-13. Table-mounted and floor-mounted stepping unit stands.

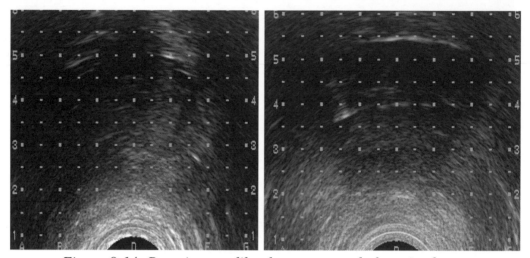

Figure 8-14. Poor images like these can result from inadequate probe pressure against the anterior rectal wall, or by gas, mucous, or feces. Passing the probe in and out of the rectum, or increasing the probe pressure against the rectal wall, will usually improve the image. It's always possible to do better than these! Don't proceed until you have a sharp image, even if it means starting over again with a new probe cover.

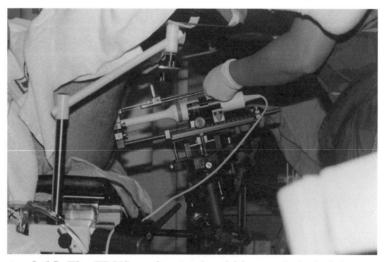

Figure 8-15. The TRUS probe tip should be angled slightly toward the floor.

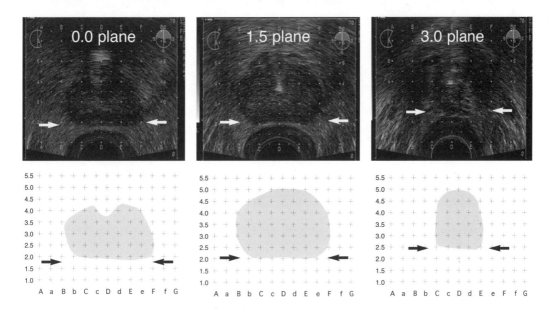

Figure 8-16. Make sure that the posterior prostatic margin aligns on the template the way that it did on the planning images. The prostate should be midline on the screen, typically with the urethra on the middle coordinate. In this case, the posterior prostate is aligned on the 2.0 template row.

ters difference between the planning images and those at the time of the procedure. After all, the entire prostate volume will be unpredictably up to 100% larger by the time you're finished with the implant (see chapter 9).

The probe tip should be angled slightly toward the floor (**Figure 8-15**). The precise angle doesn't make as much difference as you might think, because the prostate tends to follow the angle of the probe. The simplest way to get the prostate lined up properly on the grid is to make sure that the posterior margin of the mid-prostate is lined up on the template as it was on the planning images, and then to check that the base and apex also match the plan (**Figure 8-16**). To get it "perfect" you may need to tilt the probe slightly in various directions. As long as the back of the prostate aligns properly, slight differences in the anterior margin are probably clinically unimportant.(MCNEAL, ROSEN)

Once you think you've got it right, it's a good idea to step back and look at the probe's position, making sure that it is not grossly skewed in relation to the pelvic bones, increasing the chance of pubic arch interference on one side.

minimal pressure   moderate pressure   excessive pressure

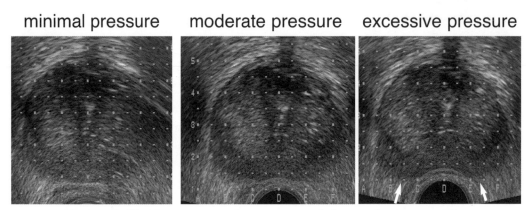

Figure 8-17. Excessive probe pressure deforms the image. These midprostatic images of the same patient were taken with minimal, moderate, and excessive probe pressure, causing artifactual "drooping" of the posterior-lateral margins (arrows).

Probe pressure

Gentle probe pressure against the prostate allows good coupling with the tissue, but too much pressure distorts the image, leading to artifactual flattening of the prostate (**Figure 8-17**). In the extreme, "dog ear" artifacts are produced. Considering that prostate tissue is very firm, these deformities are not due to actual prostatic deformation, but to image artifact.

Determine the zero plane

Once the probe is positioned so that the TRUS images match those of the preplan, you need to determine the depth at which source loading will start. The 0.0 plane, at the bladder/prostate interface, should match the corresponding plane of the planning images. The 0.0 plane can be best appreciated by ratcheting the probe through the junction of the seminal vesicles, bladder, and prostatic base. It can also be verified on sagittal imaging (**Figure 8-18**). (Remember that, when using the Mick Applicator®, the seed will be inserted beyond the tip of the needle, so that you should retract your needle tip 4–5 mm before placing a seed at the zero plane.)

NEEDLE GUIDE TEMPLATE

Once you're satisfied with the image quality and prostatic positioning on the screen grid, mount the needle-guide template on the stepping unit, near the perineum. We leave 1–2 cm of space between the skin and the template, to allow for manual adjustment of the needle direction if needed (**Figure 8-19**).

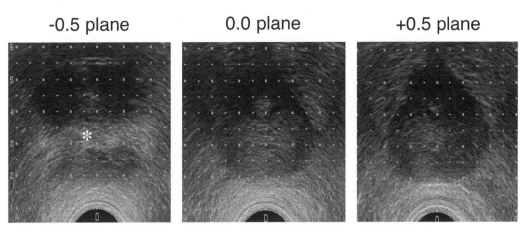

-0.5 plane   0.0 plane   +0.5 plane

Figure 8-18. Finding the zero plane can be done by stepping the probe through the prostatic base. The -0.5 plane should show seminal vesicle and some bladder, without prostate. The 0.0 plane typically shows the seminal vesicles blending into the prostate (middle upper panel). The connective tissue plane between the base of the seminal vesicles and the posterior bladder (*) is a good landmark to identify the plane above the prostatic base (-0.5). The sagittal image (left) is a good way to verify that you are at the base.

sagittal image

seminal vesicle

-0.5 plane   0.0 plane   0.5 plane

Needle insertion

Once TRUS probe positioning is set, needles are inserted through the template holes and through the perineal skin. If the skin is caught tangentially, it's difficult to pierce it—retract the needle, and pull the skin taught and reinsert. To pierce thicker skin, the needle should be pressed firmly against the skin surface and then

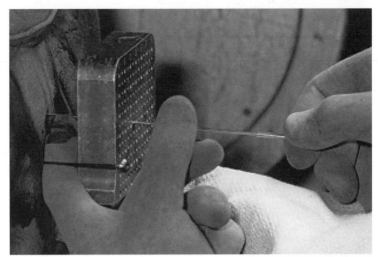

Figure 8-19. Needle-guide template, 1-2 cm from perineal skin.

advanced with a sudden, controlled thrust. Once through the skin, quick advancement will minimize needle deviations. But be careful—a rapid thrust of the tip against the pubic arch can give you a bent (or even broken) needle.

Needle deflection
Needles can be deflected by the skin, the tissue planes, or by the pubic bones. Deflection will cause the needle to appear in some spot on the TRUS image other than that predicted by the template insertion coordinate. When in doubt, deflection is usually obvious on fluoroscopy (**Figure 8-20**). When it occurs, the needle should be withdrawn several centimeters, and reinserted. If it's a peripheral needle, make sure you're not grazing the inner surface of the pubic bone. Twisting the needle during insertion may help get it through the offending tissue plane with less deflection. If deflection still occurs, withdraw the needle and check that it's straight!

Visualizing needles
Once multiple needles and sources have been inserted, image degradation typically occurs (**Figure 8-21**). Degradation may be lessened by inserting and loading the more anterior needles first and proceeding to the more posterior needles, helping to prevent the posterior needles from obscuring the more anterior ones. When in doubt, you can usually verify a needle's proper positioning on TRUS images more proximal to the template (caudal to the prostatic apex), where the image is not obscured by sources.

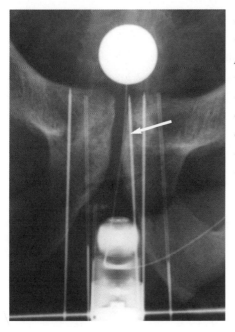

Figure 8-20. Needle deflection is usually obvious on fluoroscopy. In this patient, the most anterior needle (arrow) has deflected medially as it brushed against the pubic arch. This deflection will cause the needle tip to appear at a more medial template coordinate than intended.

Needle depth

Determining the depth of the needle is as important to proper source placement as is correct positioning in the transverse images. The simplest way to verify proper depth is to insert the needle while viewing the plane to which it is to be inserted, and stopping when you see the needle tip reach that plane. A second way is to view

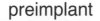 preimplant 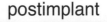 postimplant

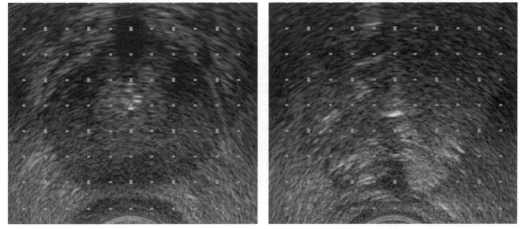

Figure 8-21. The prostate image, needles, and sources are often markedly obscured toward the end of a case, due to artifacts from sources, bleeding, and/or edema.

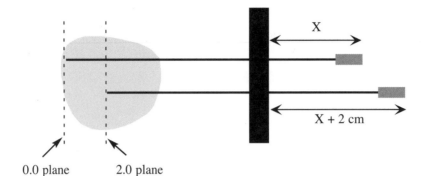

X

X + 2 cm

0.0 plane   2.0 plane

checking needle tip depth

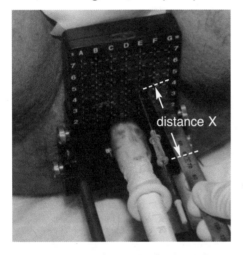

distance X

checking source/spacer number

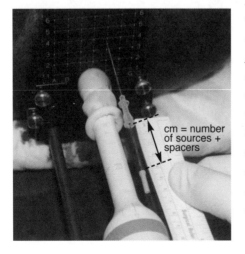

cm = number
of sources +
spacers

Figure 8-22. Needle depth can be checked by measuring how much is sticking out of the template when the needle is inserted to its proper depth. At the start of the case, the distance X is determined, with the needle tip at the 0.0 plane (top panel). All other hub measurements should be related to that of the zero plane. For instance, if the needle tip is supposed to be at the 2.0 plane for the first seed, the template-to-hub distance should be X+2. This is a quick and effective way to verify proper needle depth, but make sure to check that you're still setup to your zero plane throughout the procedure because the zero plane can shift relative to the stepper as the prostate swells or the patient moves slightly. The middle panel shows the hub measurement being made intra-operatively, to verify depth of the needle tip. The lowest panel shows a check of the number of sources/spacers loaded inside the needle, by measuring how much tro-car is sticking out of the sheath.

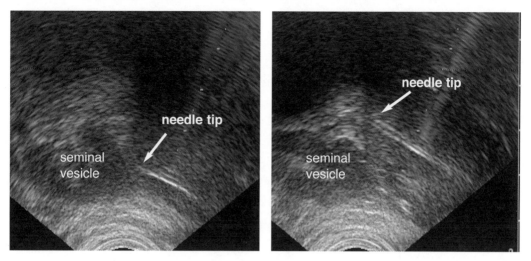

Figure 8-23. Needle depth can be checked on sagittal TRUS. but frequent switching between the transverse and sagittal views can become tedious.

the insertion with fluoroscopy, with the zero plane being at the lower edge of the catheter balloon—if the needle tip is at the base of the prostate, the tip of the needle should be within 2–4 mm of the inferior edge of the balloon (**Figure 8-4**). A third is to measure how many centimeters of the needle should be distal to the template when the needle is inserted to its proper depth (**Figure 8-22**). These methods can be combined to give extra confidence. And if still in doubt as to the proper insertion depth, sagittal imaging can be very helpful (**Figure 8-23**).

PIERCING THE URETHRA
Even with a catheter in place, the urethra is probably pierced commonly in the course of an implant procedure. Although there is no evidence that piercing it increases acute or chronic morbidity, it seems prudent to minimize doing so.

PERIRECTAL SOURCES
Using a posterior treatment margin of 3–5 mm, there should be minimal risk of serious rectal complications (see chapters 6 and 9). However, while serious rectal complications have been infrequent in modern implant series, there is a consistent 5% to 10% incidence of proctitis, with self-limited rectal bleeding.(MERRICK, HAN, GELBLUM) One technical maneuver that may contribute to proctitis is the temptation to place sources nearer the posterior prostatic margin than called for in the treatment plan. We note this tendency among ourselves and others, with the inten-

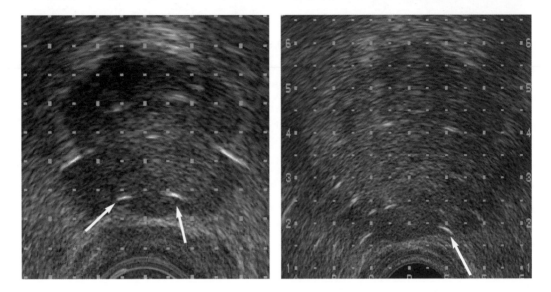

Figure 8-24. Be careful about putting sources closer to the posterior prostatic margin than called for by the plan. In the patient on the left, sources were properly placed 4 mm inside the capsule. In the patient on the right, sources were shifted back a couple mm, to just inside the capsule. This minor deviation from the plan, done with the intention of increasing the posterior treatment margin, increases the likelihood of rectal complications.(HAN, GELBLUM, MERRICK)

tion of adding "a little extra margin" for potential extraprostatic extension. Be careful—doing so will increase the likelihood of rectal morbidity (**Figure 8-24**).

PROSTATE MOTION
The prostate can be highly mobile, even when it's not being stuck by needles and shoved by an ultrasound probe, as has been well documented in the external beam radiation literature.(LATTANZI) The primary motion, in the absence of needle insertion, is in the anterior-posterior direction. During needle insertion, fluoroscopy commonly shows lateral and cephalad motion of up to 1 cm, leading to source misplacements (**Figures 8-25 through 8–27**). Anterior displacement occurs when posteriorly placed needles strike the posterior surface tangentially. Presumably, the prostate can also twist around its longitudinal axis, though the degree of twisting has not been documented. These motions can easily be viewed fluoroscopically, looking at the change in position of the catheter balloon and any sources that have already been implanted (**Figure 8-25**).

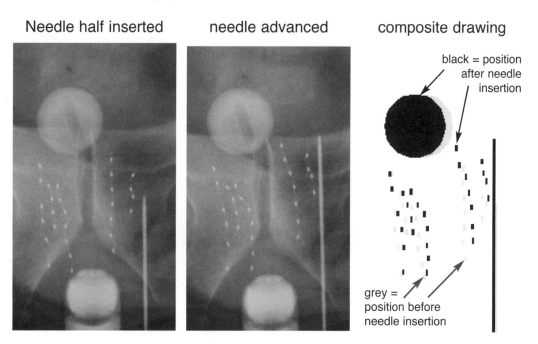

Needle half inserted   needle advanced   composite drawing

black = position after needle insertion

grey = position before needle insertion

Figure 8-25. Prostate motion as the needle is inserted is usually obvious on fluoroscopy.

Prostate mobility varies substantially from patient to patient, presumably due to differences in periprostatic fat, periprostatic veins, looseness of the pelvic tissues, or changes in the general muscle tone of the organ.

Prostatic motion is something that you need to be aware of and make adjustments for, but that you don't necessarily need to stop. If you prefer, several methods help to limit prostate motion, but none are completely effective. Tissue-gripping needles hold the prostate and decrease motion along the needle tracks. Commercially available needles are inserted on each side of the prostate, with retractable hooks to grip the tissue once inserted (**Figure 8-28**). Their clinical benefit is a matter of some dispute.(TASCHEREAU)

Another method to decrease prostate motion is insertion of two crossing needles through the posterior aspect of the prostate (**Figure 8-29**).(DATTOLI) Crossing needles limit prostate motion, by anchoring in the pelvic floor musculature at an angle. This works fairly well, but it's still important to pay attention to the prostate position during the implant procedure.

The problem: Pushing prostate cephalad, leaving source gap at base

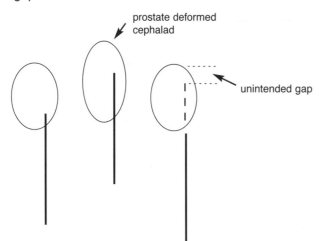

Figure 8-26. Prostate motion can lead to unintended gaps between the prostatic base and the sources, due to superior displacement of the prostate during needle insertion. The answer is to over insert the needle, then withdraw it back into the prostate before placing the sources (lower panel).

The solution: over insert, then withdraw partially

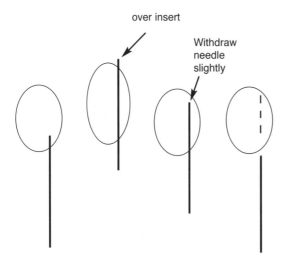

DEPOSITING SOURCES

Placement of sources can be done with a variety of tools and techniques (see chapter 5). Regardless of technique, there are ways that errant sources can occur. Sources can also wind up in unusual places by migrating in the retroperitoneal space, veins, or bladder (**Figure 8-30**). Concentration, attention to detail, and *not rushing* can make the difference between occasional versus excessive errant sources.

The problem: Pushing prostate medially from the advancing needle, leaving sources too lateral

Figure 8-27. Prostate motion can lead to unintended lateral source placement, due to medial displacement of the prostate during needle insertion. The answer is to insert the needle with a more rapid motion, with less displacement of the prostate (lower panel).

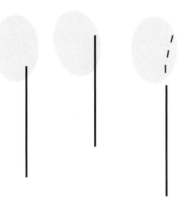

The solution: insert the needle more rapidly, to decrease displacement of the prostate.

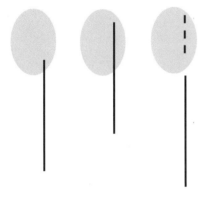

One of the most likely problems is sources sliding along the track as a needle is withdrawn (**Figures 8-31 and 32**). This is apparently a vacuum phenomenon and can be largely avoided by moving needles slowly. Watching the sources under fluoroscopy during insertion is a good way to to guard against source misplacement, because you can usually see when sources are not staying put after they're supposed to have left the needle tip. Sometimes, source displacement can be minimized with judicious reinsertion or retraction of the needles, watching under fluoroscopy.

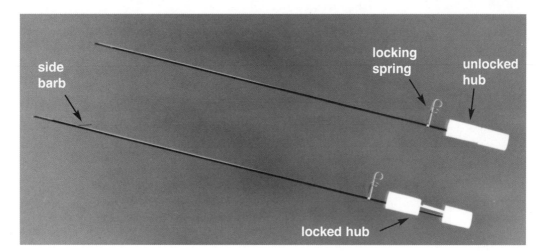

Figure 8-28. Stabilizing needles are commercially available. The Morganstern needle (MDTech Inc., Gainesville, Florida) has a single, retractable side barb that protrudes when the two-part hub is separated. The locking spring is snugged against the template to prevent the needle from sliding into or out of the template once the needle is fixed in the tissue. One needle is inserted on each side of the prostate.

PUBIC ARCH INTERFERENCE
One of the more common procedural problems is the potential for the most anterior needles to strike the pubic bones, preventing their advance or deflecting them medially. Fortunately, pubic arch interference (PAI) can usually be readily circumvented by one or more maneuvers that alter the needle path in relation to the pubic arch. The spatial relationship between the pubic arch and prostate and the alteration with pelvic rotation and needle angle have been elegantly illustrated by Tincher and colleagues.(TINCHER)

The simplest way to circumvent pubic arch interference is to change the patient to a more extended lithotomy position, either by moving the stirrups cephalad or by sliding the buttocks farther down the table (keeping the stirrups in the same place). Extending the lithotomy position rotates the pubic arch superiorly, allowing more room under it (**Figures 8-33 and 34**).

Changing the probe angulation or depressing the probe away from the prostate can help get needles under the pubic arch, but such maneuvers can simultaneously change the relationship of the probe to the prostate, shifting your alignment on the

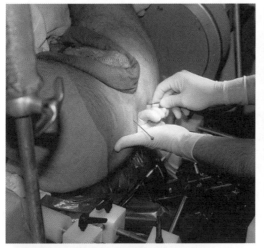 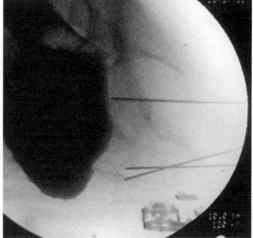

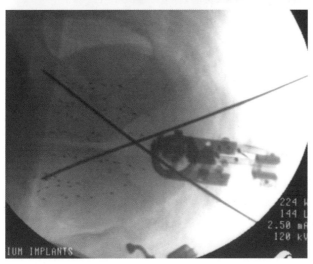

Figure 8-29. Insertion of crossing needles to stabilize the prostate. The top right photo shows a fluoroscopic view of the two crossing needles (arrow). To the left is an anterior fluoroscopic view after completion of source placement.

template grid; be sure to check the prostate's grid positioning each time you alter the probe's position.

A third way to circumvent pubic arch interference is to bend the needle tip slightly, 3 or 4 cm from the tip (**Figure 8-35**). Then insert it 0.5 or 1.0 cm medial and posterior to the intended template position with the tip pointed away from the arch and insert the tip past the arch. Then rotate the needle 180 degrees, and continue inserting. The bend will force the needle to veer away from the probe after passing the arch, often allowing the tip to reach a tissue point that would have been shielded by the pubic arch. This technique requires some finesse. And even with finesse, it often requires several passes of the needle. In addition to introducing some uncer-

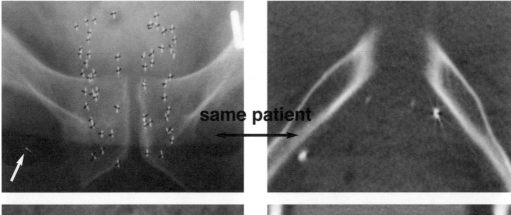

same patient

same patient

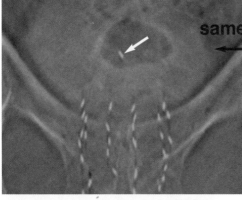

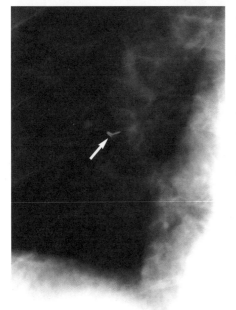

Figure 8-30. No matter how careful you are, seeds can end up in a variety of unintended places, migrating into the perirectal space (top panels), the bladder (middle panels) or the lungs (bottom left). None of the these mishaps are known to lead to any clinically significant problems, but excessive seed loss could lead to underdosing part of the prostate.(DAVIS) *While some source migration is inevitable, if you're consistently getting more than a couple of errant seeds, you may be a little too sloppy. A good way to see when and why you're getting errant sources is to use intraoperative fluoroscopy to watch the sources as they leave the needle tip.*

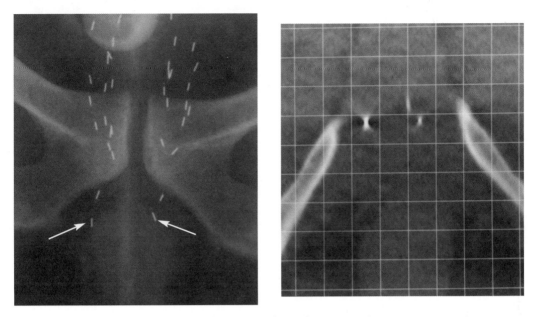

Figure 8-31. Misplaced, perineal seeds (arrows) seen on anterior fluoroscopy and corresponding CT image. Be careful that seeds are not pulled down into the perineum as you withdraw the needles.

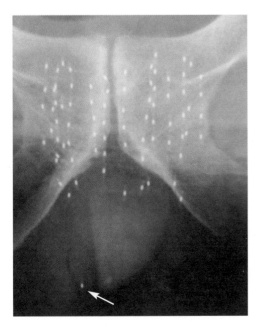

Figure 8-32. Example of source (arrow) that was pulled far down into the perineum as the needle tip was withdrawn. This is the kind of error than can be caught and minimized, if fluoroscopy is used during the procedure.

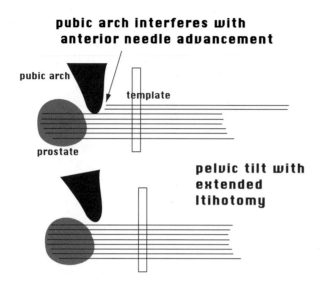

pubic arch interferes with anterior needle advancement

pubic arch

template

prostate

pelvic tilt with extended ltihotomy

Figure 8-33. By moving to the extended lithotomy position, the pubic arch is drawn back, allowing more room for anterior-lateral needles to clear the pubic bones.

tainty in the grid location of the seeds (since the needle is not completely perpendicular to the template), the technique increases tissue trauma and may, in fact, have been a contributing factor to the high post-implant urinary retention rates seen during an early period at the University of Washington.(WANG) If you're faced with an extreme case of pubic arch interference, it is possible to remove the TRUS template, and to place seeds by hand, using TRUS or anterior and lateral fluoroscopy to check for proper positioning in relation to the other sources or to the Foley catheter. This is the least desirable option, because it doesn't control for the needle trajectory relative to the template.

One saving grace, if maneuvers to circumvent pubic arch interference are not wholly successful, is that the part of the prostate underdosed is the most anterior-lateral, where cancerous tissue is less likely to be found, and where minor variations from the plan are unlikely to have any clinical significance.(ROSEN, MCNEAL)

POSTPROCEDURE CYSTOSCOPY
Postimplant cystourethroscopy has been practiced as a way to remove intravesicle or intraurethral radioactive sources or blood clots. However, in experienced hands, errant sources in the bladder or urethra are unusual, and when the situation does occur, the sources are readily identified fluoroscopically and simply pass once the urinary catheter is removed. Similarly, postimplant blood clots generally pass spontaneously—postimplant bladder irrigation is seldom necessary. Evidence to

Normal lithotomy | Extended lithotomy (right leg only)

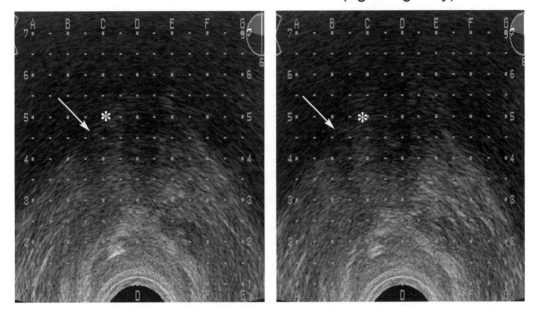

*Figure 8-34. Pubic arch interference can be reduced by extending the patient's lithotomy position. In this patient, the pubic arch (arrow) obstructed needle insertion at the C5 template position (*). By flexing the patient's right hip, the right side of the pubic arch moved away from the TRUS probe, allowing access to the C5 position. **A word of caution:** if you change a patient's leg positioning during the case, check that the prostate still aligns properly on the grid.*

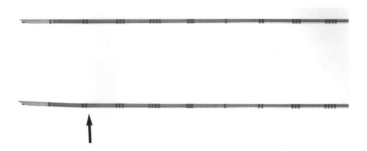

Figure 8-35. Slightly bending a needle tip (arrow) will cause the needle to veer in the direction of the bend, helping to steer it by the pubic arch.

date is that routine pre- or postimplant cystoscopy serves only to increase resource utilization and subject patients to unnecessary procedures.(GRAY, YAP, STONE)

LOTS OF CHOICES
Like we said at the beginning of this chapter, there are a lot of ways to do a good implant—keep an open mind and look at your many options. Figure out what works best for you, given your own dexterity, practice setting, and the skill level of your team.

REFERENCES
1. Dattoli M, Wallner K. A simple method to stabilize the prostate during transperineal prostate brachytherapy. Int J Rad Oncol Biol Phys 1997; 38:341-342.

2. Davis BJ, Pfeifer EA, Wilson TM, King BF, Eschelman JS, Pisansky TM. Prostate brachytherapy seed migration to the right ventricle found at autopsy following acute cardiac dysrhythmia. J Urol 2000; 164:1661.

3. Gelblum DY, Potters L. Rectal complications asociated with transperineal interstitial brachytherapy for prostate cancer. Int J Rad Oncol Biol Phys 2000; 48:119-124.

4. Gray G, Wallner K, Roof J, Corman J. Cystourethroscopic findings before and after prostate brachytherapy. Tech Urol 2000; 6:109-111.

5. Han B, Wallner K. Dosimetric and radiographic correlates to prostate brachytherapy-related rectal complications. (submitted) 2002;

6. Han BH, Demel KC, Wallner KE, Young L. Patient reported short-term complications after prostate brachytherapy. J Urol 2001; (in press):

7. Lattanzi J, McNeely S, Hanlon A, Das I, Schultheiss TE, Hanks GE. Daily CT localization for correcting portal errors in the treatment of prostate cancer. Int J Rad Oncol Biol Phys 1998; 41:1079-1086.

8. McNeal JE, Price HM, Redwine EA, Freiha FS, Stamey TA. Stage A Versus Stage B Adenocarcinoma of the Prostate: Morphological Comparison and Biological Significance. J Urol 1988; 139:61-65.

9. Merrick GS, Butler WM, Dorsey AT, Lief JH, Walbert HL, Blatt HJ. Rectal dosimetric analysis following prostate brachytherapy. Int J Rad Oncol Biol Phys 1999; 43:1021-1027.

10. Rosen MA, Goldstone L, Lapin S, Wheeler T, Scardino PT. Frequency and location of extracapsular extension and positive surgical margins in radical prostatectomy specimens. J Urol 1992; 148:331-337.

11. Stone NN, Stock RG. Dynamic cystography can replace cystoscopy following prostate seed implantation. Tech Urol 2000; 6:112-116.

12. Sylvester J, Grimm P, Blasko J, Meier R, Grier D, Heaney C, Cavanagh W. Urethral visualization during transperineal interstitial brachytherapy for early stage prostate cancer. Journal of Brachytherapy International 2000; 16:145-150.

13. Taschereau R, Pouliet J, Roy J, Tremblay D. Seed misplacement and stabilizing needles in transperineal permanent prostate implants. Radiother Oncol 2000; 55:59-63.

14. Tincher SA, Kim RY, Ezekiel MP, et al . Effects of pelvic rotation and needle angle on pubic arch interference during transperineal prostate implants. Int J Rad Oncol Biol Phys 2000; 47:361-363.

15. Wang H, Wallner K, Sutlief S, Blasko J, Russell K, Ellis W. Transperineal brachytherapy in patients with large prostate glands. Int J Cancer 2000; 90:199-205.

16. Yap J, Wallner K, Gray G. Cystourethroscopic findings and long-term urinary function after prostate brachytherapy. Journal of Brachytherapy International 2001;

9

Implant evaluation

Postimplant evaluation, or *dosimetry*, is a key part of prostate brachytherapy for several reasons (**Table 9-1**). First, postimplant dosimetry is the cornerstone of quality assurance—it provides a reasonably precise, objective evaluation of your result. Second, dosimetry is the best way to close the learning loop—it tells you how good (or bad) your technique is. Third, dosimetry is *the* legal document regarding the procedure. Taking pains to dictate a lengthy, detailed operative note isn't so important—it's where the seeds *are* that's important, not how you got them there. If a patient develops a serious complication and turns to the courts, the first thing that the lawyers (his *and* yours) will want is the postimplant dosimetry, espe-

> *Table 9-1. Why postimplant dosimetry is important.*
>
> - Quality assurance
> - Closes the learning loop
> - Legal document
> - Patient interest

cially the CT scans. If the dosimetry looks bad, you've got a serious problem. And if postimplant dosimetry wasn't done, you've got an even worse one.

One more reason to do postimplant dosimetry is that patients frequently ask about it. With prostate cancer patients' growing do-it-yourself approach and medical savviness, many will have already read extensively about brachytherapy (some will have read this book!). Patients might ask about their "DVH" or may even want to *see* their postimplant CT scan and dosimetric calculations! You'll look better if you have something to show them—otherwise they would rightly conclude that you're not interested in the quality of your work.

As data emerge regarding the clinical relevance of some basic dose parameters, prostate brachytherapy is becoming better standardized. We still have a lot of work to do in order to understand what constitutes a *good* implant as opposed to a *bad* implant. But we're getting there.

CRUDE INDICES
In the days of retropubic implants, total activity and matched peripheral dose (MPD) were the standard criteria for evaluating implant quality. Both are crude indices, at best.

The simplest way to describe an implant is to state the total amount of radioactivity implanted—a very crude quality indicator because it gives no information regarding the spatial relationship between dose and the prostate. If the activity implanted is in the usual range, it doesn't mean much. However, the total amount implanted can be telling if it is far from the norm. If very low, it would be likely that the prostate was not covered adequately (unless the gland was very small). If very high, the prostatic or normal tissue doses are likely to be excessive.

The total activity used for prostate brachytherapy has increased over the years. Current amounts are approximately double what was used for retropubic implants

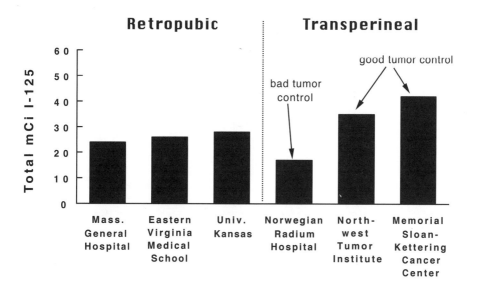

Figure 9-1. Average total activity used for retropubic and transperineal implants. Clinical results from the Norwegian Radium Hospital were abysmal—a very low amount of I-125 was used, and there was apparently no quality assurance system in place. With such low amounts of activity, the target coverage would almost certainly have been poor.(WAEHRE, DELANEY, REDDY)

in the 1970s (**Figure 9-1**). Higher activity in transperineal series probably reflects more accurate determination of prostate volume and shape with TRUS imaging, and a better match of isodose lines to the prostate periphery.

The matched peripheral dose (MPD)—not to be confused with mPD, the minimum tumor dose—is an ingenious concept that was devised by Lowell Anderson before wide availability of CT-based dosimetry.(ANDERSON) The MPD is the dose for which the isodose contour volume equals the volume of an ellipsoid having the same orthogonal dimensions as the target volume. To calculate the MPD, seed position is reproduced in three dimensions using orthogonal or stereo-shift films. Dose to a lattice of points throughout the implant volume is determined by summing the contribution from each source using computerized dose look-up tables. Several isodoses and their corresponding volumes are graphed. The MPD, corresponding to the ellipsoidal volume estimation (y-axis), is taken from the x-axis of the graph (**Figure 9-2**). The MPD isodose line can be drawn in relation to the sources, on the original set of radiographs. Points outside of the MPD volume

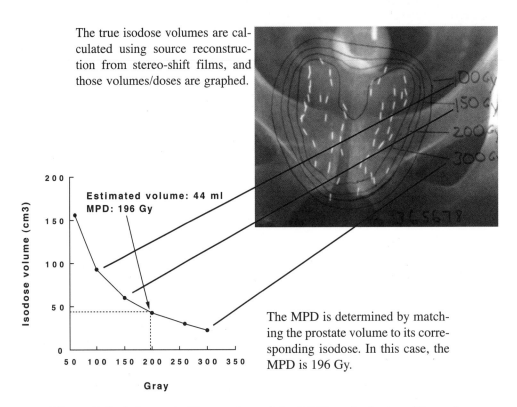

The true isodose volumes are calculated using source reconstruction from stereo-shift films, and those volumes/doses are graphed.

Estimated volume: 44 ml
MPD: 196 Gy

The MPD is determined by matching the prostate volume to its corresponding isodose. In this case, the MPD is 196 Gy.

Figure 9-2. Schematic illustration of the MPD calculation. The volumes encompassed by several isodose lines are graphed against the isodose levels. The dose to the approximation of the prostatic volume is taken from the graph, going from the y-axis to the x-axis. The target volume can be estimated from orthogonal dimensions, or determined from planar reconstruction of CT, TRUS, or MR images.

receive less than the MPD dose. While the actual isodose volumes, calculated from source positions on orthogonal films, are accurate the problem with MPD calculations is that without CT-derived prostate definition, you can't accurately compare the isodose volumes with the prostate margin.

Because MPD calculations use orthogonal dimensions to estimate the prostatic size (and shape), the MPD is an approximation of the dose to an approximation of the prostate volume—it does not accurately reflect the true dose to the prostate. This limitation of the MPD in defining an adequate implant is obvious by looking at the MPD of a 1980 retropubic implant from MSKCC (**Figure 9-3**).

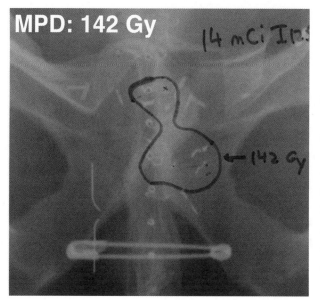

Figure 9-3. Anterior view of a 1980 retropubic implant, for which the calculated matched peripheral dose is 142 Gy. While the MPD is close to the prescription dose of 150 Gy, it's obvious that this is an awful implant; the 142 Gy iso-dose line could not possibly match the prostatic margins. But judging from the MPD alone, the implant was a good one!

Despite the inherent inaccuracy of the MPD calculation, some correlation between higher MPDs and local control rates has been reported.(FUKS) While suggesting that the MPD is a valid concept, the data itself is very suspect, being based on vague definitions of local failure. More important, the quality of the retropubic implants on which it is based was so poor by today's standards that such data are of historical interest only.

The introduction of CT-based dosimetry made the MPD concept obsolete. However, it is important to understand what it means because it has been widely reported in past brachytherapy literature, and is still sometimes mentioned.

IMAGING MODALITIES
To perform meaningful dosimetry, both the sources and the prostatic margins must be identified. The choices for postimplant imaging include TRUS, CT, and MR, each with distinct qualities (**Figure 9-4**). CT currently is the most practical dosi-metric imaging modality. Its principle advantages are wide availability and easy source identification. But CT images are only so-so for visualizing the prostatic margins. Unfortunately, typical images are not nearly as nice as the ones that make it to the cover of a textbook (**Figure 9-5**). In reality, the prostatic margins are indis-tinct, especially near the prostatic apex.

TRUS   CT   MR

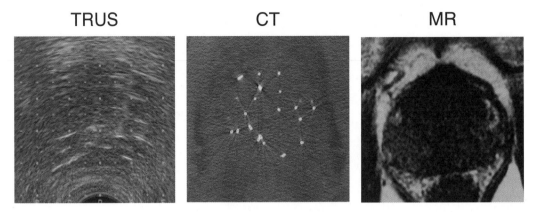

Figure 9-4. TRUS, CT, and MR each have their advantages and disadvantages as postimplant imaging modalities.(DUBOIS, AMDUR)

MR and TRUS are potential alternative to CT-based dosimetry. Compared to CT, MR typically offers better visualization of the prostatic margins, but less distinct source identification. Despite some claims that two sets of MR images are needed to separately identify the sources versus the prostate, a single set is probably sufficient, with optimal parameters.(AMDUR) Image fusion between MR and CT could optimize source location and prostatic margin definition, but such an approach makes post-implant dosimetry more cumbersome, with no demonstrable clinical benefit. A switch to MR as the standard is unlikely, due partly to its higher cost, and mostly to the fact that it is unlikely to enhance clinical outcomes.

Real-time TRUS could be the most practical postimplant imaging modality, since it is readily available intra-operatively. The problem with it is image degradation that typically occurs once a large number of sources are implanted (**Figure 9-6**). If image degradation could be avoided, TRUS could provide practical real-time dosimetry, so that an implant could be evaluated (and touched up) while the patient is still under anesthesia.

With technologic improvements, the future may bring a melding of modalities, or replacement of CT by TRUS or MR. But in the meantime, CT remains the standard of care for implant evaluation. The remainder of this chapter will focus on CT-based dosimetry.

CASUAL INSPECTION
The first step in implant analysis is to take a minute to peruse the postimplant images. Before getting into a discussion of dosimetric parameters, don't lose sight

for show   real life

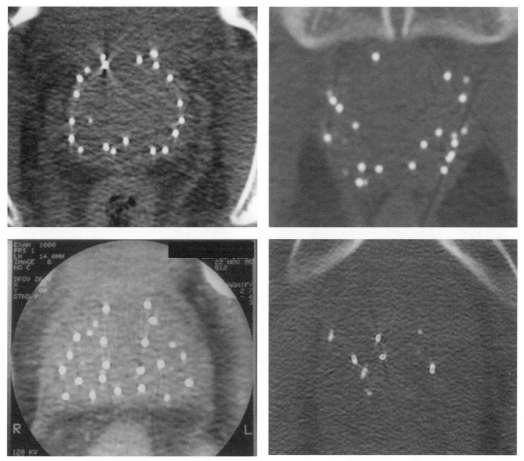

Figure 9-5. Fantasy versus reality. The CT images on the left are particularly nice ones, the kind that are typically shown in books! Unfortunately, the prostatic margins and sources frequently look more like the ones on the right. Note how indistinct the margins are near the prostatic apex, seen in the lower right panel.

of the fact that simple visual inspection of a postimplant CT scan is an important way to evaluate what you've done in the operating room. You can see, for instance, if you've placed seeds too close the the urethra, increasing the likelihood of urinary morbidity, or too posteriorly, increasing the possibility of rectal complications (**Figure 9-7**).

preimplant   postimplant

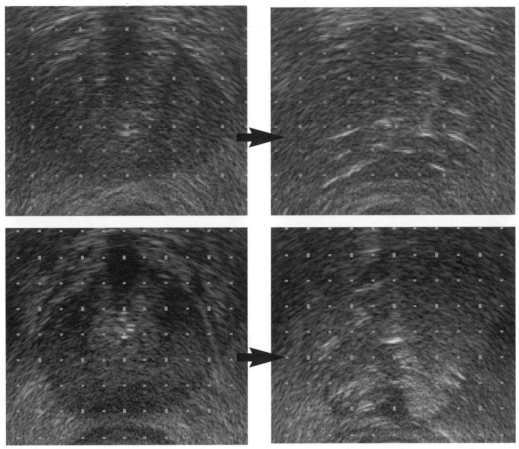

Figure 9-6. Pre- and postimplant TRUS images. Placement of sources partially obscures the prostatic margin. The postimplant margin visibility varies substantially from patient to patient, and at different levels in the same patient. These examples are fairly typical of what you'll see.

Isodose overlays

The best way to analyze an individual implant is visual inspection of the isodoses overlaid on cross sections of the prostate (**Figures 9-8 and 9-9**). By inspecting the overlays, you can determine if and where any cold spots are and get a good idea of where you may be making placement errors. For instance, if you're not inserting needles far enough, there will be insufficient coverage of the base, which is obvious from the overlays. Alternatively, if you're overly cautious posteriorly, you may be cold at the posterior capsule, a common site for cancers.

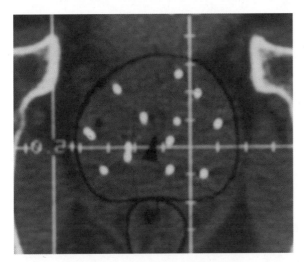

Figure 9-7. Casual inspection of a post-implant CT scan is enough to appreciate some problems. In this image, excessive periurethral sources are obvious. The first thing to do if you see something like this is to check the plan and make sure that it didn't call for it. If it did—you need to have a serious talk with your physicist. If not, then it's probably physician error.

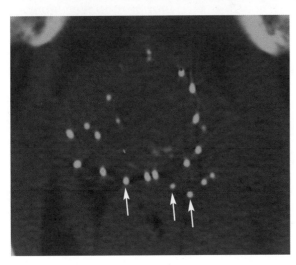

In this example, it's obvious that sources were mistakenly placed too posteriorly, on the rectal wall (arrows). This kind of mistake does not require sophisticated dosimetric evaluation to see—a quick look at the CT is enough!

Despite the emphasis on dosimetric parameters, looking at the overlays remains the best way to evaluate the clinical significance of the dose distribution. That's because dose parameters like *D90* or *V100* don't take into account where cancers are more likely to be. For instance, in a patient with a PSA less than 10, Gleason score less than 7, and a positive biopsy from the right apex only, inadequate coverage of the anterior portion of the prostate is probably of minimal or no clinical significance.(D'AMICO, DAVIS, MCNEAL)

QUANTIFYING TARGET COVERAGE
While isodose overlays are the best way to evaluate an individual patient's implant, analyzing groups of patients regarding the dose-related clinical effects

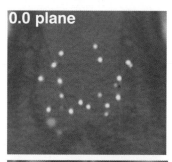

0.0 plane

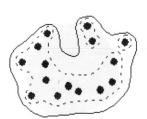

Figure 9-8. CT-based evaluation of a 115 Gy Pd-103 implant. This patient had 97% coverage of the post-implant CT-defined prostate volume, well in excess of the minimum 80% desirable. The only cold spot was at the midanterior margin, where cancer generally is less likely to be found compared to other intraprostatic locations.

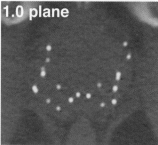

1.0 plane

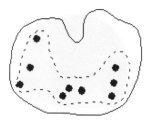

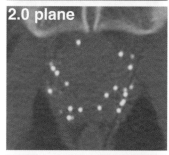

2.0 plane

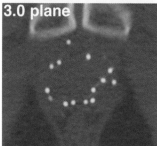

3.0 plane

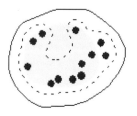

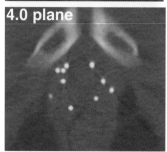

4.0 plane

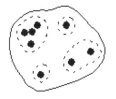

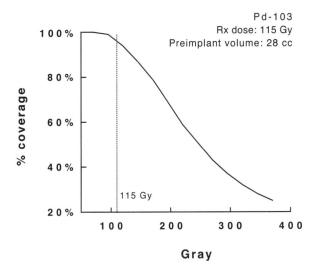

Figure 9-8 (continued). Dose-volume histogram (DVH) for the patient to the left. Target coverage by the prescription dose of 115 Gy is 97%.

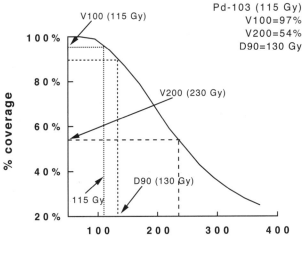

Various dosimetric parameters can be taken from the DVH.

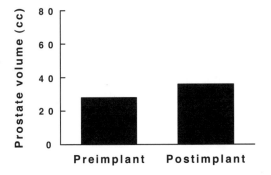

The preimplant TRUS volume was 28 cc, versus a postimplant volume of 36 cc, a fairly typical implant-related volume increase.(WILLINS 98)

9.11

0.0 plane

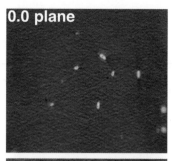

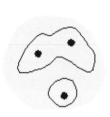

1.0 plane

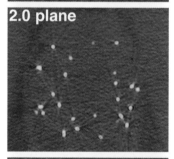

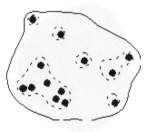

2.0 plane

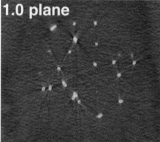

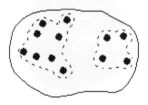

3.0 plane

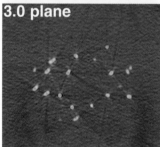

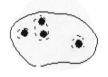

4.0 plane

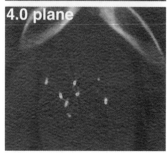

Figure 9-9. Postimplant CT-based evaluation of a 144 Gy I-125 implant. This patient had 80% coverage of the postimplant prostate volume, barely considered within the minimum 80% desirable. He had diffuse underdosed regions at the periphery, especially at the base and apex.

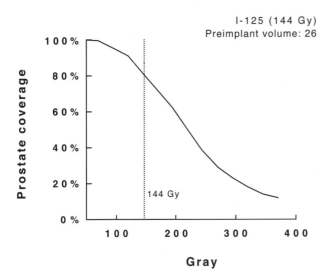

I-125 (144 Gy)
Preimplant volume: 26

144 Gy

Figure 9-9 (continued). Dose-volume histogram for the patient to the left. Prostate coverage by the prescription dose of 144 Gy (V100) was 81%. The reason for the lower V100 in this patient compared to the one in Figure 9-8 was his greater implant-related volume increase (lower panel).

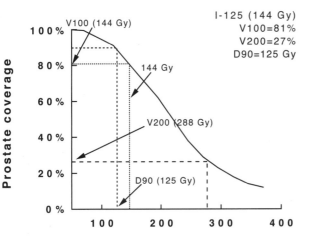

I-125 (144 Gy)
V100=81%
V200=27%
D90=125 Gy

V100 (144 Gy)

144 Gy

V200 (288 Gy)

D90 (125 Gy)

Various dosimetric parameters taken from the DVH.

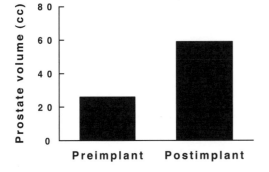

The preimplant TRUS volume was 26 cc, versus a postimplant volume of 59 cc, a relatively large implant-related increase that accounts for the lower prostate coverage in this patient.

9.13

Table 9-2. Some indices used to quantify implant quality.

V100: The percent of the prostate volume that receives the prescription dose or higher

D100: The dose that covers 100% of the prostate volume

D90: The dose that covers 90% of the prostate volume

V200: The percent of the prostate volume that receives twice the prescription dose or higher

V200/V100: The fraction of the prostate volume that receives more than twice the prescription dose

Dmin: The minimum dose delivered to any part of the prostate

requires summary dosimetric indices. The *dose-volume histogram* (DVH) graphs the percent of the target covered versus increasing doses (see **Figures 9-8 and 9-9**). A nearly endless variety of indices taken from the DVH might be used to summarize the implant quality. Probably the simplest to conceptualize DVH-derived index is the V100, or the percent of the postimplant target volume covered by the prescription dose (**Table 9-2**). Roy and colleagues were the first to use postimplant CTs to calculate V100s, reporting typical values of only about 80%.(ROY) Initially they assumed that inadequate coverage was due to source placement errors. It later dawned on them (and others) that the inadequacies were instead due primarily to implant-related prostate swelling.(WATERMAN 98, WILLINS 98) In fact, V100s of 80% to 95% are typical among experienced implant teams (**Figure 9-10**).

Stock and colleagues correlated various dosimetric parameters with PSA-based freedom from cancer relapse and found that tumor control was better with a D90 greater than 140 Gy (**Figure 9-11**). While this is far more information than anyone else has come up with so far, its relevance is limited because follow-up was short and data were accumulated during the investigators' learning curve.(STOCK 98, STOCK 00) Additionally, higher-dose patients were treated later in the series, leading to artifactual bias in favor of their PSA-based cancer control calculations.(VICINI) Still, Stock's work is the best available. And it makes sense—greater prostate coverage yields better tumor control rates!

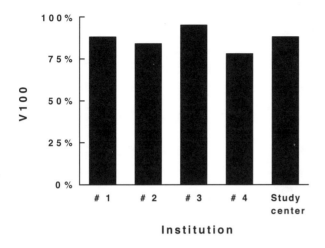

Figure 9-10. Average V100s by five prominent brachytherapy teams. Note the similarity among teams, even though their programs and policies evolved fairly independent of each other.(BICE*)*

While D90 correlated best with biochemical control, D90 and V100 are closely correlated, so that both are commonly used; the principle advantage to V100 is that it's easier to conceptualize (**Figure 9-12**). The minimum prostatic dose (Dmin) might seem a likely candidate for implant analysis, but has not proven useful by virtue of the fact that it is too sensitive to minor variations in source placement or target definitions.(ROY)

While Stock has contributed important pioneering work in defining the optimal brachytherapy doses, we need much more information about what constitutes adequate target coverage. In an effort to better define a dose response relationship, Dr. Gregory Merrick and colleagues are organizing large multicenter prospective studies, designed to accumulate large patient numbers over a short time, to correlate uniform, centrally analyzed, postimplant dosimetry with biochemical control. Initial results should be available by 2006.

HOT SPOTS
Due to the nature of the brachytherapy, whereby tissue adjacent to the sources receives extremely high doses, a substantial amount of prostate gets *far* greater than the prescription dose (**Figure 9-13**). The prescription dose is the *minimum* desired, while tissue close to the sources receive doses far in excess of that prescribed.

The clinical significance of hot spots is unclear. High-dose regions near the urethra or rectum increase the chance of morbidity, but it's unknown whether excessive dose to the parenchyma itself carry any significance. Based on the fact that

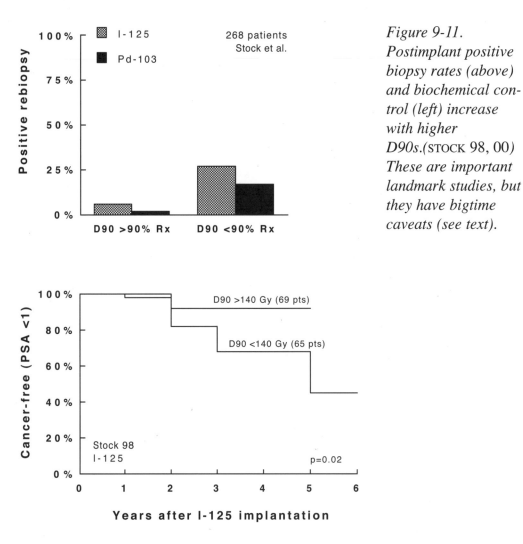

Figure 9-11. Postimplant positive biopsy rates (above) and biochemical control (left) increase with higher D90s.(STOCK 98, 00) These are important landmark studies, but they have bigtime caveats (see text).

serious complications (incontinence, rectal ulcers, or parenchymal necrosis) are unusual, hot spots are probably not all that important, at least with the peripheral loading patterns that are now standard. High-dose regions *might* have some effect on tumor control rates.(LING) With the peripheral loading patterns that are typically used, the magnitude of high-dose regions doesn't vary so markedly as it did in earlier experience, probably explaining the inability to correlate clinical outcomes with the magnitude of high-dose regions (**Figure 9-14**).(MERRICK 99, GELBLUM)

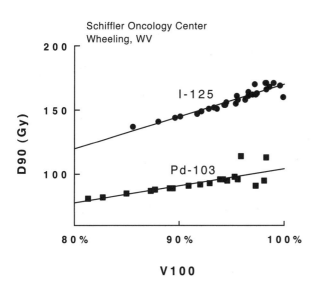

*Figure 9-12. There is a tight correlation between D90 with V100, so that the choice of one or the other probably doesn't make much difference. (*MERRICK 99*)*

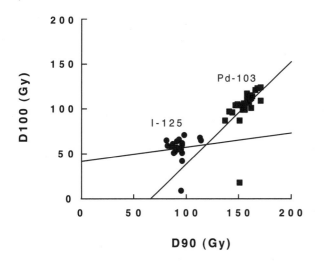

*There's little correlation correlation between D90 with D100, because a tiny portion of the prostate typically extends outside of the higher dose volumes. (*MERRICK 99*)*

PROBLEMS WITH CT-BASED DOSIMETRY

The introduction of CT-based dosimetry was a milestone in modern prostate brachytherapy. But CT has its shortcomings, the most obvious of which is fuzziness of the prostatic margins. The second major shortcoming is that the prostate size *changes* in the peri-implant period.

0.0 plane

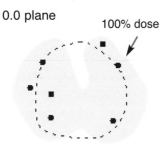
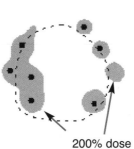
100% dose

prostate

200% dose

Figure 9-13. A substantial portion of the prostate typically receives far in excess of the prescription dose. In this typical I-125 patient, the V100 covered 94% of the prostate volume, while the V200 covered 31% and the V300 covered 8%.

1.5 plane

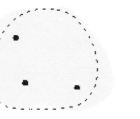
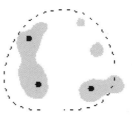

3.0 plane

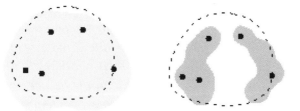

anterior view

right

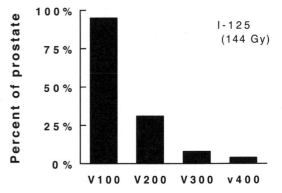

I-125
(144 Gy)

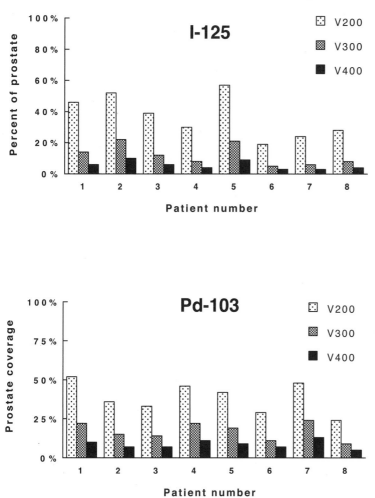

Figure 9-14. V200, V300, and V400 for ten unselected I-125 or Pd-103 patients at the Puget Sound VA. Even without particular attention to this parameter in the planning process, the degree of similarity among patients is more striking than the degree of difference. There appears to be little significance, if any, to high-dose prostatic parenchymal regions and postimplant morbidity (JONES).

Defining the prostate

The prostatic margins are not sharply delineated on CT scan, and there is substantial subjectivity defining them. It is especially difficult to delineate the prostatic apex, as it blends with the pelvic floor musculature. Also, the lateral margins can be difficult to distinguish from the puborectalis muscles (see chapter 4). Inclusion of the puborectalis or levator ani musculature in the target volume or overly generous drawing of the prostatic apex leads to falsely large prostate volume and falsely low V100s. The vagaries of prostatic margin interpretation can lead to substantial inter-observer variability in the postimplant dosimetric calculations.

Preimplant

Postimplant

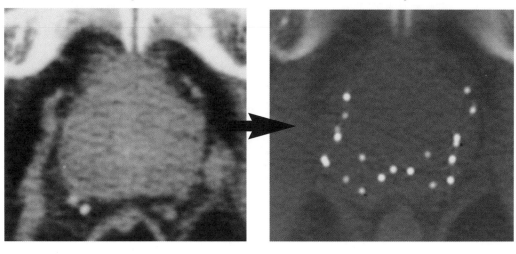

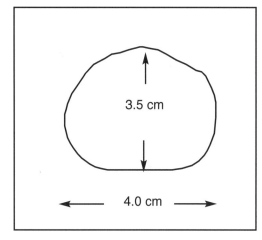

3.5 cm

4.0 cm

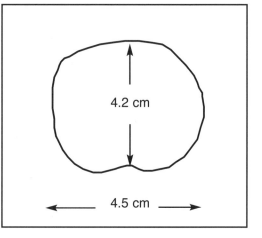

4.2 cm

4.5 cm

Figure 9-15. Typical preimplant and postimplant CT (day 0) showing greatest increase in the anterior-posterior dimension.

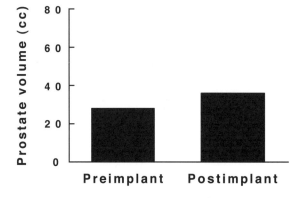

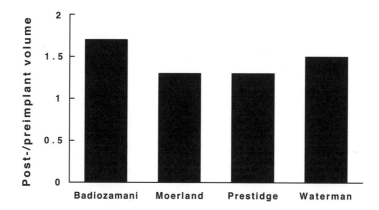

Figure 9-16. The degree of postimplant prostate swelling has been fairly consistent between reported series.(BADIOZAMANI, MOERLAND, PRESTIDGE, WATERMAN 98)

Because of the potential for substantial interobserver variability in the way CT images are interpreted, there is interest in switching to MR-based postimplant imaging, a move that is likely to become more practical in the future. But for now, CT-based dosimetry is the basis for most of what we know about implant analysis, and is considered the standard of care. Despite its image interpretation problems, it is important to point out that CT-based dosimetric studies have been fairly consistent between experienced implant groups (see **Figure 9-10**), and that CT-based dosimetry does correlate with tumor control rates.(STOCK 98 & 00)

Prostate swelling
Getting implanted is tough on a prostate. Think about it—enemas beforehand, catheterization, a DRE or two, and 20 to 100 needle jabs. Throw in a postimplant cystoscopy and you've got a pretty battered gland—it shouldn't be surprising that it's swollen by the time you're done.

Numerous investigators have shown that the prostate volume increases by approximately 25% to 50% during the implant procedure, with substantial variability between patients (**Figures 9-15 and 9-16**). And the size increase is not just a TRUS or CT artifact—it's evident when comparing pre- and postimplant CT or MR.(WILLINS 98, WATERMAN 98)

The problem that implant-related swelling causes from a dosimetric perspective is that it increases the prostate volume on which postimplant evaluation is based. A

Pre-implant   **Post-implant**

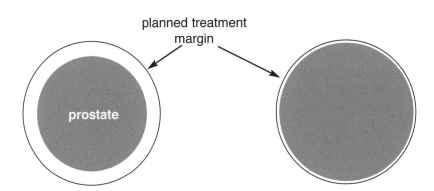

Figure 9-17. Why the postimplant prostate coverage is less affected than predicted by the degree of implant-related swelling. The planned treatment margin allows for swelling, such that most of the larger postimplant prostate volume is still within the prescription isodose volume.

bigger prostate volume makes target coverage inferior to what would be determined if it was based on the smaller, preimplant prostate size. But the effect of implant-related swelling is not as great as the volume change would suggest. Willins showed that the target coverage fell an average of only 5%, despite an average volume increase of 25%, the reason being that the addition of treatment margins in the preplan allows for a large degree of swelling, with most of the volume increase still inside of the prescription dose (**Figure 9-17**).(WILLINS 98, WATERMAN 98)

Variability in the degree of implant-related swelling among patients is an impediment to establishing uniform guidelines for dosimetric evaluation in the setting of a changing target volume, especially in extreme cases. Waterman and colleagues showed that the magnitude of the volume increase is not related to the number of needles used, the radioisotope used, or the number of sources.(WATERMAN 98) With the hope of more effectively customizing treatment planning to the individual patient, Badiozamani and colleagues compared implant-related volume changes with multiple clinical parameters, including preimplant volume, hormonal ablation, and preimplant external beam radiation in 50 patients treated at the University of Washington. Their hope was to determine which patients required a larger planning treatment margin (TM) to ensure adequate postimplant prostate coverage. Overall, the postimplant prostate volume increased by an average factor

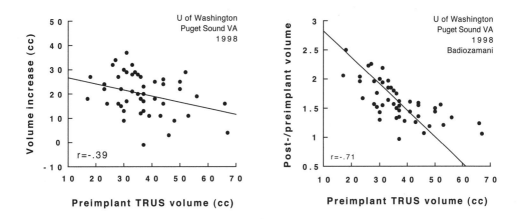

Figure 9-18. Absolute (left) and proportional (right) prostate volume increase versus preimplant TRUS volume.

of 1.7 (±0.34) compared to the preimplant volume. The absolute volume change was similar in patients with small versus large preimplant prostate volume, but the proportional change was less in patients with a larger prostate volume (**Figure 9-18**).

As expected, the degree of postimplant target coverage was less in patients with greater volume increase. Because patients with a small preimplant prostate had

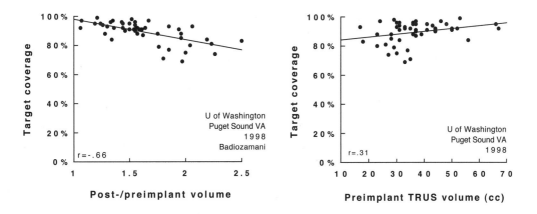

Figure 9-19. Fraction of postimplant prostate covered by prescription dose (V100) versus the degree of implant-related swelling (left) or versus preimplant volume (right).

9.23

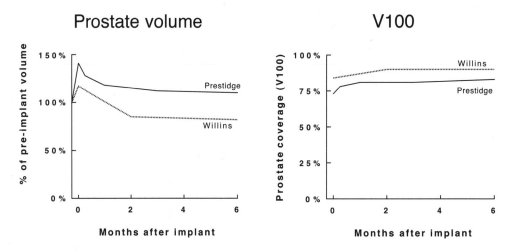

Figure 9-20. Time course of implant-related prostate swelling, and the corresponding V100s reported by two independent investigative teams.(PRESTIDGE, WILLINS 98)

proportionately greater volume increase, their postimplant target coverage was generally less (**Figure 9-19**). But while some trends regarding the degree of swelling in relation to preimplant parameters were seen, the most striking finding was the substantial scatter in the data for all parameters.

The use of an arbitrary degree of postimplant target coverage to assess implant adequacy is probably not ideal, in that it does not allow for the substantial variability in postimplant swelling. And while it is possible that with larger numbers of patients some combination of factors may correlate more closely with the degree of swelling, any such correlation would likely not be helpful for an individual patient, given the remarkable scatter in the degree of swelling.

One way to account for the degree of swelling is to base the postimplant dosimetry on the preimplant volume, somehow registered with the postimplant source locations. Doing so may be the most realistic way to assess how well the pre-plan was executed. But such a solution would likely be of little clinical utility because some of the dose will be delivered while the prostate is still larger than the pretreatment volume.

Delaying the postimplant scan
Another way to circumvent the added uncertainty of implant-related prostatic swelling is to wait one or two months to obtain postimplant dosimetry films. This

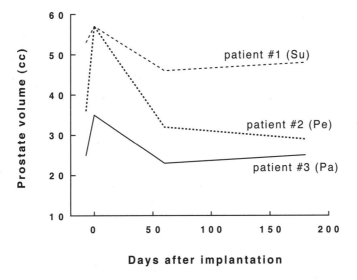

Figure 9-21. The degree of swelling and its resolution vary sub-stantially among patients, making a uniform policy regarding its consideration in postimplant dosimetry difficult, at best.(WILLINS 98)

allows time for much of the implant-related swelling to resolve. The practical lim-itation of such a policy is that if target coverage is determined at that time to be inadequate, adding sources so long after the initial procedure would probably be radiobiologically suboptimal.

Currently, in most practices postimplant scans are routinely done within twenty-four hours of the procedure, primarily out of convenience. Other reasons for doing the scan in the immediate postimplant period include the convenience of leaving a urinary catheter in place to allow urethral dose calculations, and the chance to learn quickly if an implant is inadequate and needs to be supplemented with extra sources. Finally, for teams that are new to brachytherapy, immediate scanning should help shorten the learning loop, revealing mistakes soon after the fact to make it easier to figure out ways to correct them.

Swelling resolution
The confounding effect of implant-related prostate swelling is exacerbated by the variable resolution of swelling in the postimplant period. In order to characterize the postimplant prostate volume changes, investigators have analyzed serial scans.(WILLINS 98, WATERMAN 98) In general, the prostate volume returns to its

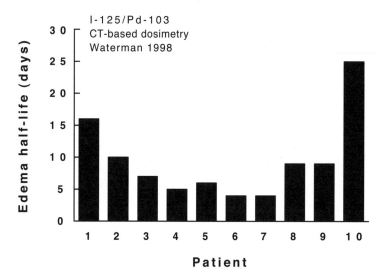

Figure 9-22. The time course of edema resolution is highly variable from one patient to the next, making the application of a standard correction factor in evaluating prostatic coverage impractical in the clinical setting.(WATERMAN 98)

preimplant size by two months, and prostate coverage increases by about 5% to 10% (**Figure 9-20**).

Elegant studies have devised formulas to account for the degree of swelling resolution over time.(CHEN) Unfortunately, such correction factors are impractical in clinical practice, because the volume changes are so inconsistent from one patient to the next (**Figures 9-21 and 9-22**).

From a practical standpoint, it would be reasonable to consider the degree of prostate swelling when interpreting postimplant prostate dose coverage. In general, a V100 of 80% or greater is considered adequate, but if a patient's prostate swells more than usual, a lesser V100 might be considered adequate. Perhaps even 60 to 70% postimplant prostate coverage should be considered adequate in cases where the prostate swells by more than a factor of 1.5. In making such a proposal it is assumed that much of the swelling will resolve early in the isotope's life, resulting in better target coverage than calculated based on films taken early after implantation. An additional ameliorating factor is that most of the swelling occurs in the anterior-posterior direction (**Figure 9-23**), so that cold spots tend to be worse anteriorly, where the likelihood of cancerous tissue is minimized. Although

9.26

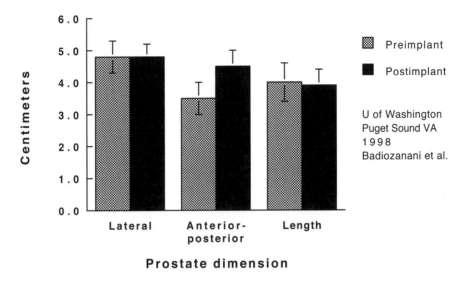

Figure 9-23. Prostatic dimensions before and after the implant procedure.

there are no actual outcomes data to support such an interpretation of postimplant images, not considering the degree of swelling can erroneously lead to the conclusion that an implant was not executed well, a source of consternation for both physician and patient. Outcomes data to test such a policy should be available in the future. In the meantime, probably the best solution is to rely primarily on the isodose overlays to assess an individual patient's implant.

PLANNED WITH TRUS, EVALUATED BY CT?
Perhaps the biggest conceptual problem with CT-based dosimetry is that it is not based on TRUS, the usual treatment planning imaging modality. One could make an argument that whatever modality is used to plan an implant should also be used to assess it. The most obvious potential problem with using different imaging modalities is the tendency to derive larger prostate volumes from CT scan, compared to TRUS. In fact, the accuracy of TRUS versus CT is still a contentious topic, and the importance of crossing imaging modalities is uncertain. However, this problem should be minimized if CTs are not overread to include the levator ani muscles with the prostatic volume (see chapter 4).

ASSESSING DOSE TO THE TUMOR ITSELF
Current practice is to assess the dose to the entire prostate, considering it to be uniformly at risk of cancerous involvement. In reality, cancers are far more likely to

A not-so-good implant

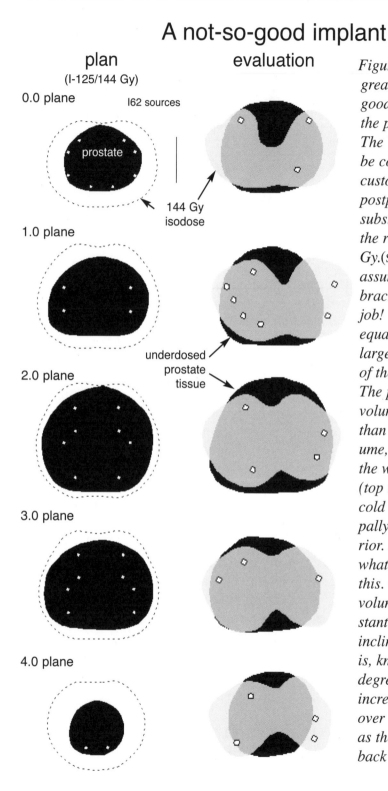

plan
(I-125/144 Gy)

0.0 plane   I62 sources

prostate

144 Gy isodose

1.0 plane

2.0 plane

3.0 plane

4.0 plane

evaluation

underdosed prostate tissue

Figure 9-24. This is a great example of a not-so-good implant, based on the postimplant dosimetry. The V100 of 78% would be considered too low, by customary standards. The postplan D90 was 115 Gy, substantially lower than the recommended 140 Gy.(STOCK 98 & 00) Don't assume that the brachytherapist did a bad job! The reasons for inadequate coverage are largely beyond the control of the brachytherapist. The postimplant prostate volume was 60% larger than the preimplant volume, due to increases in the width and thickness (top right graphs). The cold spots were principally anterior and posterior. It's tough to decide what to do in cases like this. Considering that the volume increase was substantial, we would be inclined to accept this as is, knowing that the degree of coverage will increase by about 5% over the next few weeks, as the prostate shrinks back to it original size.

9.28

A not-so-good implant (cont'd)

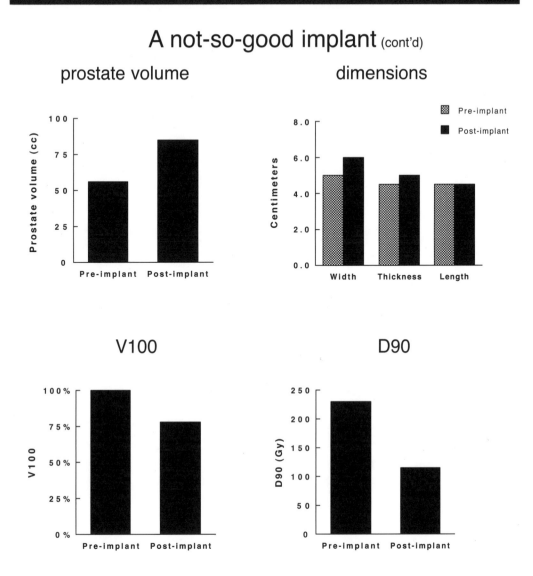

prostate volume

dimensions

V100

D90

involve the posterior portion of the prostate.(MCNEAL) While it would seem desirable to determine the dose to the tumor itself, current imaging techniques do not allow accurate delineation of cancer within the prostate.(SCHEIDLER) Even if it were possible, it would likely be best to continue to treat the entire prostate, to maximize the likelihood of eradicating microscopic synchronous cancers.

WHAT TO DO WITH AN INADEQUATE IMPLANT
Uh-oh. Regardless of one's level of experience, there will be cases in which the degree of target coverage appears insufficient. Although there are no clearly established criteria for adequate target coverage, there will be cases in which an implant

Table 9-3. Some considerations in assessing a low V100.

- Look at degree of swelling
  -if more than normal, would be more accepting of slightly inferior coverage
  -consider rescanning at one month postimplant, to let swelling resolve

- Look at where the cold spots are
  -if anterior, less significant in terms of cancer eradication

- Look at site(s) of positive biopsies
  -if positive where the implant is cold, more impetus to supplement the implant

is grossly suboptimal by customary standards. While you might quibble about the significance of a V100 of 80% versus 75%, if the V100 is down around 50%, you've got a problem that you need to address (**Table 9-3**).

The first thing to do when an implant seems inadequate is to review the site of the positive pre-treatment biopsies. If the involved portion of the prostate is covered well by the prescription dose, and the biopsies were negative elsewhere, tumor control *might* not be compromised by underdosage of the apparently uninvolved regions. Of course, this assumes that those portions of the prostate with negative biopsy tissue truly are free of cancer, a certain leap of faith, especially in a patient with a substantially elevated PSA, for whom more extensive cancer would be expected.

If the prescription dose coverage is suboptimal, and you are having trouble deciding on the adequacy of an implant, it may help to run the coverage at slightly lower dose levels—try the 80% isodose lines. It is likely that the full current prescription doses are not needed to eradicate cancer and that coverage of the cancerous regions by the 80% isodose line is adequate. But again, this is an admittedly big assumption. Another option for borderline inadequate implants is to repeat the evaluation CT one month later, to see how the coverage looks. But remember, the

Table 9-4. Ways to correct a low V100.

- Add sources
  -medically most sensical
- Supplemental external beam radiation

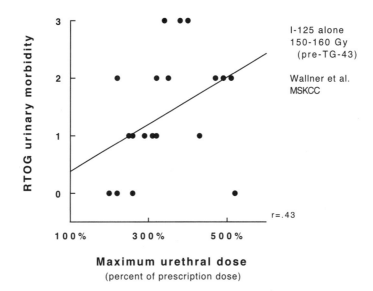

Figure 9-25. Maximum urethral dose versus RTOG post-implant urinary morbidity.(WALLNER 95)

V100 typically improves by only about 5% to 10% (see Figure 9-21). So if you have really bad coverage, a delayed CT scan is unlikely to resolve the issue.

In cases where prostatic coverage is deemed deficient, a decision is needed as to how to supplement the implant. There are two reasonable choices—either add some external beam radiation, or go back and add sources (**Table 9-4**). Adding supplemental external beam radiation is a murky proposition, which should be approached with caution. It's one thing to add supplemental external radiation to a prostate that has been treated with a relatively homogeneous implant. But it's another thing to add it to a prostate that has received a full therapeutic dose to some areas, and far less to others. Bringing the therapeutic dose to acceptable levels in the most underdosed regions may mean overtreating other regions, and possibly risking complications. Using even the most sophisticated treatment planning technique to supplement just a portion of the gland is probably not realistic.

Probably the best way to supplement an inadequate implant is to return to the operating room to add more sources to the underdosed region. To do so, use the post-implant CT to determine the dose to be delivered by the sources already implanted, and then prepare a plan to adequately supplement the underdosed regions, without excessive rectal or urethral doses.

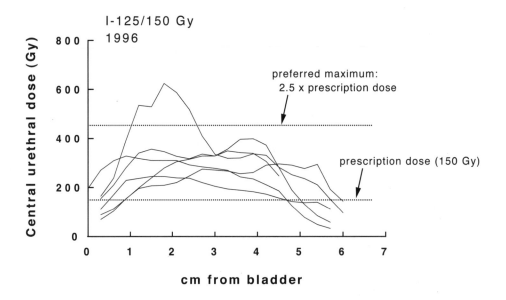

Figure 9-26. Typical I-125 urethral doses with peripheral loading pattern.

Deciding what to do about an inadequate implant is an admittedly poorly documented aspect of brachytherapy. Unfortunately, there are no data to support or refute the above guidelines—and there probably won't be for a long time.

DOSIMETRY OF NORMAL TISSUES
Everything we've covered so far in this chapter relates to *prostate* coverage. The other role of postimplant dosimetry is preventing (or explaining) the occurrence of complications, primarily of the urethra and rectum.

Urethral doses
Urethral doses have typically been calculated by leaving a urinary catheter in place to identify the urethra on postimplant CT scan images. A reasonable alternative for leaving the catheter in place, is to arbitrarily use the central prostatic point on each CT slice as the urethral dose calculation point. Waterman showed that approximating the urethral point comes very close to catheter-based calculations. In his report, use of an arbitrary point came within 5% to 10% of the catheter-based point in the higher dose ranges, where the clinical effect is most relevant.(WATERMAN) The notable exceptions would be an occasional patient with a markedly asymmet-

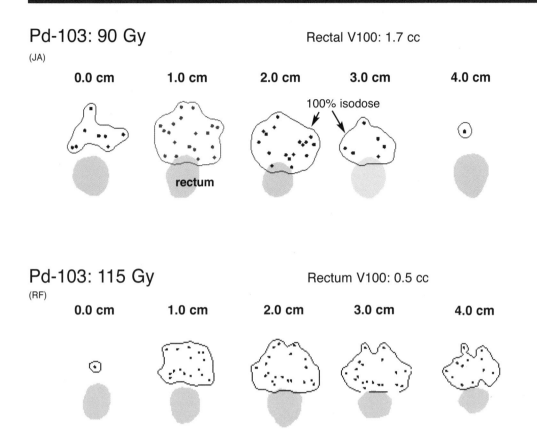

Pd-103: 90 Gy
(JA)

Rectal V100: 1.7 cc

Pd-103: 115 Gy
(RF)

Rectum V100: 0.5 cc

Figure 9-27. Examples of rectal coverage by prescription isodose. Top panels show patient with 1.7 cc rectal volume included in prescription isodose, versus 0.5 cc for patient in lower panels. The top patient is more likely to develop implant-related bleeding.(HAN)

ric urethra (see Figure 8-2). The close correlation between actual and arbitrary urethral dose calculations diminishes at the bladder neck, where the urethra tends to lie more anteriorly.

In patients implanted at MSKCC, urinary morbidity correlated fairly well with the maximal central urethral dose. Patients with a maximum I-125 urethral dose below 2.5 times the prescription dose were less likely to develop substantial urinary morbidity (**Figure 9-25**). More sophisticated calculations, including the length of urethra that received greater than 400 Gy, were no better for predicting morbidity than the simple parameter of maximum dose. The maximum desirable urethral dose for Pd-103 is presumed to be approximately 300 Gy. With a peripheral loading pat-

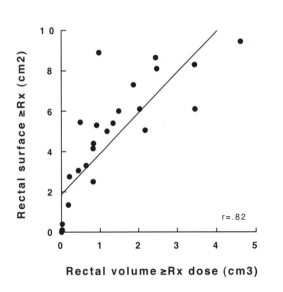

Figure 9-28. Scatter plots of rectal surface area versus rectal volume receiving greater than the prescription dose. These parameters are closely related, and it's unclear if one is more useful than the other.

tern, the central urethral dose can easily be kept well below 2.5 times the prescription dose (**Figure 9-26**).

Since the significance of excessive urethral doses was first reported in the mid-1990s, peripheral loading patterns have become standard. Accordingly, excessive urethral doses, like those seen in the early experience of Blasko and colleagues and Wallner and colleagues, are uncommon. In fact, with peripheral loading patterns, no relationship between urethral doses and morbidity has been described, probably because the range in urethral doses is too limited.(MERRICK 99) Within a narrower dose range, differences in urethral morbidity are more likely related to individual physical or biologic factors than to radiation dose. Accordingly, urethral doses are currently not routinely calculated by most implant teams.

The desirable maximal urethral dose when brachytherapy is combined with beam radiation has also not yet been documented. Extrapolating from the early report of Wallner and colleagues, and in the absence of data to the contrary, keeping it below 2.5 times the brachytherapy prescription dose seems prudent and practical.

RECTAL DOSES
Rectal bleeding, ulcerations, and fistulas are the most worrisome implant-related complications, potentially requiring major corrective surgery. The good news is that serious rectal complications are uncommon. The bad news is that because they are uncommon, little data exist regarding rectal tolerance doses and how to mini-

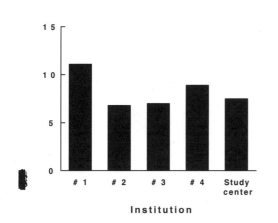

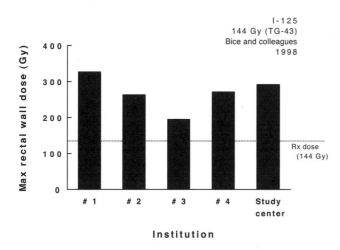

Figure 9-29. Average rectal surface area receiving greater than 100 Gy (I-125) (top panel) and maximum rectal surface dose (bottom panel), reported from five high-profile implant teams. Note the similarity among centers, even though their programs and policies evolved fairly independent of each other.(BICE) Remember, these are averages, so that many patients received doses far in excess of these, with a apparently low likelihood of rectal complications.

mize rectal morbidity. The most pressing practical issue is how generous the posterior treatment margin can safely be made.

In some cases, the cause of a rectal complication is obvious—for example, when several sources are placed in the rectal wall (see **Figure 15-11**). But most of the time, it's not so obvious why a particular patient develops a problem. To date, dosimetry has given only part of the answer.

There are a variety of ways to quantify rectal doses. Transverse isodose overlays are probably the most illustrative of the variability in rectal wall doses (**Figure 9-27**). Han and colleagues showed that rectal surface and volume doses are closely

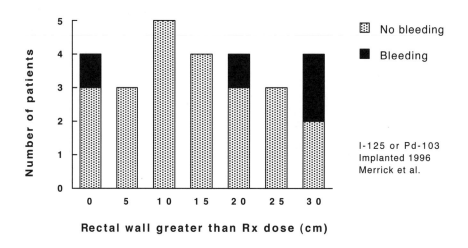

Figure 9-30. Rectal bleeding versus length of rectal wall treated to prescription dose or higher.(MERRICK 99)

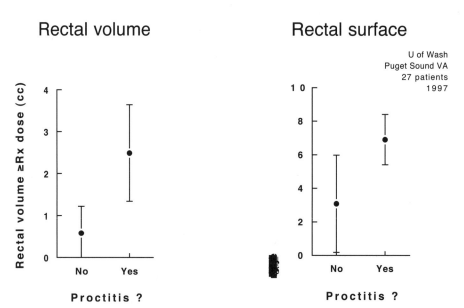

Figure 9-31. Rectal volume or rectal surface area receiving greater than the prescription dose is greater in patients with postimplant rectal bleeding.(HAN)

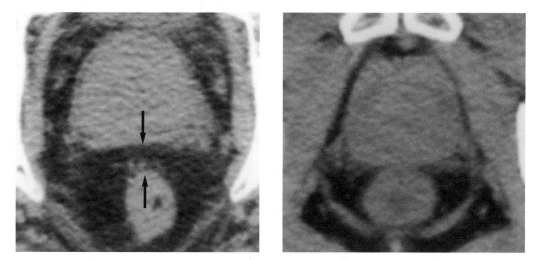

Figure 9-32. Patients with lesser degrees of perirectal fat are more likely to receive excessive rectal doses. The patient on the left has ample fat between his anterior rectal wall and prostate. In contrast, the patient on the right has far less fat, leaving the rectum closer to the prostate (and the radioactive sources). Han and colleagues showed that patients like those on the right were more prone to develop postimplant proctitis. (HAN)

correlated and that all are predictive of implant-related proctitis (**Figure 9-28**).(HAN)

Just how high is *too* high for rectal wall doses is unclear. Bice and colleagues summarized dosimetry from five experienced implant groups, all with an allegedly low incidence of rectal complications. The maximum rectal wall doses were approximately twice the prescription dose (**Figure 9-29**). Probably more important than the maximum dose on the rectal wall is the amount of rectum treated to higher doses.

Several investigators have compared rectal wall doses with complications. Wallner and colleagues found a loose correlation between rectal bleeding or ulceration and doses in excess of 100 Gy.(WALLNER 95) While there was a statistical correlation, rectal complications were only partially explained by higher doses—some patients who developed ulcerations did not appear to have excessive rectal wall doses, and most patients with higher doses did not suffer complications. Surprisingly, high dose regions within the implant have not correlated with the likelihood of complications.(HOWARD) There are, apparently, other unexplained

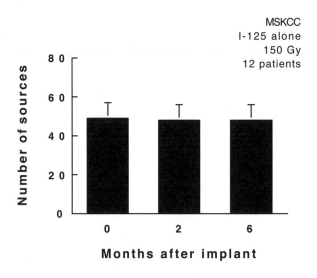

Figure 9-33. Source loss at two and six months after implantation. (WILLINS 98)

factors that contributed to rectal morbidity. In a more recent study, Merrick and colleagues found little relationship between the likelihood of complications and the length of the rectal wall receiving more than the prescription dose (**Figure 9-30**).(MERRICK 99)

In a preliminary look at nine patients with rectal bleeding among 147 patients treated in 1997 at the University of Washington, Han and colleagues showed a fairly good correlation between bleeding and the rectal volume treated to higher doses (**Figure 9-31**).(HAN) They also noted that some patients may be predisposed to higher rectal doses due to a limited amount of perirectal fat, placing their rectum in closer proximity to the prostate (**Figure 9-32**).

While there is some statistical correlation between rectal doses and morbidity, any relationship seems loose, at best. Although rectal dose contributes to the likelihood of complications, it appears that some patients are predisposed to complications, perhaps by virtue of a limited rectal wall blood supply, or some other normal variant. But such predisposing factors remain to be determined. This theory is supported by the lack of correlation between severe rectal complications and dosimetric calculations.(HOWARD)

SOURCE LOSS
Sources can migrate into the retroperitoneum, lungs, or heart (see Figure 8-30). Migration to the perineum seems to occur only by being pulled down with the

withdrawing needle tip (see Figures 8-31 and 8-32). But despite commonly raised concerns about the possibility of source loss or *migration*, it typically occurs with only one or two sources, and is inconsequential dosimetrically.

Sommerkamp and colleagues reported that 90% of patients implanted retropubically lost an average of two sources, usually within the first month after implantation.(SOMMERKAMP) In patients treated by Willins and Wallner and followed with CT scans at two and six months, source loss was minimal. From the time of the implant, patients lost an average of one source in the first two months, and only one of six patients lost an additional source between two and six months follow-up (**Figure 9-33**). Merrick and colleagues reported a similar low incidence of source migration despite the fact that they place a large percentage of sources outside the prostatic periphery.(MERRICK 00)

Source migration to the pulmonary vasculature occurs in 11% to 25% of patients.(STEINFELD, TAPEN) However, no morbidity from pulmonary sources has been described, and routine follow-up chest Xrays are not warranted. The only significant problem posed by source migration to the lungs is the loss of those sources' dose contribution to the implant—if you're losing more than one or two sources per patient, you need to work on your technique (see chapter 8).

REAL LIFE DOSIMETRY
Admittedly, dosimetric analysis is time-consuming and expensive, adding about $1,000 to $2,000 in patient charges. However, the price of quality assurance is still small compared to the overall costs of care.(WALLNER 00) Adequate prostate coverage *should* be verified in every patient, as part of a meaningful quality assurance procedure.

In the early part of your brachytherapy experience, it would be prudent to do more extensive dosimetric analysis including urethral and rectal doses, to be sure that your implants meet generally acceptable guidelines in regards to the risk of complications. Once you're confident that urethral and rectal doses are being kept within acceptable limits while still achieving adequate prostate coverage, some corner-cutting is in order. In contrast to target coverage, routine calculation of urethral and rectal doses in every patient is probably not necessary. Detailed dosimetric studies correlating dosimetry with urinary and rectal complications were valuable in helping to establish dosimetry guidelines. In current practice, however, serious rectal and urinary complications are very low if implants are executed by the general guidelines outlined in chapter 6, and it seems reasonable to limit routine dosimetric analysis to the degree of prostate coverage. We limit our urethral and rectal dose calculations to patients enrolled in research trials, or the occasional patient who develops a serious complications, in which case doses are calculated at the time the complication is discovered—typically long after the implant procedure.

REFERENCES

1. Amdur RJ, Gladstone D, Leopold KA, Harris RD. Prostate seed implant quality assessment using MR and CT image fusion. Int J Radiat Oncol Biolo Phys 1999; 43:67-72.

2. Anderson LL. Brachytherapy planning and evaluation. Endo/Hyper Oncol 1991; 7:139-146.

3. Badiozamani K, Wallner K, Sutlief S, Ellis W, Blasko J, Russell K. Anticipating prostatic volume changes due to prostate brachytherapy. Radiat Oncol Invest 1999; 7:360-364.

4. Bice WS, Prestidge BR, Grimm PD, et al . Centralized multiinstitutional postimplant analysis for interstitial prostate brachytherapy. Int J Rad Oncol Biol Phys 1998; 41:921-927.

5. Chen Z, Yue N, Wang X, Roberts KB, Peschel R, Nath R. Dosimetric effects of edema in permanent prostate seed implants: A rigorous solution. Int J Rad Oncol Biol Phys 2000; 47:1405-1419.

6. D'Amico AV, Davis A, Vargas SO, Renshaw AA, Jiroutek M, Richie JP. Defining the implant treatment volume for patients with low risk prostate cancer: does the anterior base need to be treated? Int J Rad Oncol Biol Phys 1999; 43:587-590.

7. Davis BJ, Pisansky TM, Wilson TM, Rothenberg HJ, Pacelli A, Hillman DW, Sargent DJ, Bostwick DG. The radial distance of extraprostatic extension of prostate carcinoma: implications for prostate brachytherapy. Cancer 1999; 85:2630-2637.

8. DeLaney TF, Shipley WU, O'Leary MP, Biggs PJ, Prout GR. Preoperative irradiation and 125-Iodine implantation for patients with localized carcinoma of the prostate. Int J Radiat Oncol Biol Phys 1986; 12:1779-1785.

9. Dubois FD, Prestidge BR, Hotchkiss LA, Bice WS, Prete JJ. Source localization following permanent transperineal prostate intersititial brachytherapy using magnetic resonance imaging. Int J Radiat Oncol Biol Phys 1997; 39:1037-1041.

10. Fuks Z, Leibel SA, Wallner KE, Begg CB, Fair WR, Anderson LL, Hilaris BS, Whitmore WF. The effect of local control on metastatic dissemination in carcinoma of the prostate: Long term results in patients treated with 125-I implantation. Int J Radiat Oncol Biol Phys 1991; 21:337-347.

11. Gelblum DY, Potters L, Ashley R, Waldbaum R, Wang X, Leibel S. Urinary morbidity following ultrasound-guided transperineal prostate seed implantation. Int J Rad Oncol Biol Phys 1999; 45:59-67.

12. Han B, Wallner K. Dosimetric and radiographic correlates to prostate brachytherapy-related rectal complications. (submitted) 2002;

13. Howard A, Wallner K, Han B, Schneider B, et al . Rectal fistulas after prostate brachytherapy. Journal of Brachytherapy International 2001; (in press):

14. Jones S, Wallner K, Merrick G, Cavanagh W, Butler W. Clinical correlates of high brachytherapy dose regions within the prostate. (submitted) 2002;

15. Ling CC, Roy J, Sahoo N, Wallner K, Anderson L. Quantifying the effect of dose inhomogeneity in brachytherapy: Application to permanent prostatic implant with 125-I seeds. Int J Rad Oncol Biol Phys 1994; 28:971-978.

16. McNeal JE, Price HM, Redwine EA, Freiha FS, Stamey TA. Stage A Versus Stage B Adenocarcinoma of the Prostate: Morphological Comparison and Biological Significance. J Urol 1988; 139:61-65.

17. Merrick GS, Butler WM, Dorsey AT, Lief JH. Potential role of various dosimetric quality indicators in prostate brachytherapy. Int J Rad Oncol Biol Phys 1999; 44:717-724.

18. Merrick GS, Butler WM, Dorsey AT, Lief JH, Benson ML. Seed fixity in the prostate/periprostatic region following brachytherapy. Int J Rad Oncol Biol Phys 2000; 46:215-220.

19. Merrick GS, Butler WM, Dorsey AT, Lief JH, Walbert HL, Blatt HJ. Rectal dosimetric analysis following prostate brachytherapy. Int J Rad Oncol Biol Phys 1999; 43:1021-1027.

20. Merrick GS, Butler WM, Dorsey AT, Walbert HL. Influence of timing on the dosimetric analysis of transperineal ultrasound-guided, prostatic conformal brachytherapy. Radiat Oncol Invest 1998; 6:182-190.

21. Moerland MA, Wijrdeman HK, Beersma R, Bakker CJG. Evaluation of permanent I-125 prostate implants using radiography and magnetic resonance imaging. Int J Radiat Oncol Biol Phys 1997; 37:927-933.

22. Nag S, Vivekanandam S, Martinez-Monge R. Pulmonary embolization of permanently implanted radioactive palladium-103 seeds for carcinoma of the prostate. Int J Rad Oncol Biol Phys 1997; 39:667-670.

23. Prestidge BR, Bice WS, Kiefer EJ, Prete JJ. Timing of computed tomography-based postimplant assessment following permanent transperineal prostate brachytherapy. Int J Radiat Oncol Biolo Phys 1998; 40:1111-1115.

24. Reddy EK, Krishnan L, Mebust WK, Weigel JW. External beam radiation vs Iodine-125 implantation in localized prostatic cancer. Endocurie/Hyper Oncol 1991; 7:179-183.

25. Roy JN, Wallner KE, Harrington PJ, Ling CC, Anderson LL. A CT-based evaluation method for permanent imlants: Application to prostate. Int J Radiat Oncol Biol Phys 1993; 26:163-169.

26. Scheidler J, Hricak H, Vigneron DB, Yu KK, Sokolov DL, Huang LR, et al . Prostate cancer: Localization with three-dimensional proton MR spectroscopy imaging—clinicopathologic study. Radiol 1999; 213:473-480.

27. Sommerkamp H, Rupprecht M, Wannenmacher M. Seed loss in interstitial radiotherapy of prostatic carcinoma with I-125. Int J Radiat Oncol Biol Phys 1988; 14:389-392.

28. Steinfeld AD, Donahue BR, Plaine L. Pulmonary embolization of iodine-125 seeds following prostate implantation. Urol 1991; 37:149-150.

29. Stock RG, Stone NN, Kao J, Ianuzzi C, Unger P. The effect of disease and treatment-related factors on biopsy results after prostate brachytherapy. Cancer 2000; 89:1829-1834.

30. Stock RG, Stone NN, Tabert A, Iannuzzi C, DeWyngaert JK. A dose-response study for I-125 prostate implants. Int J Rad Oncol Biol Phys 1998; 41:101-108.

31. Tapen EM, Blasko JC, Grimm PD, et al . Reduction of radioactive seed embolization to the lung following prostate brachytherapy. Int J Rad Oncol Biol Phys 1998; 42:1063-1067.

32. Vicini FA, Kestin LL, Martinez AA. The importance of adequate follow-up in defining treatment success after external beam irradiation for prostate cancer. Int J Rad Oncol Biol Phys 1999; 45:553-561.

33. Waehre H, Amellem O, Stenwig AE, Tvera K, Juul M, Pettersen EO, Fossa SD. Deoxyribonucleic acid cytometry and histological findings before and after 125-Iodine implantation of primary prostate cancer. J Urol 1992; 148:838-842.

34. Wallner KE. SmartMedicine: How to cut medical costs and cure cancer. Seattle: SmartMedicine Press, 2000.

35. Wallner KE, Roy J, Harrison L. Dosimetry guidelines to minimize urethral and rectal morbidity following transperineal I-125 prostate brachytherapy. Int J Radiat Oncol Biol Phys 1995; 32:465-471.

36. Waterman FM, Dicker AP. Effect of post-implant edema on the rectal dose in prostate brachytherapy. Int J Rad Oncol Biol Phys 1999; 45:571-576.

37. Waterman FM, Dicker AP. Determination of the urethral dose in prostate brachytherapy when the urethra cannot be visualized in the postimplant CT scan. Med Phys 2000; 27:448-451.

38. Waterman FM, Yue N, Corn BW, Dicker AP. Edema associated with I-125 or Pd-103 prostate brachytherapy and its impact on post-implant dosimetry: an analysis based on serial CT acquistion. Int J Rad Oncol Biol Phys 1998; 41:1069-1077.

39. Willins J, Wallner K. CT-based dosimetry for transperineal I-125 prostate brachytherapy. Int J Rad Oncol Biol Phys 1997; 39:347-353.

40. Willins J, Wallner KE. Time-dependent changes in CT-based dosimetry of I-125 prostate brachytherapy. Radiat Oncol Invest 1998; 6:157-160.

10

Postoperative Care

One of the major advantages of brachytherapy is that perioperative care is relatively simple. Serious complications or hospital readmissions after brachytherapy are infrequent.(HAN) However, patients typically experience marked urinary and rectal symptoms and need ready access to medical advice, even if only by phone. There is a wide range of acceptable ways to manage patients postoperatively with little data to support one approach over another. The pages ahead mostly summarize our own experience and biases.

SKIN CARE

After withdrawing the last needle, the perineum should be cleaned with a damp cloth. Povidine-iodine solutions or other cleansing agents are better saved for the OR staff than the patient. The value of postimplant perineal icepacks is questionable. Application of a perineal dressing is impractical. Patients are instructed to shower with soap after returning home, several hours after the implant. Neither John Blasko, Michael Dattoli, nor Kent Wallner has ever seen an implant-related perineal infection, regardless of what perineal care is used.

CATHETER REMOVAL

A urinary catheter is commonly used for the implant procedure. There is no known relation between catheter removal time and the risk of postimplant urinary retention. At the Seattle Prostate Institute, University of Washington, and Puget Sound VA, the catheter is removed upon completion of the procedure. M. Dattoli prefers to keep it in overnight, a policy that prevents some patients from being recatheterized for short-term retention.

Patients who are able to pass a urine stream within several hours after the implant will almost certainly not develop acute retention later, although urination is typically frequent and uncomfortable. Occasionally a patient will urinate spontaneously immediately after catheter removal, but still go on to develop urinary retention over the next twenty-four hours. If a patient has not urinated within six hours of catheter removal, he will usually need to to be catheterized. But the need for catheterization should be individualized.

URINARY RETENTION

Urinary retention is the most common acute implant-related complication and it is almost impossible to predict (see chapter 12). Fortunately, it typically resolves rapidly (**Figure 10-1**). In preliminary, uncontrolled studies, prophylactic alpha-1 blockers have not been shown to decrease the need for short-term catheterization (see chapter 12).

Postimplant retention usually resolves spontaneously within twenty-four hours. Patients who still cannot urinate the next day will need longer catheterization. How you manage prolonged retention in these less fortunate patients can make a big difference in their postimplant experience.

A better option than reinserting an indwelling catheter is to instruct patients in self-catheterization—those patients willing to give it a try generally prefer it over an indwelling catheter. Intermittent catheterization avoids the irritation of the constant presence of a catheter, and allows a more normal lifestyle. It also allows

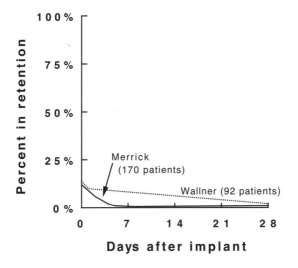

Figure 10-1. Resolution of retention after I-125 or Pd-103 implantation. Most patient were managed with intermittent catheterization or an indwelling catheter with intermittent voiding trials. We prefer now to proceed sooner to intermittent self-catheterization.(WALLNER 96, MERRICK 00)

patients to urinate spontaneously as they improve, rather than waiting for a voiding trial. Considering that most patients do well with intermittent self-catheterization, a suprapubic catheter should be reserved only for those who cannot or will not self-catheterize or can't tolerate an indwelling catheter.

Nearly all cases of postimplant retention resolve spontaneously within a few days of implantation. Surgical intervention, including transurethral resection or incision of the prostate (TURP or TUIP) or a suprapubic tube, should be avoided in favor of longer term intermittent self-catheterization or indwelling Foley catheter (see chapter 15).(HU, LANDIS)

HEMATURIA
Most patients have a minor degree of postimplant gross hematuria, lasting for 1 to 14 days. Occasional patients will pass clots for a longer time. The amount of bleeding is usually minimal, but patients occasionally pass larger amounts, possibly from a urethral tear or minor bladder injury. When that happens, a Foley catheter can be placed and irrigated until clear. Hemodynamically significant postimplant bleeding is rare. Catheter placement usually tamponades and stops the

bleeding immediately. We typically leave the catheter in for three days. Diagnostic cystoscopy or any surgical intervention is usually not necessary.

DYSURIA IN THE FIRST POSTOPERATIVE WEEK

Patients typically experience substantial dysuria in the immediate postoperative period, presumably due to needle-related trauma. This initial dysuria subsides substantially within twenty-four hours. Taking nonsteroidal anti-inflammatory drugs (NSAID) within several hours after implantation can help with acute discomfort. Bleeding problems, even with immediate use of NSAIDs, are rare. Narcotics generally do not help to alleviate the acute dysuria. Prophylactic alpha-1 blockers are routinely prescribed by some brachytherapists, but their benefit in the immediate postoperative period is unclear.

Patients are instructed not to drink extra fluids during the first few hours following implantation, because it can exacerbate their already troublesome urinary problems. They should start drinking extra fluids the morning after the implant, and continue doing so for three days, possibly decreasing the likelihood of a urinary infection.

GOING HOME

Patients are typically sent home after recovery from anesthesia. They are usually asked to stay within a one-hour drive of the hospital, unless arrangements can be made to be seen in local emergency room if an acute problem develops. If a patient lives more than an hour away, it is probably best that they stay in a hotel close to the hospital.

SCROTAL BRUISING

Patients commonly develop scrotal and perineal bruising several days after the procedure. It resolves spontaneously, but it should be mentioned beforehand because its unexpected appearance can be disconcerting. Application of an ice pack to the perineum may decrease the likelihood of bruising.

INFECTION

Perioperative urinary infections are unusual, regardless of whether antibiotics are used (see chapter 7).(WALLNER 96, DICKER) Late infections occur occasionally, and should be treated appropriately.

PAIN

Postoperative pain (apart from dysuria) is usually limited to minor perineal discomfort. More significant post-operative pain is unusual. Narcotic analgesics

Table 10-1. Alpha blockers.

Generic	Brand	Tablet strength	Approximate Cost/tablet
doxazosin	Cardura™	1, 2, 4, 8 mg	$1.10
tamsulosin	Flomax™	0.4 mg	$1.40
terazocin	Hytrin™	1, 2, 5, 10 mg	$1.10

should not be routinely prescribed. Patients who experience pain requiring narcotics should be carefully assessed for an unusual circumstance.

DYSURIA AFTER THE FIRST WEEK
Nearly all patients develop symptoms of radiation prostatitis, including dysuria, daytime frequency, nocturia, and urgency. Radiation-related symptoms generally start one to two weeks following implantation, and are due to *urethral* inflammation, not to *cystitis*.

If no medications are routinely prescribed, about half of patients do not have severe enough urinary symptoms to request medication.(WALLNER 96) The other half are symptomatic enough to prefer treatment. Selective alpha-1 adrenergic blockers are by far the most effective treatment for radiation prostatitis (**Table 10-1**). Terazocin (Hytrin™), doxazosin (Cardura™), or tamsulosin (Flomax™) are remarkably effective in relieving radiation-related obstructive symptoms, usually within an hour or two of ingestion.

The usual starting dose for Hytrin™ or Cardura™ is 1 or 2 mg at night, and 0.4 mg for Flomax™. There is a risk of hypotension, especially when first starting alpha blockers. Hypotensive episodes are probably more likely in older, thin patients, but patients should be warned about this when first starting the medication. Hypotension and fatigue seem to be least likely with Flomax.

Some patients do well taking the drugs once daily. Although all three drugs are said to have twenty-four-hour action, patients often do better if they take two or more daily doses. In general, the total daily dose of prazocin or terazocin should be kept below 10 mg; above that, patients commonly experience fatigue. Flomax™

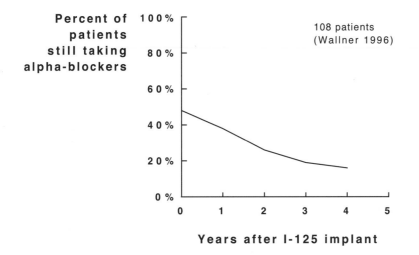

Figure 10-2. Percent of patient still using alpha-blockers after I-125 implantation.(WALLNER 96)

(0.4 mg) can usually be given up to three times daily with little chance of side effects.

Radiation prostatitis begins to remit within several months of implantation, and at some point most patients stop their alpha-blockers (**Figures 10-2 & 10-3**). Patients can try decreasing their medication for one or two days. If symptoms of radiation prostatitis persist, alpha-blockers can be restarted and stopped again in a month or two. There is much variability among patients in their time to resolution of radiation-related symptoms and in their response to medication, so that patients and physicians should be flexible regarding the way that mediations are taken (**Figure 10-4**). To keep things in perspective regarding the 20% of patients still using alpha-blockers at one year, keep in mind that many men in the prostate cancer age range are on alpha-blockers even without having had an implant.

It is fairly common for patients to have an exacerbation of their prostatitis symptoms around the one-year mark after implantation, about the same time they frequently experience a temporary rise ("bump") in their PSA (see chapter 13). The mechanism for these temporary symptom exacerbations (or benign PSA bumps) is unknown, but temporary reinstitution of alpha-blockers may be called for. While late urinary infections are distinctly uncommon, urine cultures should be done as clinically indicated.

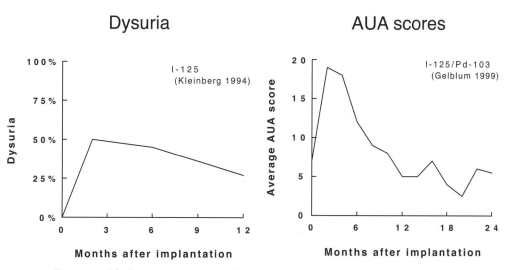

Figure 10-3. Dysuria and AUA scores in the postimplant period.(KLEINBERG, GELBLUM*)*

PHYSICAL ACTIVITY

Patients are instructed to avoid strenuous physical activity for one to two days following implantation. After that, all restrictions are lifted. This policy seems prudent in the post-anesthesia setting, with some possibility of bleeding. Having said that, however, many patients have ignored our advice to limit their activity and we have rarely seen any problem even remotely related to rigorous activity in the perioperative period.

Physical activity generally alleviates urinary obstructive symptoms, the mechanism of which is unclear. Regular exercise should be encouraged as part of the treatment for postimplant obstructive urinary symptoms (and for other good reasons as well). Some patients experience discomfort with perineal pressure, and avoid activities like bicycling. The authors are unaware, however, of any adverse effects from perineal pressure.

SEXUAL ACTIVITY

There is no published information regarding ill effects from sexual activity in the postimplant period. Surprisingly, some patients engage in sex the night of the implant, and we're unaware of any problems with that apart from some discomfort with ejaculation (see chapter 16).

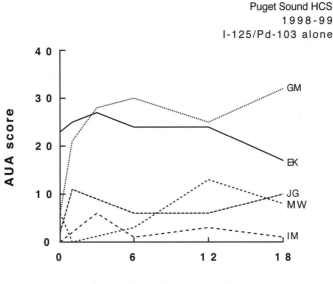

Puget Sound HCS
1998-99
I-125/Pd-103 alone

Figure 10-4. Postimplant AUA scores in different patients. Patients vary tremendously in how quickly their symptoms resolve—be flexible in regard to alpha-blocker use. Many patients don't need them at all, and others need higher doses for extended periods of time.

Theoretically, one or more sources could be passed with the ejaculate, although this is apparently very rare. However, it may be prudent to recommend condom use for four months after I-125 and one month after Pd-103.

RECTAL BLEEDING
Patients may have a slight amount of bright red blood per rectum in the immediate postoperative period, presumably due to inadvertent piercing of the rectal mucosa or to procedure-related hemorrhoidal exacerbation. Bleeding due to radiation itself is extremely unlikely in the first six postimplant months (see chapter 15).

RADIATION PROTECTION
Radiation detectable at the skin surface is low. The dose rate at the skin surface immediately following a full dose I-125 implant is approximately 2–10 mR/hour. The typical exposure at skin surface with full dose Pd-103 implant is 1–5 mR/hour. There is no data regarding the risk to humans from such low exposure rates. Extrapolating from much higher dose rates, regulations have been advanced

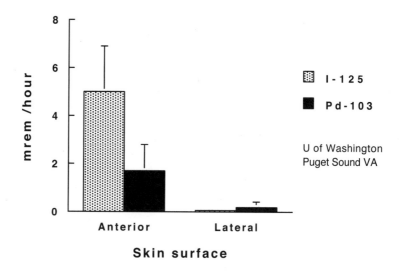

Figure 10-5. Exposure rates at the anterior and lateral skin surfaces with I-125 versus Pd-103.(SMATHERS)

limiting the total annual dose to 0.1 mR/hour for the general public. Accordingly, the *safe* total exposure time at the anterior skin surface would be approximately 20 hours for I-125 and 50 hours for Pd-103 (**Figures 10-5 & 10-6**). Of course, the "safe" exposure times would increase with each radionuclide half-life that passes.

Exposure to others can be decreased with increased distance from the patient. The exposure at one meter from the pelvic skin surface is virtually undetectable with a conventional clinical ionization chamber. Exposure to others can be almost eliminated by wearing a lead apron fabricated from lead-lined sheeting or purchased from a radiology supply company (**Figure 10-7**).

PSA DETERMINATIONS
The proper timetable for postimplant PSA determination is still unclear. Until recently, it was common to get the first follow-up PSA one month after the procedure. However, PSA values taken before two years will not be used to make a clinical decision, because readings commonly rise between one and two years, and then fall again (see chapter 13). Even if a PSA were continuously rising, a follow-up biopsy would not be recommended until two years, because of the higher rate of false positives before that time (see chapter 13). One could even make an argument to wait to get a PSA until two years have passed. Understandably, some patients are anxious to "get some results" sooner, but any PSA taken before then

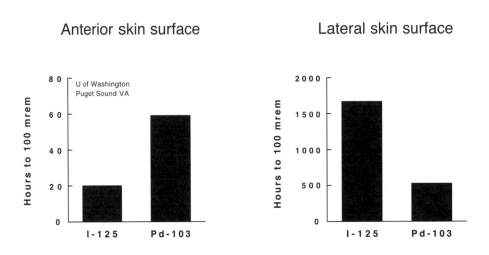

Figure 10-6. Approximate exposure times at anterior and lateral skin surfaces needed to reach NRC annual limits for the general public (100 mrem).(SMATHERS)

will not be of much clinical use. And if the PSA happens to "bounce" up, the patient may suffer considerable anxiety while waiting for the next value.

Patients with markedly elevated pretreatment PSA or elevated prostatic acid phosphatase should probably be monitored at six-month intervals from the day of implantation, because they are at higher risk of having metastatic disease. A rapidly rising PSA would be an indication to obtain a bone scan to look for possible bone metastases, which may warrant early hormonal ablation.

A reasonable compromise between patients' desire for information about their course and the fact that early PSAs usually don't mean much, is to get PSAs every six months for the first two years, and annually thereafter. If the PSA is greater than 1.0 ng/ml at the two-year mark and is not falling, a repeat prostate biopsy should be considered, providing the patient is a potential candidate for salvage therapy.

IT'S USUALLY EASY
In general, there is minimal need for physician intervention in the postoperative period. Problems that do occur typically can be managed over the telephone. Low-tech interventions such as listening, providing explanations and reassurance, and the liberal use of alpha-blockers are generally all that is needed. Surgical intervention is rarely required. Tincture of time is the best remedy for nearly all implant-related problems. It's important, however, that patients have easy access

Lead underwear (Radiation Guard)

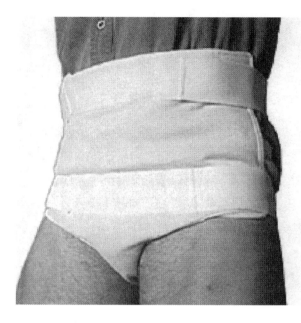

Figure 10-7. Lead-lined shield to be worn over underwear will stop more than 95% of I-125 emissions and 99% of Pd-103 emissions (Atlantic Nuclear, Canton, MA, 800-878-9118).

to a physician or nurse clinician for advice in coping with postimplant symptoms. Second and third opinions should be sought before proceeding with any surgical intervention for seemingly intractable implant-related problems.

REFERENCES
1. Dicker AP, Figura AT, Waterman FM, et al . Is there a role for antibiotic prophylaxis in transperineal intersitial permanent prostate brachytherapy? Tech Urol 2000; 6:104-108.

2. Gelblum DY, Potters L, Ashley R, Waldbaum R, Wang X, Leibel S. Urinary morbidity following ultrasound-guided transperineal prostate seed implantation. Int J Rad Oncol Biol Phys 1999; 45:59-67.

3. Han BH, Demel KC, Wallner KE, Young L. Patient reported short-term complications after prostate brachytherapy. Int J Rad Oncol Biol Phys 2000; 48 (supp):77.

4. Hu K, Wallner KE. Urinary incontinence in patients who have a TURP/TUIP following prostate brachytherapy. Int J Radiat Oncol Biol Phys 1998; 40:783-786.

5. Kleinberg L, Wallner K, Roy J, Zelefsky M, Arterbery VE, Fuks Z, Harrison L. Treatment-related symptoms during the first year following transperineal I-125 prostate implantation. Int J Radiat Oncol Biol Phys 1994; 28:985.

6. Landis D, Wallner K, Locke J, Ellis W, Russell K, Cavanuagh W, Blasko J. Late urinary morbidity after prostate brachytherapy. (submitted) 2002;

7. Merrick GS, Butler WM, Lief JH, Dorsey AT. Temporal resolution of urinary morbidity following prostate brachytherapy. Int J Radiat Oncol Biolo Phys 2000; 47:121-128.

8. Smathers S, Wallner KE, Lai K, Bergasagel K, Hudson R, Sutlief S, Blasko J. Radiation safety parameters following prostate brachytherapy. Int J Radiat Oncol Biol Phys 1999; 45:397-399.

9. Wallner KE, Roy J, Harrison L. Low risk of perioperative infection without pro-phylactic antibiotics for transperineal prostate brachytherapy. Int J Radiat Oncol Biol Phys 1996; 36:681-683.

10. Wallner KE, Roy J, Harrison L. Tumor control and morbidity following transperineal I-125 implantation for Stage T1/T2 prostatic carcinoma. J Clin Oncol 1996; 14:449-453.

11

Supplemental Beam Radiation

Some patients may not be candidates for brachytherapy, due to general health or urologic conditions. But from an oncologic perspective, nearly all early-stage patients can be appropriately treated with brachytherapy, either alone or combined with external beam radiation. A combination of brachytherapy plus supplemental external beam radiation has long been used successfully in the definitive therapy of cervical, endometrial, and tongue cancers, the rationale being that brachytherapy eradicates large central tumor masses while beam radiation eradicates microscopic disease outside of the implant volume.

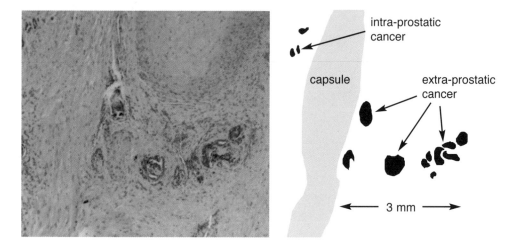

Figure 11-1. Advanced EPE—in this prostatectomy specimen, cancer has penetrated the capsule, extending approximately 3 mm outside of capsular margin. The cancer is still within the margin of resection (not visible here). This degree of EPE probably would be included within the cancercidal isodose of an implant (see Figure 11-3) (courtesy of Dr. L. True).

Supplemental beam radiation has been used with Ir-192 prostate implants with substantial success.(SYED, MATE, MARTINEZ) So when TRUS-based transperineal I-125 and Pd-103 brachytherapy emerged in the late 1980s, the concept of combining brachytherapy with external beam radiation was similarly adopted for many patients. The external beam fields typically used are just large enough to cover the prostate, with a 2–4 cm margin (see chapter 6).

For a while, there was general agreement as to which patients should receive supplemental external radiation—those with a pretreatment PSA above 10 or a Gleason score above 6. While the tumor control rates with this policy have been favorable, two areas of clinical investigation have reopened the question of the need for supplemental beam radiation. First, results with implant alone, even in patients with higher PSA and Gleason scores, have been remarkably good in experienced hands.(BLASKO 00, ZELEFSKY, MERRICK 01, SHARKEY) Second, detailed pathology studies have revealed that the radial extent of extraprostatic cancer extension, even in patients with higher PSA and Gleason scores, is surprisingly limited.(DAVIS, SOHAYDA) It turns out that the role of supplemental external radiation is one of the least understood aspects of prostate brachytherapy.

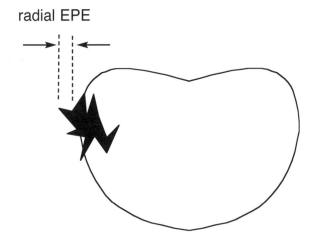

Figure 11-2. As cancer breaches the prostatic capsule, it extends laterally and radially. The potential for radial extension is the rationale for seeking greater peripheral coverage with supplemental external beam radiation.

RATIONALE FOR BEAM RADIATION

There are three rationales for using supplemental external beam radiation:

1. *enhance coverage of the periprostatic tissue*
2. *escalate dose to intraprostatic tumor*
3. *make up for a technically inadequate implant*

In practice, there is substantial overlap between the rationales.

EPE

The primary rationale for supplemental beam radiation is to increase the coverage of the periprostatic region, helping to sterilize extraprostatic cancer extension (EPE) (**Figure 11-1**). The prostatic capsule is a collection of fibrous layers of variable thickness and without a distinct margin, and cancers commonly achieve varying degrees of extraprostatic extension by the time of diagnosis (**Figure 11-2**).(SAKR, SATTAR) Patients with early EPE are still curable, providing the extracapsular tumor can be eradicated. The most compelling evidence for their curability is that cure rates following radical prostatectomy are still possible in the setting of EPE, assuming that the surgical margins are clear of cancer (**Figure 11-3**). And considering the high cure rates with radiation, the same must hold true—patients with minimal capsular penetration are still curable if the cancercidal radiation dose

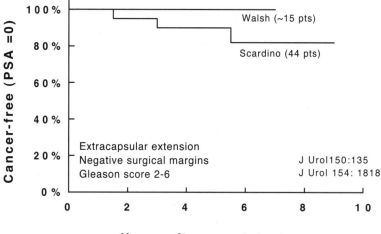

Figure 11-3. Disease-free survival for T1/T2 prostatectomy patients with limited ECE and negative margins. Such patients are still highly curable surgically, despite the presence of EPE.(OHORI, EPSTEIN)

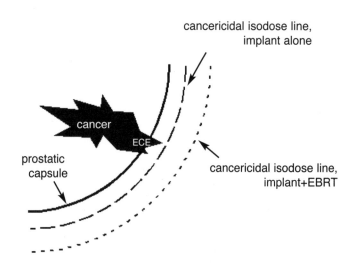

Figure 11-4. A major theoretical issue regarding the need for supplemental beam radiation is whether it is needed to assure that the cancercidal isodose encompasses EPE.

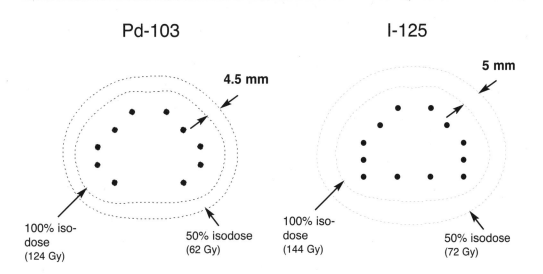

Figure 11-5. It's not known exactly how much extra therapeutic margin supplemental beam radiation provides, but a perusal of two typical plans gives an estimate. Assuming that 45 Gy beam radiation brings the 50% brachytherapy isodose up to a cancericidal level, then beam radiation would increase the treatment margin by about 4–5 mm.

encompasses all EPE. Unfortunately, the precise cancercidal margin with implant alone or combined with supplemental beam radiation is unclear, partly because no one knows precisely what the cancericidal dose is! Assuming the cancericidal isodose line of an implant combined with beam radiation is somewhere between that of a half-dose and a full-dose implant, supplemental beam radiation should increase the therapeutic margin by approximately 4 mm (**Figures 11-4, 11-5 & 11-6**).

Guidelines for adding supplemental beam radiation were initially extrapolated from surgical pathology studies, whereby the likelihood of EPE was correlated with pretreatment PSA and Gleason score (**Figure 11-7**). Although the likelihood of EPE is a continuum with increasing parameters, the generally accepted cutoff for adding beam radiation has been a PSA of 10 or a Gleason score of 7. Stage has been a lesser-used criterion, due to the subjectivity of the digital rectal exam and the fact that the majority of patients diagnosed currently have nonpalpable disease (**Figure 11-8**).

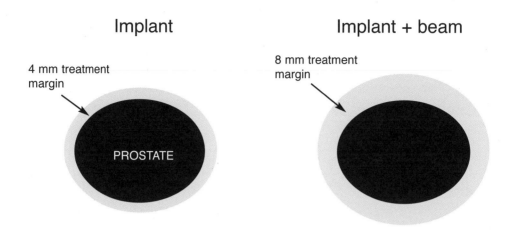

Figure 11-6. Schematic representation of the therapeutic margin with an implant alone versus an implant plus supplemental external radiation, assuming the brachytherapy treatment margin is increased from 4 mm to 8 mm.

The limitation of most pathology studies regarding EPE is that they address only its *incidence*, not its radial distance from the prostatic capsule. The *Partin Tables*, for instance, have been misinterpreted by doctors and patients alike to equate EPE with incurability (**Box 11-1**).(PARTIN) More recent studies of the *radial* extent of EPE have rekindled the debate regarding its clinical significance and the rationale for supplemental beam radiation.

Using prostatectomy specimens, Dr. Brian Davis from the Mayo Clinic and Dr. Chris Sohayda from Cleveland Clinic correlated radial EPE with pretreatment PSA and Gleason score (**Figures 11-9 & 11-10**). In what came as a real surprise to most oncologists, EPE is limited to within 3 mm of the prostatic edge in nearly all patients. Accordingly, a radiation treatment margin (TM) of 3 mm should suffice. Since brachytherapy alone can consistently achieve a TM of 3 mm or more, the rationale for adding beam radiation to achieve a wider treatment margin has been reopened to debate (**Figure 11-11**).(MERRICK 02)

> **Box 11.1 Why the Partin Tables are unduly frightening**
>
> The Partin Tables have been misinterpreted by both physicians and patients to mean that patients with EPE are not curable. In fact, a large percentage of patients with EPE are still curable, surgically or with brachytherapy, provided that the EPE is still encompassed within the surgical margins, or within the cancercidal dose range. This should be stressed to patients, who otherwise believe that their high likelihood of EPE is synonymous with a high likelihood of treatment failure.

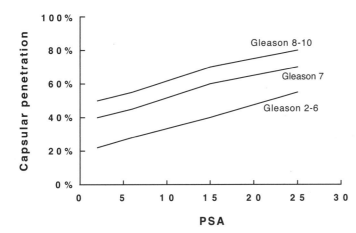

Figure 11-7. Likelihood of EPE in patients with Stage T1c-T2a tumors, versus Gleason score and PSA, based on data from JHU. (PARTIN)

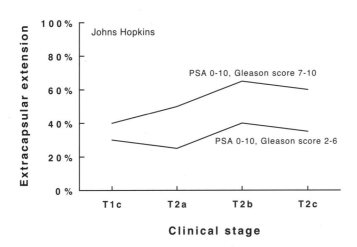

Figure 11-8. In comparison to PSA and Gleason score, the effect of clinical stage on the likelihood of EPE is minor, due to subjective nature of the exam and because palpable abnormalities are likely to be unrelated to cancer. (PARTIN)

Dose escalation

The second rationale for adding beam radiation to an implant is to increase the intraprostatic radiation dose. Unfortunately, simple addition of implant and beam doses is not wholly radiobiologically legitimate. Orton and colleagues have estimated dose translations between modalities, but such estimates are plagued by ignorance of in vivo radiobiologic parameters used in such calculations.(ORTON) Simpler estimates, expressed as percent of full monotherapy doses, suggest that the biological effect of combined modality is higher than standard brachytherapy or beam doses alone (**Figure 11-12**).

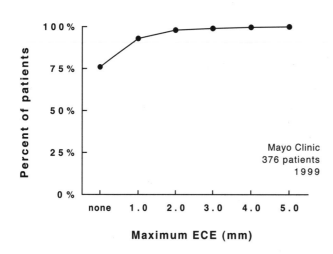

Figure 11-9. Nearly all cases of EPE are limited to within 3 mm of the prostatic capsule.(DAVIS)

Radial extent of EPE

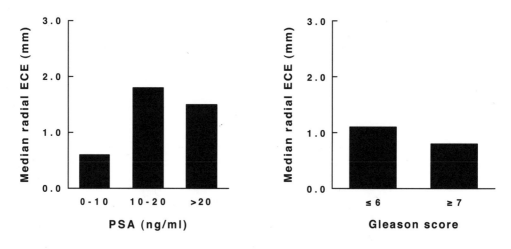

Figure 11-10. The magnitude of EPE, measured perpendicular to the prostatic capsule, versus pretreatment PSA or Gleason score.(SOHAYDA)

11.8

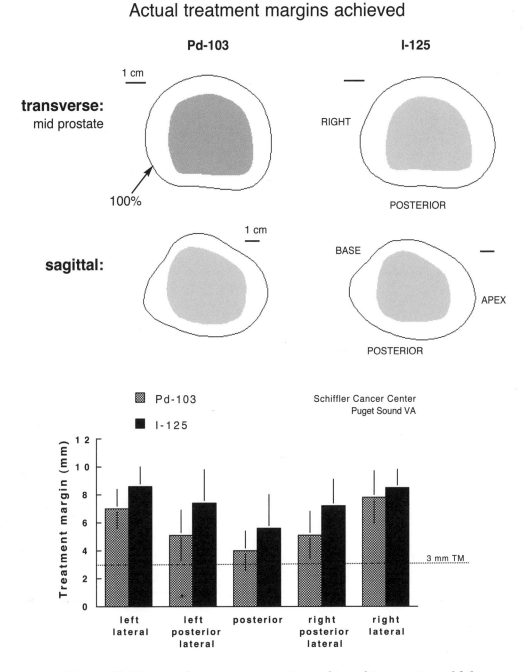

Figure 11-11. Actual treatment margins achieved in a series of 26 patients treated as part of a randomized I-125 versus Pd-103 protocol. The TMs, measured from postimplant day 0 CT, based on a total of 13,104 data points, exceeded the minimum 3 mm desirable in nearly all patients.(MERRICK 02)

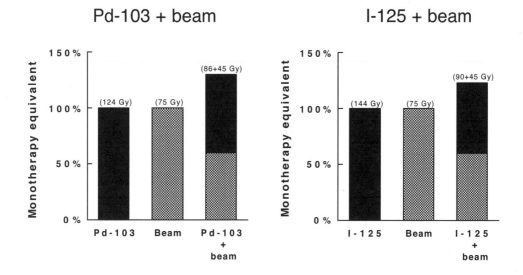

Figure 11-12. Approximation of biologically effective doses of brachytherapy therapy alone versus brachytherapy combined with supplemental external beam radiation, based on simple proportions of monotherapy doses.

But like the arguments for increasing the treatment margins with beam radiation, the rationale for using combined modality therapy for dose escalation is highly questionable. Based on the high rates of negative postimplant biopsies that have been consistently reported, it does not appear that intraprostatic dose escalation is needed—the real problem is the possibility of metastatic disease, not local tumor eradication.(PRESTIDGE, SHARKEY)

Inadequate implants

There are two causes of a technically inadequate implant—poor technique or implant-related prostate swelling. Poor technique is something that should be uncommon, now that more brachytherapists have gained experience. But implant-related swelling is something that we can't predict or control. (BADIOZAMANI, PRESTIDGE, MERRICK 00) One way to minimize its impact is to use greater treatment planning margins to allow

> **Box 11-2. Why brachytherapy may be more effective than surgery**
>
> The potential for capsular penetration extending beyond the surgical margins is part of the theoretical appeal of brachytherapy. Patients with capsular penetration extending beyond the likely surgical margin, may have a higher likelihood of cure with the wider therapeutic margin achieved with brachytherapy (**Figure 12-4**).

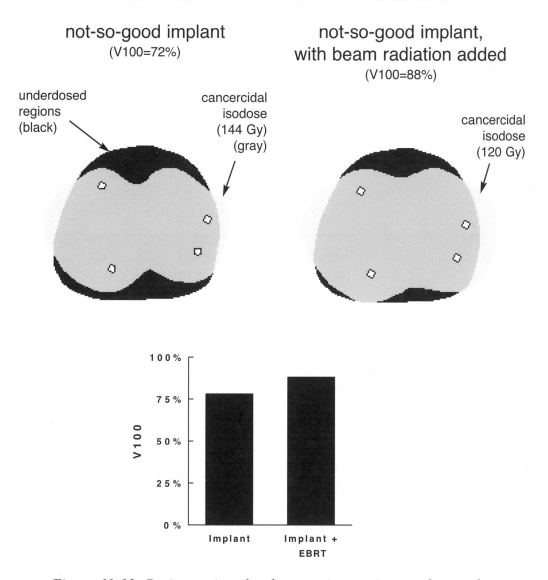

Figure 11-13. By increasing the therapeutic margin, supplemental external beam radiation improves prostatic coverage by an inadequate implant. In this case, taken from the inadequate implant from chapter 9 (Figure 9-24) only 72% of the postimplant prostate volume was covered by the 144 Gy prescription dose (top left). If supplemental beam radiation (45 Gy) had been added to this inadequate implant, and assuming that the new cancercidal isodose was the 120 Gy brachytherapy isodose, approximately 3 mm would be added to the treatment margin (top right). Accordingly, the V100 would increase from 72% to 88%.

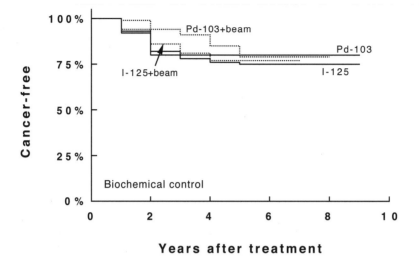

Figure 11-14. Biochemical tumor control for patients with pre-treatment PSA of 10 to 20 ng/ml, treated with brachytherapy, with or without supplemental beam radiation.(ZELEFSKY, BLASKO 00, CRITZ, DATTOLI) *The most striking finding, apart from the fact that all of the curves level off at relatively high levels, is that they are all so similar. (Although the biochemical endpoints differ between studies, with longer follow-up the definition of biochemical failure makes little difference.*[LU, KESTIN]*)*

for swelling and still achieve adequate coverage (see chapter 6). But even with larger treatment margins, some portion of the prostate may end up with less than a 3 mm cancericidal dose margin. Adding supplemental beam radiation should increase the periprostatic coverage by several millimeters, decreasing the clinical impact of a technically inadequate implant (**Figure 11-13**).

The necessity for the increased treatment margin afforded by supplemental beam radiation depends on one's level of skill and the treatment planning margins used. For a novice brachytherapist who's not yet up to speed with technique, use of beam radiation is more appealing than to someone who's already highly skilled. Brachytherapists who consistently achieve 3 mm treatment margins are unlikely to need the extra margin afforded by supplemental beam radiation.(HAN, MERRICK 02)

Supplemental beam dose trial

(Wallner, Merrick, Butler, Cavanagh, et al.)

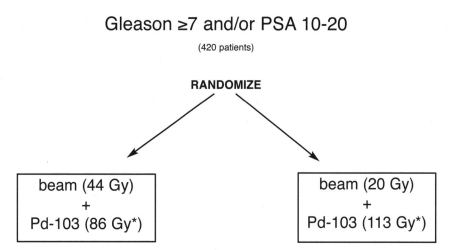

Figure 11-15. Design of ongoing trial to compare moderate- versus low-dose supplemental external beam radiation (180 patients randomized as of May 2001). (*NIST-99 doses)

Clinical results

The use of supplemental beam radiation remains a subject of intense theoretical debate. In the meantime, emerging clinical data are also casting doubt on the routine use of supplemental beam radiation. Outcomes data with implant alone versus implant plus beam radiation appear similar. Fairly mature series with Pd-103 or I-125, used alone or with beam radiation, show similar 5-year freedom from failure rates, regardless of the use of beam radiation (**Figure 11-14**).(BLASKO 00)

Sensing that the debate regarding supplemental beam radiation would rage forever in the absence of controlled trials, Wallner, Merrick, and colleagues are conducting a large, prospective randomized study comparing moderate-dose versus low-dose supplemental beam radiation for intermediate-risk patients (**Figure 11-15**). If this study shows no difference between treatment arms, their next study will compare low dose supplemental beam with *no* supplemental beam, akin to Wilms' tumor studies performed in the 1980s, in which the doses of beam radiation were gradually decreased through a series of randomized trials.(THOMAS)

DIAGNOSTIC IMAGING

Right or wrong, the general consensus has been to use PSA and grade as the principle criteria by which to use supplemental external beam radiation, even though

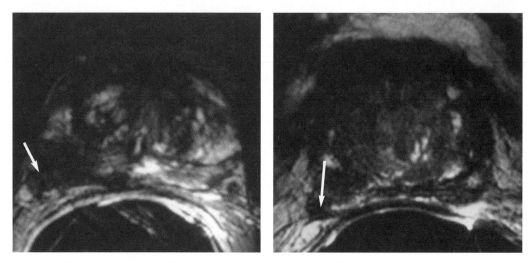

Figure 11-16. Examples of extraprostatic cancer extension (arrows) on transverse MR (courtesy of Dr. Daniel Clarke).

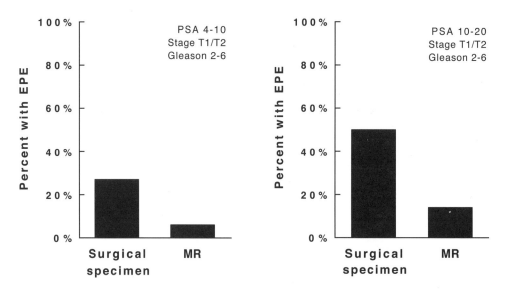

Figure 11-17. Likelihood of detecting EPE on pathology specimen versus presurgical MR in T1/T2 prostate cancer. In patients with PSA less than 10 ng/ml, the likelihood of detecting EPE with MR is so small that its routine use is questionable. The likelihood of detecting EPE is higher for patients with PSA greater than 10 (estimated from D'AMICO).

11.14

MR and EPE

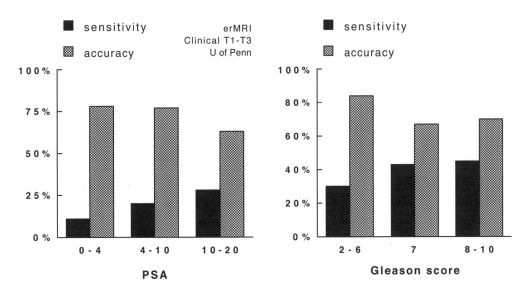

Figure 11-18. Sensitivity and accuracy of MR in detecting EPE, based on pretreatment PSA or Gleason score. With a low PSA or Gleason score, there is little likelihood of detecting EPE. Although sensitivity is greater at higher PSA, those patients should be assumed to have substantial ECE even if not detected radiographically. So it's unclear that MR really adds to their management.(D'AMICO)
sensitivity =true-positive/(true-positive+false negative)
accuracy=(true-positive + true-negative)/total patients

such criteria are plagued by their imprecision in predicting radial EPE. Diagnostic imaging is a potentially more precise way to determine the need for supplemental external radiation, with the rationale being that EPE identified on imaging would be an indication for the wider treatment margins afforded by beam radiation. Unfortunately, CT and TRUS are remarkably unreliable ways to diagnose EPE, with investigators unanimously concluding that the sensitivity and accuracy are insufficient to evaluate EPE or seminal vesicle invasion.(ENGELER, PLATT, RIFKIN)

MR scanning is much more likely to provide useful information about the presence and extent of EPE, allegedly capable of detecting 3 mm of EPE (**Figure 11-16**).(SCHIEBLER) Because patients with ECE of less than 3 mm should be highly

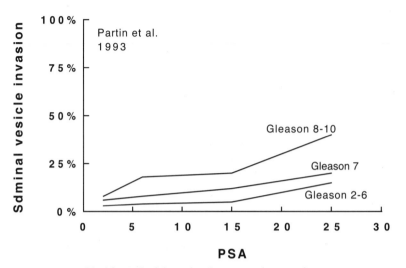

Figure 11-19. Likelihood of seminal vesicle invasion in patients with Stage T1c-T2a tumors versus Gleason score and PSA.(PARTIN)

curable with the cancercidal dose margin of an implant alone, it seems logical that if MR does not reveal EPE, monotherapy would be appropriate. Conversely, those patients with MR-detected EPE presumably have greater than 3 mm radial extent and might benefit from supplemental radiation (or larger implant treatment margins that deliver full doses to all ECE disease). Following this strategy, Clarke and colleagues reported high cure rates with beam radiation plus seeds for MR-based T3 disease. Their treatment strategy includes extraprostatic implantation of all MR-detected ECE.(CLARKE)

D'Amico and coworkers have made considerable efforts to define which patients are most likely to benefit from MR staging.(D'AMICO) The problem with routine MR scanning in low-risk patients is that only a small percent of them will have their treatment altered by the test findings. The incidence of EPE on pathology specimens is only 20% to 30%, and of those, only approximately 10% will be detected by MR (**Figures 11-17 & 11-18**). MR has higher sensitivity for EPE in patients with high-grade cancer or high PSA, presumably because their magnitude of ECE is greater and hence more readily detected.

The ability to evaluate the presence and extent of EPE would go a long way to making more rational use of supplemental external beam radiation. Unfortunately, all imaging modalities are of limited or unproven value for diagnosis of EPE, and

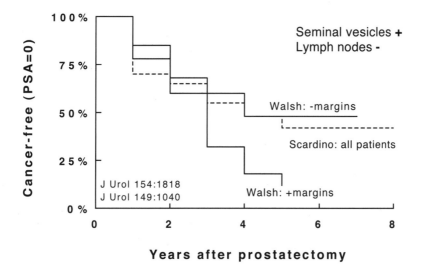

Figure 11-20. Freedom from failure for patients with seminal vesicle involvement. It appears that a small proportion of patients may be cured, if the lymph nodes and surgical margins are negative.

especially in evaluating its radial extent. The principle limitation with MR studies to date is that they may not distinguish between minimal EPE, which should be highly curable with implant alone, versus more substantial EPE, which may call for supplemental external radiation to enhance the cancercidal treatment margin. Proper studies to address these issues would require correlating radial EPE measurements on prostatectomy specimens with presurgical MR findings.

Seminal vesicles

Invasion of the perivesicle tissue or the muscular wall of the seminal vesicles related to PSA and Gleason score, and is associated with a high likelihood of post-prostatectomy recurrence (**Figures 11-19 &20**). (EPSTEIN 93) However, judging from prostatectomy series some patients with early seminal vesicle involvement are still surgically curable, and the same is likely true for radiation.

The seminal vesicles, irregular structures that change their shape and position as the bladder expands and contracts, cannot be treated adequately with brachytherapy alone, due to rapid dose fall-off outside of the prostate.(STOCK) Sources cannot be reliably placed in the seminal vesicle because the vesicles move when

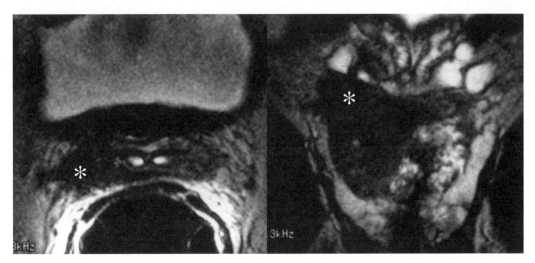

Figure 11-21. MR showing right-sided seminal vesicle invasion (*)
on transverse and coronal view (courtesy of Dr. Daniel Clarke).

pushed by a needle tip, and sources tend to migrate after being ejected in their vicinity.

Perhaps the best use of preimplant diagnostic imaging is to rule out seminal vesicle invasion, a task for which MR is highly accurate (**Figure 11-21**).(D'AMICO) But even so, questions remain as to MR's relevance in relation to therapy. Early seminal vesicle invasion, still compatible with cure, is frequently limited to within a few mm of the prostatic capsule, potentially well covered by implant alone.(DAVIS) More extensive seminal vesicle invasion, beyond the high-dose region of an implant, may well be synonymous with distant disease, so that adding external beam radiation would have no impact on a patient's ultimate prognosis. Like the case for EPE, the accuracy of MR needs to be correlated with the *degree* of vesicle invasion before a stronger argument can be made for its routine use as a pre-brachytherapy staging modality.

CURRENT PRACTICE
While the role of supplemental beam radiation is likely to be debated for years to come, the generally accepted criteria for treatment with implant alone are PSA≤10, Gleason score ≤6 and clinical stage T1-T2b (**Table 11-1**). Patients with a PSA >10, Gleason ≥7 or T3 tumor on digital rectal exam have typically been given supplemental beam radiation. In borderline cases, extensive tumor in the biopsy sample or the presence of perineural invasion would favor the use of supplemental beam radiation, on the assumption that they are associated with increased radial extent

MR and seminal vesicles

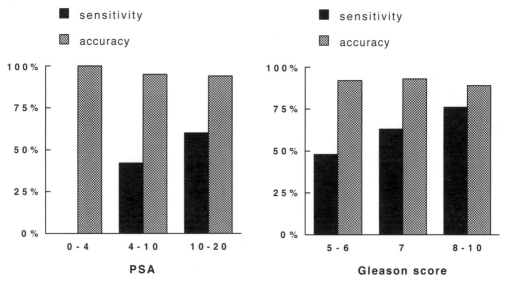

Figure 11-22. Sensitivity and accuracy of MR in detecting seminal vesicle invasion, based on pretreatment PSA or Gleason score (lower panel). With a low PSA or Gleason score, there is little likelihood of detecting SV invasion. Although sensitivity is greater at higher PSA and Gleason scores, those patients should be assumed to have SV invasion, even if not detected radiographically. So it's unclear that MR really adds to their management. (D'AMICO)

sensitivity=true-positive/(true-positive+false negative)
accuracy=(true-positive + true negative)/total patients studied

of EPE. It is clear, however, that the criteria for adding beam radiation needs to be clarified through more rigorous pathological and clinical studies.

REFERENCES

1. Badiozamani K, Wallner K, Sutlief S, Ellis W, Blasko J, Russell K. Anticipating prostatic volume changes due to prostate brachytherapy. Radiat Oncol Invest 1999; 7:360-364.

2. Blasko JC, Grimm PD, Sylvester JE, Badiozamani KR, Hoak D, Cavanagh W. Palladium-103 brachytherapy for prostate carcinoma. Int J Rad Oncol Biol Phys 2000; 46:839-850.

Table 11-1. Criteria for adding supplemental beam radiation.

Generally accepted: PSA >10
Gleason ≥7
clinical T2c/T3

Less accepted: extensive tumor in biopsy (>10 mm)
bilateral positive biopsies
perineural invasion
ECE by MR

3. Blasko JC, Grimm PD, Sylvester JE, Cavanagh W. The role of external beam radiotherapy with I-125/Pd-103 brachytherapy for prostate carcinoma. Radiother and Oncol 2000; 57:273-278.

4. Clarke DH, Banks SJ, Wiederhorn AR, Klousia JW, Lissy JM, Able AA, Artilles C, Hindle WV, Blair DN. The role of endorectal coil MRI in patient selection and treatment planning for prostate seed implants. Int J Rad Oncol Biol Phys 2000; 48 (supplement):146.

5. Critz FA, Williams WH, Benton JB, Levinson AK, Holladay CT, Holladay DA. Prostate specific anitgen bounce after radioactive seed implantation followed by external beam radiation for prostate cancer. J Urol 2000; 163:1085-1089.

6. D'Amico AV, Whittington R, Malkowicz SB, Schultz D. Critical analysis of the ability of the endorectal coil magnetic resonance imaging scan to predict pathologic stage, margin status, and postoperative prostate-specific antigen failure in patients with clinically organ-confined prostate cancer. J Clin Oncol 1996; 14:1770-1777.

7. Dattoli M, Wallner K, True L, Sorace R, Koval J, et al . Prognostic role of serum prostatic acid phosphatase for 103-Pd-based radiation for prostatic carcinoma. Int J Rad Oncol Biol Phys 1999; 45:853-856.

8. Davis BJ, Pisansky TM, Wilson TM, Rothenberg HJ, Pacelli A, Hillman DW, Sargent DJ, Bostwick DG. The radial distance of extraprostatic extension of prostate carcinoma: implications for prostate brachytherapy. Cancer 1999; 85:2630-2637.

9. Engeler CE, Wasserman NF, Zhang G. Preoperative assessment of prostatic carcinoma by computerized tomography: Weakness and new perspectives. Urol 1992; 40:346-350.

10. Epstein JI, Carmichael M, Walsh PC. Adenocarcinoma of the prostate invading the seminal vesicle: definition and relation of tumor volume, grade and margins of resection to prognosis. J Urol 1993; 149:1040-1045.

11. Epstein JI, Carmichael MJ, Pizov G, Walsh PC. Influence of capsular penetration on progression following radical prostatectomy: A study of 196 cases with long-term followup. J Urol 1993; 150:135-141.

12. Han B, Wallner K, Aggarwal S, Armstrong J, Sutlief S. Treatment margins for prostate brachytherapy. Sem in Urol Oncol 2000; 18:137-141.

13. Kestin LL, Vicini FA, Ziaja EL, Stromberg JS, Frazier RC, Martinez AA. Defining biochemical cure for prostate carcinoma patients treated with external beam radiation therapy. Cancer 1999; 86:1557-1566.

14. Lu J. Statistical aspects of evaluating treatment and prognostic factors for clinically localized prostate cancer. Sem in Urol Oncol 2000; 18:83-92.

15. Martinez AA, Kestin LL, Stromberg JS, et al . Interim report of image-guided conformal high-dose-rate brachytherapy for patients with unfavorable prostate cancer: the William Beaumont Phase II dose-escalating trial. Int J Rad Oncol Biol Phys 2000; 47:343-352.

16. Mate TP, Gottesman JE, Hatton J, et al . High dosed-rate after-loading iridium-192 prostate brachytherapy: feasibility report. Int J Rad Oncol Biol Phys 1998; 41:525-533.

17. Merrick GS, Butler WM, Dorsey AT, et al . Influence of prophylactic dexamethasone on edema following prostate brachytherapy. Tech Urol 2000; 6:117-122.

18. Merrick GS, Butler WM, Lief JH, Galbreath RW. Five year biochemical outcome after prostate brachytherapy for hormone-naive men ≤62 years of age. Int J Rad Oncol Biol Phys 2001; (in press):

19. Merrick GS, Butler WM, Wallner KE, Burden LR, Dougherty JE. Extracapsular dose distribution following permanent prostate brachytherapy. (submitted) 2002;

20. Ohori M, Wheeler TM, Kattan MW, Goto Y. Prognostic significance of positive surgical margins in radical prostatectomy specimens. J Urol 1995; 154:1818-1824.

21. Orton CG, Webber BM. Time-dose factor (TDF) analysis of dose rate effects in permanent implant dosimetry. Int J Radiat Oncol Biol Phys 1977; 2:55-60.

22. Partin AW, Kattan MW, Subong ENP, Walsh PC. Combination of prostate-specific antigen, clinical stage, and Gleason score to predict pathological stage of localized prostate cancer. JAMA 1997; 277:1445-1451.

23. Platt JF, Bree RL, Schwab RE. The accuracy of CT in the staging of carcinoma of the prostate. AJR 1987; 149:315-318.

24. Prestidge BR, Hoak DC, Grimm PD, Ragde H, Cavanagh W, Blasko JC. Posttreatment biopsy results following interstitial brachytherapy in early-stage prostate cancer. Int J Radiat Oncol Biol Phys 1997; 37:31.

25. Rifkin MD, Zerhouni EA, Gatsonis CA, Quint LE. Comparison of magnetic resonance imaging and ultrasonography in staging early prostate cancer. NEJM 1990; 323:621-626.

26. Sakr WA, Wheeler TM, Blute M, et al . Workgroup 2: Staging and reporting of prostate cancer–sampling of the radical prostatectomy specimen. Cancer 1996; 78:366-368.

27. Sartor CI, Strawderman MH, Lin X, Kish KE, McLaughlin PW, Sandler HM. Rate of PSA rise predicts metastatic versus local recurrence after definitive radiotherapy. Int J Rad Oncol Biol Phys 1997; 38:941-947.

28. Sattar AA, Noel J-C, Vanderhaeghen J-J, Schulman CC, Wespes E. Prostate capsule: Computerized morphometric analysis of its components. Urol 1995; 46:178-181.

29. Schiebler ML, Schnall M, Pollack HM, et al . Current role of MR imaging in the staging of of adenocarcinoma of the prostate. Radiol 1993; 189:339.

30. Sharkey J, Chovnick SD, Behar RJ, Perez R, et al . Minimally invasive treatment for localized adenocarcinoma of the prostate: Review of 1048 patients treated with ultrasound-guided palladium-103 brachytherapy. J Endourol 2000; 14:343-350.

31. Sohayda C, Kupelian PA, Levin JS, Klein EA. Extent of extracapsular extension in localized prostate cancer. Urol 2000; 55:382-386.

32. Stock RG, Lo Y, Gaildon M, Stone NN. Does prostate brachytherapy treat the seminal vesicles: A dose-volume histogram analysis of seminal vesicles in patients undergoing combined Pd-103 prostate implantation and external beam irradiation. Int J Rad Oncol Biol Phys 1999; 45:385-389.

33. Stone NN, Stock RG, Unger P. Indications for seminal vesicle biopsy and laparoscopic pelvic lymph node dissection in men with localized carcinoma of the prostate. J Urol 1995; 154:1392-1396.

34. Syed AM, Puthawala A, Austin P, Cherlow J. Temporary iridium-192 implant in the management of carcinoma of the prostate. Cancer 1992; 69:2515-2524.

35. Thomas PRM, Tefft M, Compaan PJ, et al . Results of two radiation therapy randomizations in the third National Wilms' Tumor Study. Cancer 1991; 68:1703.

36. Wallner K, Merrick G, True L, Kattan M, Cavanagh W, Simpson C, Butler W. I-125 versus Pd-103 for low risk prostate cancer: Preliminary urinary functional outcomes from a prospective randomized multicenter trial. Journal of Brachytherapy International 2000; 16:151-155.

37. Zelefsky MJ, Hollister T, Raben A, Matthews SM, Wallner KE. Five-year biochemical outcome and toxicity with transperineal CT-planned permanent I-125 prostate implantation for patients with localized prostate cancer. Int J Rad Oncol Biol Phys 2000; 47:1261-1266.

12

Who Can't Have One

There is no question that certain patients are not good candidates for brachytherapy, based on the fact that some experience substantial implant-related morbidity. Particular pretreatment conditions *may* predispose patients to implant-related problems; unfortunately, we still lack a reliable set of criteria to determine beforehand who is going to develop trouble. Age, prostate size, and urinary obstructive symptoms are among myriad alleged selection criteria (**Table 12-1**). However, currently perceived criteria are generally based on physicians' assumptions rather than an objective look at the data. This lack of data has fueled the proliferation of opinions regarding contraindications to brachytherapy (**Figure 12-1**).

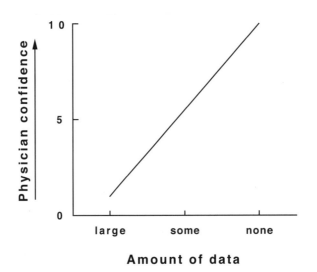

Little data = strong opinions

Figure 12-1. Lack of data has not impeded the proliferation of opinions regarding contraindications to prostate brachytherapy.

The next thirty pages is a review of the evidence (or lack thereof) regarding the validity of current selection criteria.

AGE

There has been a reluctance among oncologists to recommend brachytherapy for younger patients, primarily due to the lack of long-term tumor control data. There are mixed reports regarding the effect of age on postprostatectomy cancer recurrence.(OBEK, GRONBERG) Similarly, age itself has no consistent effect on the the likelihood of cure following brachytherapy or external beam radiation (**Figure 12-2**).(FREEDMAN, MERRICK 01)

There has been some concern that younger patients, who are typically destined to live longer, may be at risk for

Table 12-1. Alledged contraindications to brachytherapy.

- young age
- pubic arch interference
- risk of urinary retention
- AUA score
- prostate volume
- prior prostatitis
- penile prosthesis
- median lobe hypertrophy
- adverse pathologic features on biopsy
- prostatic calculi
- obesity
- inflammatory bowel disease
- prior pelvic surgery
- prior radiation

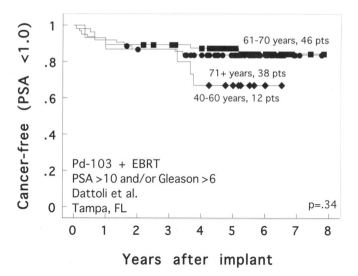

Figure 12-2. Likelihood of biochemical cancer control in high-risk patients treated with Pd-103 plus supplemental external beam radiation. There is no consistent difference between age groups, but longer follow-up is needed.

secondary malignancies due to radiation exposure. To date, no excess incidence of radiation-related malignancies has been reported following retropubic implants from the 1970s, but longer follow-up data are needed to properly address this concern.

Another issue regarding brachytherapy and age is whether older patients will live long enough to benefit from eradication of prostate cancer. Because of its long natural history, patients with low-grade cancer or low PSA should have a life expectancy of ten years or more to justify treatment of their cancer. The *ten-year rule* is used because the likelihood of dying from low-grade, untreated prostate cancer is less than 10% at ten years, and probably even lower for patients with initial PSA less than 10 ng/ml.(ADOLFSSON) In reality, North American men in their 70s generally have a life expectancy of ten years or more, so that therapy for low-risk prostate cancer (PSA <10 ng/ml) is still reasonable (**Figure 12-3**). Patients with high-grade cancer or higher PSA at initial presentation are at risk of cancer death earlier and should be considered for treatment even if their life expectancy is less than ten years.

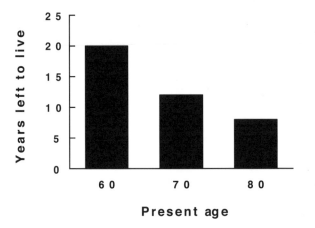

Figure 12-3. Approximate life expectancy for U.S. males versus present age.

Although not well documented in the literature, older patients *may* not tolerate radiation prostatitis as well as younger men. The possibility of a more difficult postimplant course should be considered when deciding between brachytherapy and external beam radiation for older patients.

PUBIC ARCH INTERFERENCE
Perhaps the most widely alleged contraindication to brachytherapy is pubic arch interference (PAI), whereby a relatively narrow pubic arch interferes with anterior needle insertion.(WALLNER 91, TINCHER) Preimplant pelvic CT scans have been used to check for potential pubic arch interference, with the largest prostate cross section overlaid on the narrowest region of the arch (**Figure 12-4**). If there is substantial overlap of the pubic arch over the lateral or anterior prostate margins, it may be difficult to place needles in the shielded portion of the prostate using standard techniques. TRUS images can usually be substituted for CT-based arch assessment (**Figures 12-5 & 12-6**).(WALLNER 99)

In general, blockage of 25% of the prostate diameter, or more than 1 cm of prostate, has been considered excessive, with the patient being declined for implantation or given the option of preimplant hormonal downsizing. But like nearly all alleged contraindications to prostate brachytherapy, there are limited data regarding the incidence and significance of PAI. In order to clarify the routine use of CT assessment of the potential for PAI, Bellon and colleagues analyzed the preimplant TRUS volumes and CT-based pubic arch studies of 97 unselected

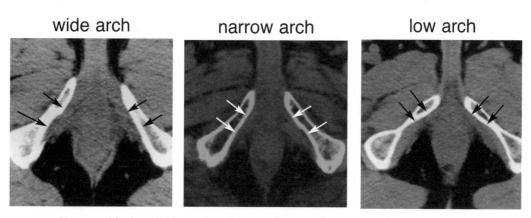

Figure 12-4. CT-based pubic arch visualization. There is a wide variety of arch anatomy, from narrow to wide. Some patients have a low-lying arch, whereby even if wide, it may interfere with placement of anterior needles (top, right panel).

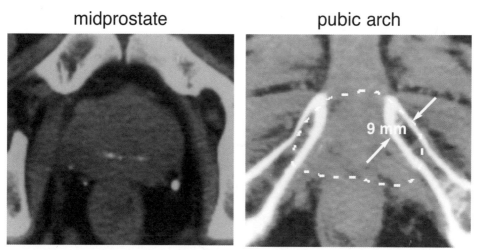

Figure 12-5. To assess the degree of pubic arch interference by CT, the largest prostate cross section can be overlaid on the image with the narrowest-appearing the pubic arch, using the CT scale as a registration point (not visible in figures here). This patient has 9 mm pubic arch interference.

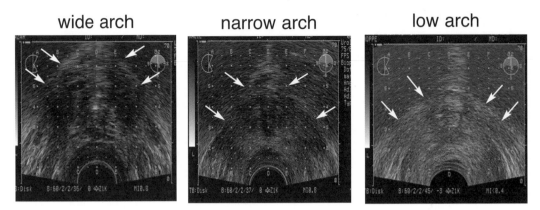

Figure 12-6. TRUS is usually adequate to assess the likelihood of pubic arch interference.

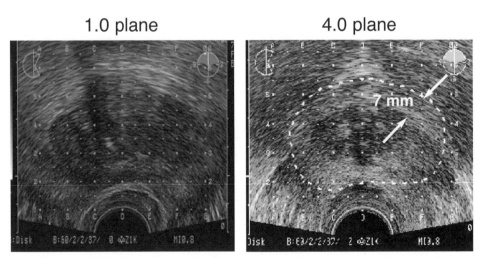

Figure 12-7. To assess the degree of pubic arch interference by TRUS, the largest prostate cross section (left) is overlaid on the image with the narrowest-appearing the pubic arch. This patient has 7 mm pubic arch interference.

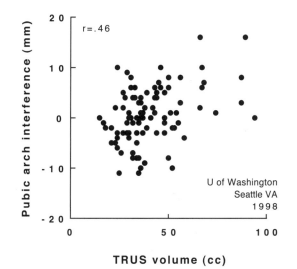

Figure 12-8. Prostate volume versus the degree of pubic arch interference.(BELLON*)*

patients.(BELLON) As expected, there was considerable variability in pubic arch interference ranging from -11 mm to 12 mm. Patients with larger prostate volumes generally had more pubic arch interference, but the degree of interference was only loosely related to the prostate volume (**Figure 12-8**). The poor correlation between PAI and prostate volume in Bellon's series calls into question the "50 cc rule," whereby patients with a prostate volume greater than 50 cc are denied brachytherapy or placed on preimplant hormonal downsizing. In fact, prostate volume is a poor predictor of PAI. Even patients with very large prostate volumes are readily implantable, if they have a wide pubic arch. Alternatively, some patients with very small prostate glands have substantial PAI, due to a very narrow pubic arch.

While the potential for pubic arch interference has received a lot of attention, its clinical significance is highly questionable. Several maneuvers, such as placing the patient in the extended lithotomy position or "steering" needles around the arch, usually circumvents interference (see chapter 8). Using such strategies, nearly all patients can be implanted successfully, regardless of prostate size or the degree of PAI.

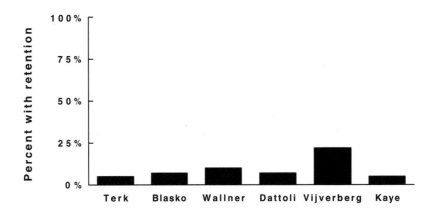

Figure 12-9. Likelihood of acute, postimplant urinary retention reported by various investigators.(TERK, BLASKO, WALLNER 96, DATTOLI, VIJVERBERG, KAYE)

RISK OF URINARY RETENTION
Postimplant urinary retention is the most common acute morbidity of prostate brachytherapy, occurring in about 5% to 10% of patients (**Figure 12-9**). In most cases retention lasts only a few days and is of no long-term consequence.(LANDIS, SHERERTZ) However, a small percentage of patients develop refractory retention, which might make them regret having chosen brachytherapy. Being able to identify those at high risk of refractory retention would be a big help in counseling prospective patients regarding their expected treatment-related complications. In fact, a dizzying array of criteria have been proposed as risk factors for urinary retention (**Table 12-2**). Unfortunately, no single factor is associated with a risk of more than 20% to 30%.

Table 12-2. Potential risk factors for postimplant urinary retention.

- high AUA score
- large prostate
- small prostate
- older age
- median lobe hypertrophy
- large postvoid residual
- low maximum flow rate

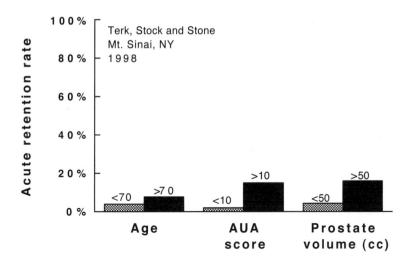

Figure 12-10. Likelihood of acute, postimplant urinary retention, versus age, AUA scores, and prostate volume. In multivariate analysis, only AUA score was predictive of retention.(TERK)

Although patients with substantial preimplant obstructive symptoms are at some-what higher risk of developing postimplant urinary retention, the relationship between preimplant obstructive symptoms and postimplant urinary obstruction is loose, at best. Terk, Stock, and Stone showed that AUA scores are only a weak pre-dictor of postimplant urinary obstruction (**Figure 12-10**). In a series of 62 patients followed prospectively at the University of Washington, there was little correlation between AUA score and acute urinary obstruction. While patients who developed retention tended to have higher preimplant AUA scores, there was a remarkable range of scores among those who did or did not develop retention (**Figure 12-11**). Based on the loose statistical correlations of Terk and colleagues and the scatter in the University of Washington data, it is safe to say that AUA scores, in themselves, are *not* a good way to predict the likelihood of retention for an individual patient.

Prostate size has long been believed to be a predictor of postimplant retention. In the Terk series, large prostate size was correlated with retention risk in univariate but not in multivariate analysis (**Figure 12-10**). Like the case for AUA scores, patients who developed retention tend to have larger preimplant prostate volumes, but there's so much scatter in the data that prostate volume is *not* a useful para-meters to predict an individual patient's risk of retention (**Figure 12-12**).

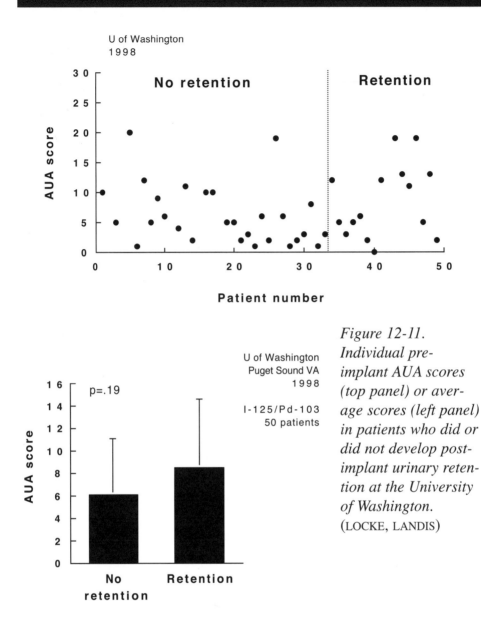

Figure 12-11. Individual pre-implant AUA scores (top panel) or average scores (left panel) in patients who did or did not develop post-implant urinary retention at the University of Washington. (LOCKE, LANDIS)

Age was not well correlated with the risk of retention in either the Terk series (**Figure 12-10**) or in the University of Washington data (**Figure 12-13**). Nor do urodynamic studies, postvoid residual urine volume or maximum flow rate appear to predict for postimplant retention (**Figures 12-14 & 12-15**). Similarly, there was no apparent relationship between the use of pre-implant alpha-blockers or androgen blockade and the likelihood of postimplant retention (**Figure 12-16**).

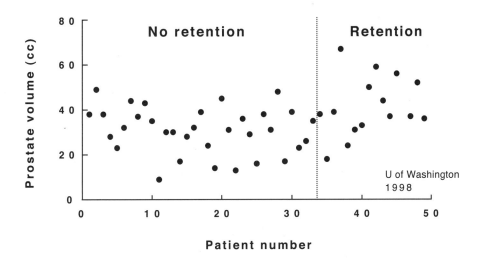

Figure 12-12. Preimplant prostate volumes in patients who did or did not develop postimplant urinary retention at the University of Washington.(LOCKE, LANDIS)

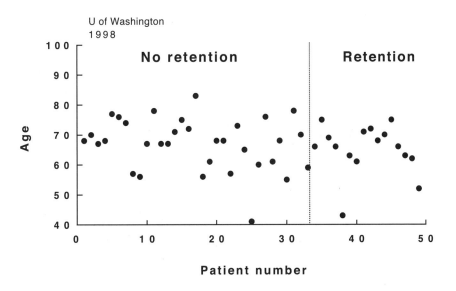

Figure 12-13. Ages of patients who did or did not develop post-implant urinary retention.(LOCKE, LANDIS)

12.11

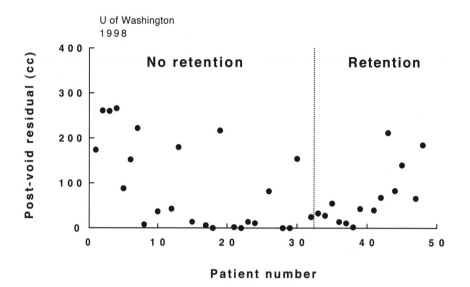

Figure 12-14. Preimplant postvoid residual urine volumes in patients who did or did not develop postimplant urinary retention.(LOCKE, LANDIS)

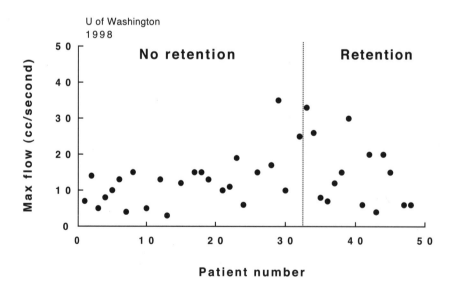

Figure 12-15. Preimplant maximum urinary flow rates in patients who did or did not develop postimplant urinary retention.(LOCKE, LANDIS)

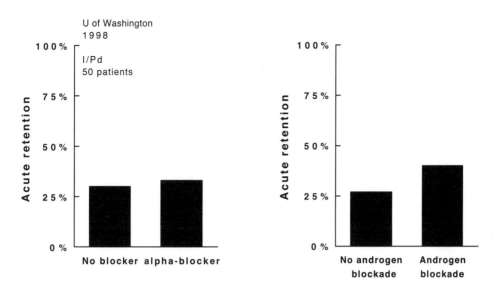

Figure 12-16. Acute postimplant urinary retention in patients taking alpha-blockers or androgen ablation prior to implantation.

Preimplant cystourethroscopy has been proposed as a way to predict the risk of postimplant retention, with the assumption that the degree of physical obstruction predisposes patients to retention. To test that assumption, Gray and colleagues, at the Puget Sound VA Hospital, prospectively performed pre- and postimplant cystourethroscopy on 15 implant patients. Their degree of pre-implant obstruction was rated using a 3-point scale, with the patients' preimplant cystourethroscopic findings ranging from minimal to complete occlusion (**Figure 12-17**).(DIN) Nearly all patients had some increased physical obstruction following completion of the procedure, but only eight of fourteen had an increase in their obstruction grade. Six patients were completely obstructed at the completion of the implant procedure, only one of whom developed urinary retention. Three patients developed postimplant urinary retention. One patient required a one-time catheterization the night of the implant, and had no further urinary retention. The second patient developed urinary retention 10 days after implantation, could not tolerate self-catheterization, and required a suprapubic catheter. At 18 months after implantation, he is able to urinate spontaneously, but still drains his bladder through the suprapubic catheter prior to bedtime. He is improving, and it is anticipated that he will not need the suprapubic catheter much longer. A third patient developed late retention, and is scheduled to undergo a TURP (**Figure 12-18**). The investigators concluded that any correlation between cystourethroscopically identified obstruction and postimplant urinary retention that might be discerned in a larger patient sampling would

grade 1
(minimal)

grade 2
(moderate)

grade 3
(severe)

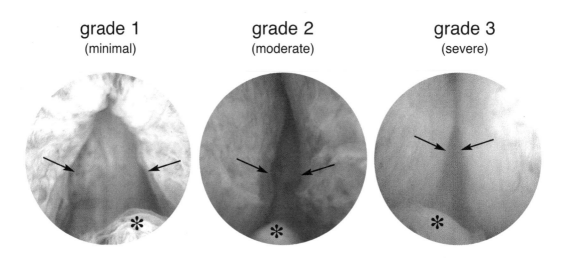

*Figure 12-17. Cystourethroscopic view from verumontanum (*)
with minimal, moderate, and severe obstruction (arrows point to
medial margins of lateral lobes).*

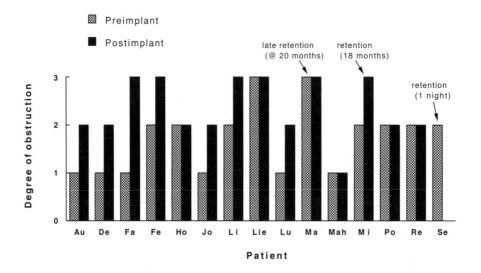

*Figure 12-18. Pre- and postimplant cystoscopic urethral obstruc-
tion among 15 brachytherapy patients at the Puget Sound Health
Care System, VA.*(GRAY, YAP)

likely be too weak to be used as a reliable predictor of postimplant retention in individual patients.

While there is no dearth of conjectures regarding the risks for postimplant retention, the best that can be said with any certainty is that the risk of retention is low, retention is typically short-lived, and that acute retention has no relationship to long-term urinary dysfunction.(LANDIS) Patients at high risk of retention are not reliably identifiable with known risk factors, but it is possible that some clinically useful combination of risk factors may be devised in the future.

BIG PROSTATES

Large prostate size is widely believed to be a relative contraindication to brachytherapy, due to technical concerns and the perception that such patients are at a higher risk of morbidity. Accordingly, patients with prostate volumes greater than 50–60 cc are commonly advised against brachytherapy or are placed on hormonal therapy prior to implant to shrink their gland. To help clarify the use of large prostate size as a contraindication to prostate brachytherapy, Wang and colleagues reviewed the dose volume histograms and postimplant course of 33 patients with a preimplant prostate volume greater than 50 cc, which comprised 7% of the implants performed at the University of Washington. Despite typical implant-related volume increases of 2% to 50%, the V100 was at least 80% in all patients (**Figure 12-19**).

One concern in treating patients with large prostates is that the anterior/lateral portion of the prostate may not be adequately covered due to pubic arch interference of needle placement. In fact, five of the 33 patients' postimplant CT scans showed some degree of incomplete target coverage of the anterior/lateral prostate margin. However, the dosimetric parameters were still well within the recommended range. Stock and colleagues also reported adequate prostate coverage for larger prostate glands.(STONE)

Twelve of the 33 patients from the University of Washington developed acute post-implant urinary retention, all developing within twenty-four hours of implantation. However, 85% of patients were catheter-free by one month and 96% were catheter-free by one year (**Figure 12-19**). Most patients eventually returned to more normal urinary function, even following prolonged intermittent self-catheterization.(SHERERTZ) The only disconcerting finding was that two of the 33 patients developed rectal fistulas. Oddly enough, detailed dosimetric analysis of these two cases showed relatively *low* rectal radiation doses.(HOWARD) One patient's fistula was likely related to a postimplant interstitial laser procedure. The second patient's

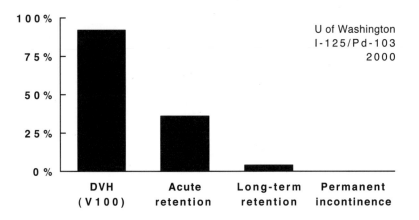

Figure 12-19. Long-term outcomes in 33 brachytherapy patients with prostate volumes greater than 50 cc.(WANG, SHERERTZ)

fistula remains unexplained, but since his prostate was only 53 cc, volume per se was probably *not* related to his complication.

Although more data is needed, patients with larger prostate volume appear to have acceptable morbidity and satisfactory technical outcome, and the perception of large prostate volume being a contraindication to therapy is highly questionable.

SMALL PROSTATES
Very small prostate volumes have been considered by some to be a contraindication to brachytherapy (**Figure 12-20**), the speculative rationale including the possibilities that small prostate glands lack sufficient tissue to hold enough sources, sources inadvertently placed outside of the prostate would migrate, or that small prostate volumes might predispose patients to urinary complications.

To assess the impact of small prostate volume in brachytherapy patients, Loblaw and colleagues reviewed the clinical course of 30 consecutive, unselected patients with prostate gland volumes less than 20 cc, comprising 8% of patients treated at the University of Washington Medical Center.(LOBLAW) The median implant-related volume increase was 63%, somewhat higher than usual, but the median V100 was 92%. To calculate the incidence of source migration, the number of sources placed at the time of implant was compared with the number identified on postimplant Xrays (**Figure 12-21**). Patients lost an average of two sources, consistent with prior reports not limited to patients with small prostate volumes.(WILLINS, SOMMENKAMP, MERRICK 00) Concerns regarding the possibility of excessive

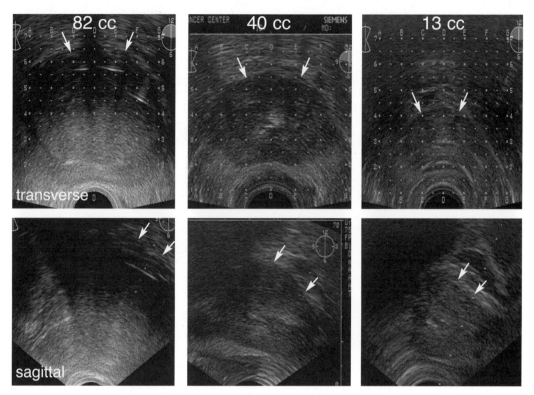

Figure 12-20. Transverse and sagittal TRUS images of base, middle, and apex of 82 cc, 40 cc, and 13 cc prostate glands. Even at the tiny volume of 13 cc, there's plenty of room for sources (arrows indicate anterior prostatic margin).

source migration from small prostates were unfounded, despite the fact that a median of 31 sources appeared to be outside of the prostatic margins, as identified on postimplant CT scan.

Of the 23 patients with longer follow-up information available, only one developed acute postimplant urinary retention, which resolved within two weeks of implantation. At last follow-up, patients' pre- and postimplant AUA scores were not substantially different, with the median AUA score rising from 7 to 8. Two patients reported mild, temporary postimplant urinary urge incontinence, lasting up to six months, but no patient had persistent incontinence (**Figure 12-22**). No serious rectal morbidity was encountered.

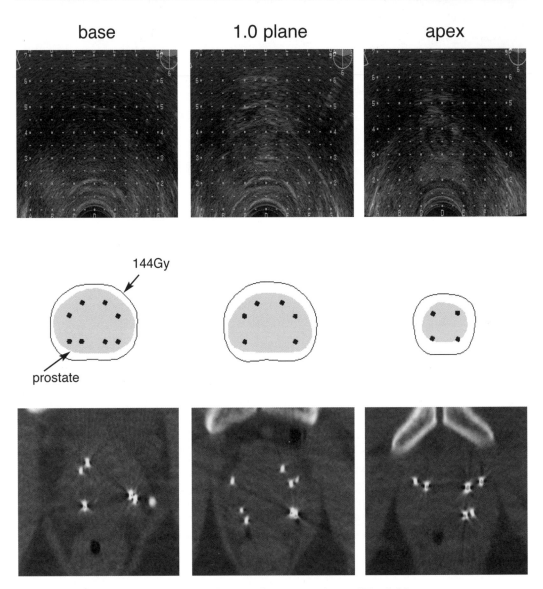

Figure 12-21. TRUS, plan and post-implant CT of 13 cc prostate. *Although all sources were at the edge of or inside the prostate on the plan, we moved most of them more peripherally at the time of the implant, knowing that the central doses would still be well above the prescription dose. Fluoroscopy was used during the procedure to make sure that sources were staying in place after being deposited.*

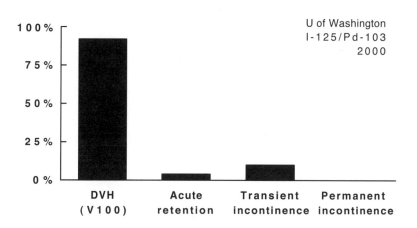

Figure 12-22. Short-term outcomes in 23 brachytherapy patients with prostate volumes less than 20 cc.(LOBLAW)

Patients with small prostate volumes appear to have acceptable morbidity and dose coverage, such that a small prostate volume should *not* be considered a con-traindication to brachytherapy.

PROSTATITIS
Prostatitis is a poorly understood condition, often treated empirically with antibi-otics. The diagnosis is usually based on clinical symptoms, unsubstantiated by biopsy or culture. A prior history of prostatitis has been considered by some to be a contraindication to brachytherapy. Aggarwal and colleagues summarized five brachytherapy patients with preimplant clinical or pathologic evidence of prosta-titis (**Figure 12-23**).(AGGARWAL) Two of the five patients developed postimplant urinary retention requiring short-term catheterization; both resolved sponta-neously, and there was no other unusual morbidity in these patients.

In a more methodical study of the role of prostatitis as a contraindication to brachytherapy, Hughes and colleagues compared preimplant clinical or patholog-ical findings of prostatitis with patients' postimplant course.(HUGHES) No relation was seen between acute and chronic urinary morbidity (**Figure 12-24**).

Because radiation prostatitis and infectious prostatitis are both associated with fre-quent, painful urination and occasionally with acute urinary retention, it would seem logical that a prior history of infectious prostatitis would be a relative con-traindication to prostate brachytherapy. However, available evidence fails to sup-

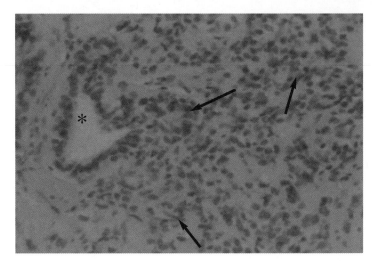

Figure 12-23. Diffuse, intense inflammatory infiltrate in pre-implant prostatic biopsy. Dense dark bands of infiltrating lympho-cytes (arrows) are seen between the glands (*).

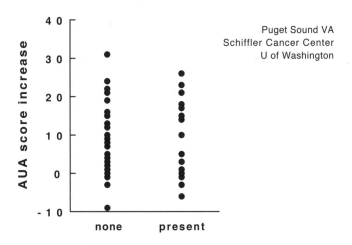

Figure 12-24. AUA score changes at one month following implant in patients with or without histologic evidence of prostatitis on pre-implant biopsy.(HUGHES)

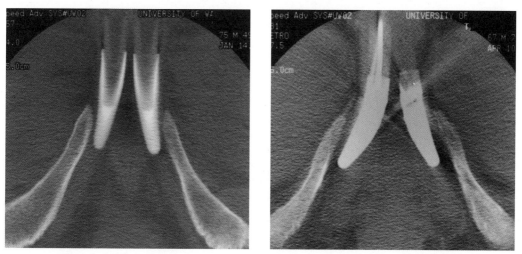

Figure 12-25. CT images showing penile prostheses near transperineal needle path.

port a policy of withholding brachytherapy on the basis of clinical or histologic evidence of prostatitis. Even the benefit of prophylactic antibiotics in patients with preexisting prostatitis remains unclear.(HUGHES)

PENILE PROSTHESIS

The presence of a penile prosthesis is a potential contraindication to brachytherapy, due to the possibility of periprosthetic infection or physical damage to the prosthesis. Li and colleagues reviewed five brachytherapy patients with a previously placed prosthesis, four of whom had semirigid, malleable implants and one of whom had a three-piece inflatable prosthesis.(LI) Pretreatment computed tomography scans of the pelvis were reviewed to rule out significant pubic arch interference (**Figures 12-25 and 12-26**) and a broad spectrum intravenous antibiotic was administered. None of the four patients available for follow-up experienced prosthesis-related pain or infection in the first postbrachytherapy year. One patient, who had a three-piece implant 7 years prior to brachytherapy, reported a malfunction in his prosthesis 13 months after seed implantation. At the time of replacement, a connector tubing leak at the abdominal reservoir site was found, probably unrelated to the brachytherapy procedure. A fifth patient was lost to follow-up after the 24-hour postoperative period, but the implant procedure itself was uneventful. Based on this limited number of patients, it appears that concerns over prosthesis-related complications may be exaggerated. In fact, the prosthetic infection rate unrelated to brachytherapy has averaged only about 2%. And while late hematogenous seeding has been reported, nearly all prosthetic infections have

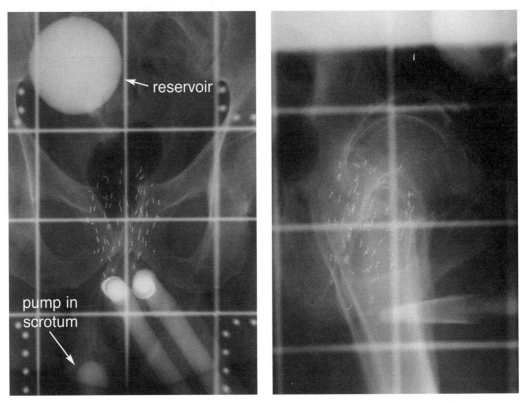

Figure 12-26. Postimplant plain films of a patient with an inflatable penile prosthesis.

been limited to the time of prosthesis placement.(CARSON, MANTAGUE, RADOMSKI, THOMALLA, DAVIS 92, SCHANNE, TIGUERT)

While brachytherapy appears to be safe in the setting of a penile prosthesis, several maneuvers may help prevent complications. First, preoperative, CT-based assessment of the pelvic anatomy can help evaluate the likelihood of pubic arch interference or striking the prosthesis. Additionally, using the extended lithotomy position and taping the genitalia and scrotum anteriorly should help move the prosthesis anteriorly, away from the needle paths. Unfortunately, intraoperative TRUS is not of much help monitoring the position of the needles in relation to the prosthesis, because the prosthesis is not well visualized. Accordingly, patients should be warned that implant-related infectious or mechanical complications could arise.

TURP
There is continued controversy regarding brachytherapy in patients with prior transurethral resection of the prostate (TURP). In early reports from Blasko,

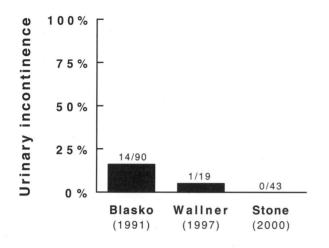

Figure 12-27. Incidence of postimplant urinary incontinence in patients with a prior TURP.(BLASKO, WALLNER 97, STONE)

Grimm, and Ragde, approximately 50% of such patients developed postimplant incontinence (see chapter 15). In more recent experience, however, the risk of incontinence in TURP patients has been low (**Figure 12-27**), probably explained by the adoption of peripheral source loading patterns that avoid excessive urethral doses (see chapter 6).(WALLNER 97, STONE) Using the homogeneous loading patterns typical of the early practice of Blasko and colleagues, urethral doses can easily exceed three times the prescription dose. In contrast, urethral doses of 150% to 200% of the prescription are routinely attainable with a modified peripheral source placement.(MERRICK 00)

If brachytherapy is performed for a patient with prior TURP, there should probably be at least a 1.0 cm rim of tissue left around the defect, to ensure sufficient tissue to hold the sources. CT or TRUS are generally adequate to assess remaining tissue (**Figure 12-28**). A waiting interval of at least four weeks after TURP has been suggested, to allow adequate time for reepitheliazation of the urethral lining, a recommendation based on experimental murine data.(SEYMORE) The risk of incontinence, if excessive urethral doses are avoided, is probably low. However, prospective patients with a prior TURP might be cautioned that they *could* be at higher risk of incontinence.

MEDIAN LOBE HYPERPLASIA
Median lobe hyperplasia (MLH) refers to protrusion of transitional zone tissue into the bladder (**Figure 12-29**).(DIN, WATSON, WALLNER 00) It has been suggested that MLH, or *intravesical prostatomegaly*, might be a contraindication to

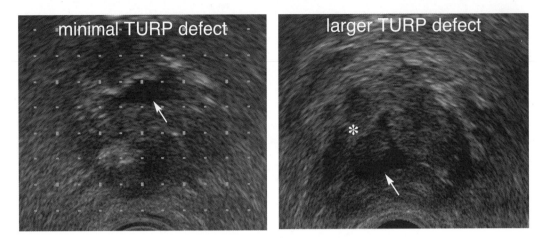

Figure 12-28. TURP defects (arrows) on TRUS. The patient on the right has a larger defect, possibly placing him at higher risk of incontinence or source loss due to the narrower rim of tissue (*) around the defect.

brachytherapy, either by increasing the risk of postimplant urinary morbidity or because of technical difficulties implanting the intravesicle tissue. Wallner and colleagues reviewed the clinical course of eight brachytherapy patients with radiographic evidence of MLH.(WALLNER 00) There was no apparent association between the degree of MLH and preimplant prostate volume or AUA score. Intraoperatively, MLH could be readily viewed by TRUS, and there was no particular difficulty placing sources in the MLH tissue. Based on postimplant CT-based dosimetry, the base of the prostate, including the median lobe tissue, was completely covered by the prescription isodose in all cases. Two of the eight patients developed prolonged postimplant urinary retention and have been slow to improve. Longer-term follow-up is suggesting that such patients may also be slow to return to their baseline urinary function **(Figure 12-30)**.(NGUYEN)

Despite some concern regarding brachytherapy in the setting of MLH, such patients don't appear to be at a substantially increased risk of postimplant urinary morbidity or inadequate target coverage. Considering that most MLH patients do well in the long term, there is little justification for prophylactic resection of hypertrophic tissue.

ADVERSE PATHOLOGIC FEATURES
High Gleason score, perineural invasion, and extensive tumor in the biopsy specimen have all been correlated with a higher likelihood of extraprostatic cancer

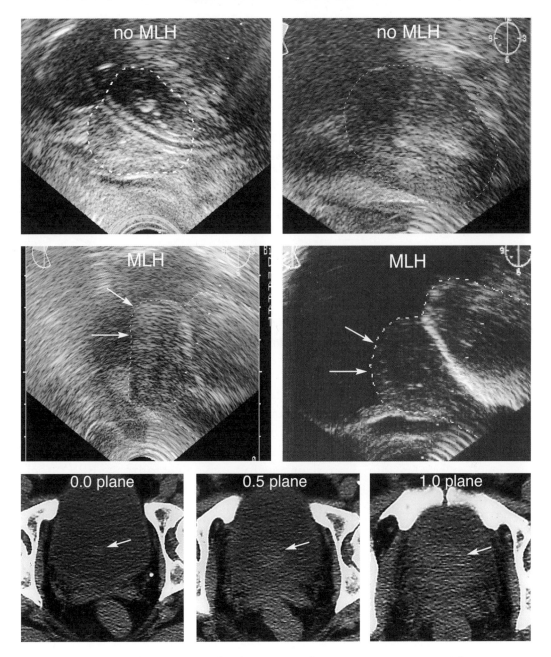

Figure 12-29. Top panels show normal prostatic contours, without median lobe hyperplasia. Middle panels show sagittal TRUS examples of median lobe hypertrophy (arrows). The lower panels show the intravesicle component of prostatic hyperplasia on CT scan (arrows).

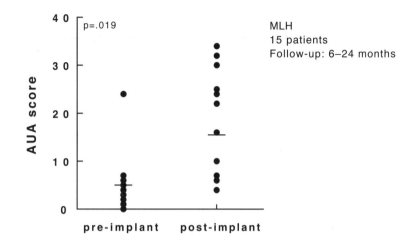

Figure 12-30. Pre- and post-implant AUA scores in patients with MLH. There is a suggestion that such patients are slower than usual to return to their baseline urinary function.(NGUYEN)

extension and of treatment failure, regardless of the modality used.(BASTAKY, GRANN, PARTIN, BOSTWICK, VILLERS) Although adverse pathologic features are associated with a higher likelihood of early extraprostatic extension (EPE), such patients are apparently still highly curable. Brachytherapy, with or without supplemental external beam radiation, appears to be able to sterilize the EPE associated with adverse pathologic features (**Figure 12-31**), consistent with reports that nearly all cases of EPE are limited to within 3 mm of the prostatic capsule and readily covered by an implant alone.(DAVIS 99, SOHAYDA) Unfortunately, no studies compare the presence of adverse pathologic features to the degree of radial EPE, the feature most relevant to brachytherapy. While there is no basis for using adverse pathologic features as a contraindication to brachytherapy, their presence has been used as an indication for adding supplemental external beam radiation (see chapter 11).

LYMPH NODES
Patients with cancerous lymph nodes are at very high risk of treatment failure, and radiation of involved lymph nodes has not been found to increase the cancer control rates.(ASBELL) Patients with PSA <20 and Gleason ≤7 have a very low likelihood of lymph node involvement, and routine staging lymph node dissection is generally not warranted (**Figure 12-32**). In patients with a pretreatment PSA above 20 ng/ml, lymph node dissection should be seriously considered, because the find-

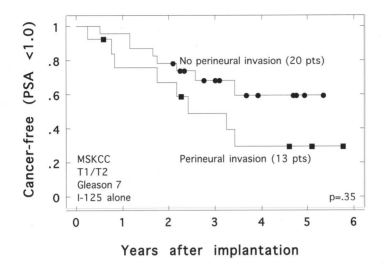

Figure 12-31. Freedom from biochemical recurrence for patients with or without perineural invasion.(GRANN)

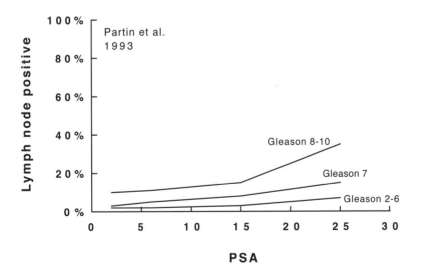

Figure 12-32. Likelihood of lymph node invasion in patients with stage T1c-T2a tumors, versus Gleason score and PSA.(PARTIN)

12.27

ing of positive lymph nodes is generally considered a contraindication to definitive local therapy. However, recent studies suggesting a benefit from radical prostatectomy in lymph node-positive patients warrants a reappraisal of the role of brachytherapy in the setting of positive lymph nodes.(GHAVAMIAN, MESSING)

CALCIUM DEPOSITS

Prostatic calcium deposits (*calculi*) might be a (relative)contraindication to brachytherapy, either by interfering with needle insertion or the potential for dosimetric perturbations. In fact, needle penetration is not substantially impeded by calculi (**Figure 12-33**). The possibility of substantial dose attenuation due to absorption of low energy gamma radiation, however, remains to be elucidated.

OBESITY

Considering the high prevalence of obesity, surprisingly little has been reported regarding treatment of prostate cancer in obese patients. There is some evidence to suggest that obesity confers a better prognosis, perhaps due to hormonal influences.(DANIELL) However, obesity can present technical difficulties, especially for prostatectomy and external beam radiation. Obese patients are more likely to develop postoperative complications, and are generally discouraged from surgery. They are more difficult to set up properly for external radiation, potentially increasing the risk of complications and decreasing the likelihood of cure using limited conformal radiation ports. In contrast, obesity poses a relatively minor problem for brachytherapy.(ROCKHILL) Operative setup can take longer, and there is less room to maneuver between the patient's legs, but this has not presented a huge problem (**Figures 12–34 & 12–35**). Standard 20 cm brachytherapy needles are almost always sufficient to reach the prostate, but 25 cm needles are commercially available.

INFLAMMATORY BOWEL DISEASE

The term *inflammatory bowel disease* (IBD) includes both ulcerative colitis and regional enteritis (Crohn's disease), which are chronic idiopathic inflammatory disorders of the gastrointestinal tract. While there is a widespread, scantily substantiated belief that IBD patients are at higher risk for radiation-related complications, there are only widely scattered mentions of bowel complications from external beam radiation in IBD patients with prostate cancer.(LEIBEL, WILLETT) Presumably, IBD patients are commonly referred for prostatectomy due to concern about an increased risk of radiation-related complications.

As an alternative to surgery, some IBD patients have been referred for brachytherapy, the rationale being that less rectal surface area would be irradiated (See

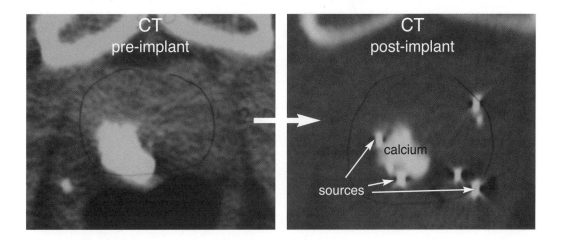

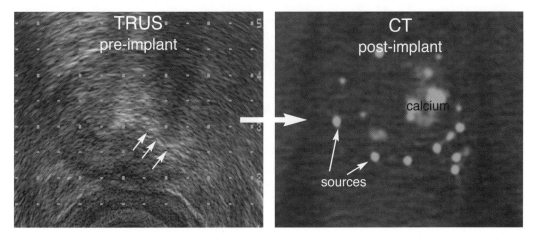

Figure 12-33. Calcium deposits. Top panels show pre- and post-implant CT images of a prostate with a large, dense deposit in the right side, that did not appear to interfere with source placement. The lower panels show a large calculus on TRUS (arrows) that did not interfere with source placement, as seen on postimplant CT.

Chapter 3). Grann and Wallner reported six patients treated with I-125, none of whom experienced unusual gastrointestinal morbidity.(GRANN) M. Dattoli has been routinely treating such patients with supplemental beam radiation, with no perceived unusual complications (data unpublished), although caution is advised until more data become available.

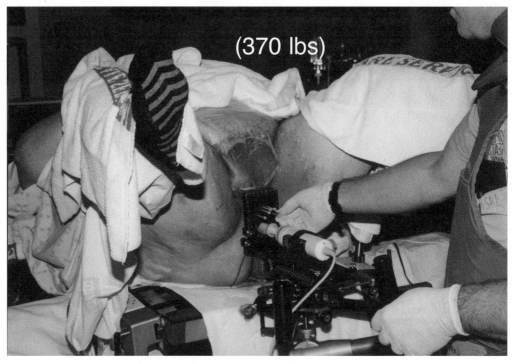

(370 lbs)

Figure 12-34. The implant procedure is not much different for massively obese patients. However, fluoroscopic images are of poorer quality in such patients.

PRIOR SURGERY

Prior pelvic surgery places patients at higher risk for external beam radiation-related bowel complications, presumably due to fixation of bowel within the abdomen or pelvis.(LANCIANO, WHELAN) Brachytherapy is probably less likely to cause bowel complications in patients with prior surgery, because it would entail less radiation to the bowel wall (see chapter 3), but no data are available.

PRIOR RADIATION

Patients with prior therapeutic pelvic radiation are presumably at higher risk for radiation-related complications. The most common scenarios are patients previously treated with intermediate-dose radiation for seminoma, or higher-dose radiation for colorectal carcinoma. If the dose to the rectal wall was greater than 40 Gy, brachytherapy would likely carry a moderate to high risk of significant complications, regardless of the time since the prior radiation. Prostatectomy may be preferable in these cases. However, because radiation may also increase the risk of surgery-related complications, such patients present unique and challenging situations, with no clearly "right" answer. The authors have treated a number of

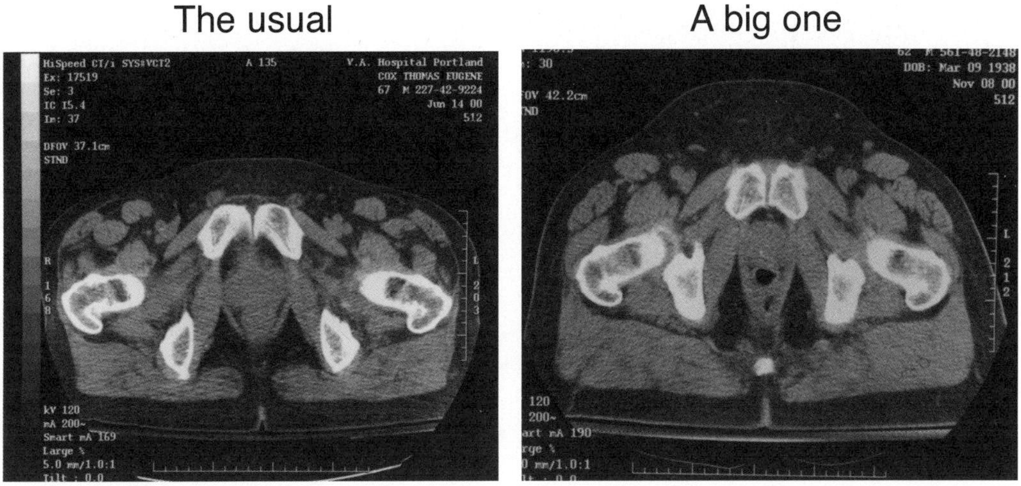

The usual

A big one

Figure 12-36. CTs of thin versus massively obese patients illustrating how much more tissue must be traversed to deliver external beam radiation., especially from the anterior and posterior directions.

patients in this setting, with no recollection of subsequent serious complications, but few reports have appeared to specifically document the incidence of morbidity.(BATTERMANN) Reirradiation in other sites has generally been better tolerated than predicted radiobiologically, and it is likely reasonably safe in the setting of prostate cancer.(WONG, DE CREVOISIER) Our current policy is generally to offer brachytherapy to patients with prior pelvic radiation, but with an explanation and warning regarding the potential risk.

REALLY BAD NUMBERS
Patients with a markedly elevated PSA or prostatic acid phosphatase have a very high likelihood of failing any treatment. Although their chance of cure is low, most brachytherapy series show some evidence of a plateau on the freedom-from-failure curve, such that there is likely a finite percentage of patients who are curable (see chapter 14). Accordingly, if such patients otherwise have a life expectancy of more than five years, aggressive brachytherapy-based treatment is warranted once a reasonable effort to rule out distant metastases and lymph node metastases has been made.

RELATIVE VERSUS ABSOLUTE CONTRAINDICATIONS
While there is no shortage of opinions regarding the contraindications to brachytherapy, most are baseless. Reports to date have failed to establish any firm

contraindication. That's not to say that all patients are great candidates for the procedure. Some factors, like prior urethral surgery, advanced age, obstructive symptoms, MLH, and pubic arch interference might be considered *relative* contra-indications, especially in the hands of novice brachytherapists. But even in situations where patients present with alleged contraindications, brachytherapy may still be their best choice, compared to the alternatives.

REFERENCES

1. Adolfsson J, Carstensen J, Lowhagen T. Deferred treatment in clinically localised prostatic carcinoma. Br J Urol 1992; 69:183-187.

2. Aggarwal S, Wallner KE, True LD, Russell K, Sutlief S, Blasko J, Ellis W. Prostate brachtherapy in patients with prior evidence of prostatitis. Int J Radiat Oncol Biolo Phys 1999; 45:867-869.

3. Asbell SO, Krall JM, Pilepich MV, Baerwald H. Elective pelvic irradiation in stage A2, B carcinoma of the prostate: Analysis of RTOG 77-06. Int J Radiat Oncol Biol Phys 1988; 15:1307-1316.

4. Bastacky SI, Walsh PC, Epstein JI. Relationship between perineural tumor invasion on needle biopsy and radical prostatectomy capsular penetration in clinical stage B adenocarcinoma of the prostate. Am J Surg Path 1993; 17:336-341.

5. Battermann JJ. Feasibility of permanent implants for prostate cancer after previous radiotherapy in the true pelvis. Radiother Oncol 2000; 57:297-300.

6. Bellon J, Wallner K, Ellis W, Cavanagh W, Blasko J. Use of pelvic CT scanning to evaluate pubic arch interference of transperineal prostate brachytherapy . Int J Radiat Oncol Biol Phys 1999; 43:579-581.

7. Blasko JC, Ragde H, Grimm PD. Transperineal Ultrasound-Guided Implantation of the Prostate: Morbidity and Complications. Scand J Urol Nephrol Suppl 1991; 137:113-118.

8. Bostwick DG, Qian J, Bergstralh E, Dundore P, Dugan J, Myers RP, Oesterling JE. Prediction of capsular perforation and seminal vesicle invasion in prostate cancer. J Urol 1996; 155:1361-1367.

9. Carson CC, Robertson CN. Late hematogenous infection of penile prosthesis. J Urol 1988; 139:50-52.

10. Daniell HW. A better prognosis for obese men with prostate cancer. J Urol 1996; 155:220-225.

11. Dattoli M, Wallner K, Sorace R. Pd-103 brachytherapy and external beam irradiation for clinically localized, high-risk prostatic carcinoma. Int J Radiat Oncol Biol Phys 1996; 35:875-879.

12. Davis BE, DeBrock BJ, Lierz MF, Weigel JW. Management of preexisting inflatable penile prosthesis during radical retropubic prostatectomy. J Urol 1992; 148:1198-1200.

13. Davis BJ, Pisansky TM, Wilson TM, Rothenberg HJ, Pacelli A, Hillman DW, Sargent DJ, Bostwick DG. The radial distance of extraprostatic extension of prostate carcinoma: implications for prostate brachytherapy. Cancer 1999; 85:2630-2637.

14. De Crevoisier R, Bourhis J, Domenge C, Wibault P, et al. Full-dose reirradiation for unresectable head and neck carcinoma: experience at the Gustave-Roussey Institute in a series of 169 patients. J Clin Oncol 2001; 16:3556-3562.

15. Din K, Wildt M, Wijkstra H, Debruyne F, Rosette J. The correlation between urodynamic and cystoscopic findings in elderly men with voiding complaints. J Urol 1996; 155:1018-1022.

16. Dunsmuir WD, Kirby RS. Conservation of inflatable penile prosthesis during radical retropubic prostatectomy. Br J Urol 1997; 79:283-284.

17. Freedman GM, Hanlon AL, Lee WR, Hanks GE. Young patients with prostate cancer have an outcome justifying their treatment with external beam radiation. Int J Radiat Oncol Biol Phys 1996; 35:243-250.

18. Ghavamian R, Bergstralh EJ, Blute ML, Slezak J, Zincke H. Radical retropubic prostatectomy plus orchiectomy versus orchietomy alone for pTxN+ prostate cancer: A matched comparison. Cancer 1999; 161:1223-1228.

19. Grann A, Gaudin PB, Raben A, Wallner KE. Pathologic features from prostate needle biopsy and prognosis after I-125 brachytherapy. Radiat Oncol Invest 1998; 6:170-174.

20. Grann A, Wallner K. Prostate brachytherapy in patients with inflammatory bowel disease. Int J Radiat Oncol Biol Phys 1998; 40:135-138.

21. Gray G, Wallner K, Roof J, Corman J. Cystourethroscopic findings before and after prostate brachytherapy. Tech Urol 2000; 6:109-111.

22. Gronberg H, Damber J, Jonsson H, Lenner P. Patient age as a prognostic factor in prostate cancer. J Urol 1994; 152:892-895.

23. Howard A, Wallner K, Han B, Schneider B, et al . Rectal fistulas after prostate brachytherapy. Journal of Brachytherapy International 2001; (in press):

24. Hu K, Wallner KE. Urinary incontinence in patients who have a TURP/TUIP following prostate brachytherapy. Int J Radiat Oncol Biol Phys 1998; 40:783-786.

25. Hughes S, Wallner K, Miller G, Miller S, True L. Pre-existing histologic evidence of prostatitis is unrelated to post-implant urinary morbidity. (submitted) 2001;

26. Kaye KW, Olson DJ, Payne JT. Detailed preliminary analysis of 125 iodine implantation for localized prostate cancer using percutaneous approach. J Urol 1995; 153:1020.

27. Lanciano RM, Martz K, Montana GS, Hanks GE. Influence of age, prior abdominal surgery, fraction size, and dose on complications after radiation therapy for squamous cell cancer of the uterine cervix. Cancer 1992; 69:2124-2130.

28. Landis D, Wallner K, Locke J, Ellis W, Russell K, Cavanuagh W, Blasko J. Late urinary morbidity after prostate brachytherapy. (submitted) 2002;

29. Leibel SA, Heimann R, Kutcher GJ. Three-dimensional conformal radiation therapy in locally advanced carcinoma of the prostate: preliminary results of a phase I dose-escalation study. Int J Radiat Oncol Biol Phys 1993; 26:55-65.

30. Li P, Wallner K, Ellis W, Blasko J, Corman JM. Prostate brachytherapy in patients with a penile prosthesis. Br J Urol 2001;

31. Loblaw DA, Wallner K, Dibiase S, Russell K, Blasko J, Ellis W. Brachytherapy in patients with small prostate glands. Tech Urol 2000; 6:64-69.

32. Locke J, Ellis W, Wallner K, Cavanagh W, Blasko J. Risk factors for acute urinary retention requiring temporary intermittent catheterization after prostate brachytherapy: A prospective study. (submitted) 2001;

33. Merrick GS, Butler WM. Modified uniform seed loading for prostate brachytherapy: rationale, design, and evaluation. Tech Urol 2000; 6:78-84.

34. Merrick GS, Butler WM, Dorsey AT, Lief JH, Benson ML. Seed fixity in the prostate/periprostatic region following brachytherapy. Int J Rad Oncol Biol Phys 2000; 46:215-220.

35. Merrick GS, Butler WM, Lief JH, Galbreath RW. Five year biochemical outcome after prostate brachytherapy for hormone-naive men ≤62 years of age. Int J Rad Oncol Biol Phys 2001; (in press):

36. Messing EM, Manola J, Sarosdy M, Wilding G, Crawford ED, Trump D. Immediate hormonal therapy compared with observation after radical prostatectomy and pelvic lymphadenectomy in men with node-positive prostate cancer. NEJM 1999; 341:1781-1788.

37. Montague DK. Periprosthetic infections. J Urol 1987; 138:68-69.

38. Nguyen J, Wallner K, Han B, Ellis W, Sutlief S. Increased long-term urinary morbidity in brachytherapy patients with median lobe hyperplasia. (submitted) 2002;

39. Obek C, Lai S, Sadek S, Civantos F, Soloway MS. Age as a prognositic factor for disease recurrence after radical prostatectomy. Urol 1999; 54:533-538.

40. Partin AW, Kattan MW, Subong ENP, Walsh PC. Combination of prostate-specific antigen, clinical stage, and Gleason score to predict pathological stage of localized prostate cancer. JAMA 1997; 277:1445-1451.

41. Partin AW, Yoo J, Carter HB, Pearson JD, Chan DW, Epstein JI, Walsh PC. The use of prostate specific antifen, clinical stage and Gleason score to predict pathological stage in men with localized prostate cancer. J Urol 1993; 150:110-114.

42. Radomski SB, Herschorn S. Risk factors associated with penile prosthesis infection. J Urol 1992; 147:383-385.

43. Rockhill J, Wallner K, Hoffman C, Hummel S, Arthurs S. Prostate brachytherapy in massively obese patients. (submitted) 2002;

44. Schanne FJ, Carpiniello V, Chaiken D. Radical prostatectomy in patients with indwelling inflatable penile prosthesis. Urol 1998; 52:715-716.

45. Seymore CH, El-Mahdi AM, Schellhammer PF. The effect of prior transurethral resection of the prostate on post radiation urethral strictures and bladder neck contractures. Int J Radiat Oncol Biol Phys 1986; 12:1597-1600.

46. Sherertz T, Wallner K, Wang H, Sutlief S, Russell K. Long-term urinary function after transperineal brachytherapy for patients with large prostate glands . (submitted) 2002;

47. Sohayda C, Kupelian PA, Levin JS, Klein EA. Extent of extracapsular extension in localized prostate cancer. Urol 2000; 55:382-386.

48. Sommerkamp H, Rupprecht M, Wannenmacher M. Seed loss in interstitial radiotherapy of prostatic carcinoma with I-125. Int J Radiat Oncol Biol Phys 1988; 14:389-392.

49. Stone NN, Ratnow ER, Stock RG. Prior transurethral resection does not increase morbidity following real-time ultrasound-guided prostate seed implantation. Tech Urol 2000; 6:123-127.

50. Terk MD, Stock RG, Stone NN. Identification of patients at increased risk for prolonged urinary retention following radioactive seed implantation of the prostate. J Urol 1998; 160:1379-1382.

51. Thomalla JV, Thompson ST, Rowland RG, Mulcahy JJ. Infectious complications of penile prosthetic implants. J Urol 1987; 138:65-67.

52. Tiguert R, Hurley PM, Gheiler EL, Tefilli MV, Gudziak MR, Dhabuwala CB, Pontes JE, Wood DP. Treatment outcome after radical prostatectomy is not adversely affected by a pre-existing penile prosthesis. Urol 1998; 52:1030-1033.

53. Tincher SA, Kim RY, Ezekiel MP, et al . Effects of pelvic rotation and needle angle on pubic arch interference during transperineal prostate implants. Int J Rad Oncol Biol Phys 2000; 47:361-363.

54. Vijverberg PLM, Kurth KH, Blank LECM, Dadhoiwala NF, de Reijke THM, Koedooder K. Treatment of localized prostatic carcinoma using the transrectal ultrasound guided transperineal implantation technique. Eur Urol 1992; 21:35-41.

55. Villers A, McNeal JE, Redwine EA, Freiha FS. The role of perineural space invasion in the local spread of prostatic adenocarcinoma. J Urol 1989; 142:763-768.

56. Wallner K, Ellis W, Russell K, Cavanagh W, Blasko J. Use of TRUS to predict pubic arch interference of prostate brachytherapy. Int J Rad Oncol Biol Phys 1999; 43:583-585.

57. Wallner K, Lee H, Wasserman S, Dattoli M. Low risk of urinary incontinence following prostate brachytherapy in patients with a prior TURP. Int J Radiat Oncol Biol Phys 1997; 37:565-569.

58. Wallner KE, Chiu-Tsao S, Roy J, Arterbery VE, Whitmore W, Jain S, Minsky B, Russo P, Fuks Z. An Improved Method for Transperineal Prostate Implants. J Urol 1991; 146:90-95.

59. Wallner KE, Roy J, Harrison L. Dosimetry guidelines to minimize urethral and rectal morbidity following transperineal I-125 prostate brachytherapy. Int J Radiat Oncol Biol Phys 1995; 32:465-471.

60. Wallner KE, Roy J, Harrison L. Tumor control and morbidity following transperineal I-125 implantation for Stage T1/T2 prostatic carcinoma. J Clin Oncol 1996; 14:449-453.

61. Wallner KE, Smathers S, Sutlief S, Corman J, Ellis W. Prostate brachytherapy in patients with median lobe hyperplasia. Int J Cancer 2000; 90:152-156.

62. Wang H, Wallner K, Sutlief S, Blasko J, Russell K, Ellis W. Transperineal brachytherapy in patients with large prostate glands. Int J Cancer 2000; 90:199-205.

63. Watson LR. Ultrasound anatomy for prostate brachytherapy. Sem in Urol Oncol 1997; 13:391-398.

64. Whelan TJ, Dembo AJ, Bush RS, Sturgeon JFG, Fine S, Pringle JF, Rawlings GA, Thomas GM, Simm J. Complications of whole abdominal and pelvic radio-

therapy following chemotherapy for advanced ovarian cancer. Int J Rad Oncol Biol Phys 1992; 22:853-858.

65. Willett CG, Ooi C, Zietman AL, Menon V, Goldberg S, Sands BE, Podolsky DK. Acute and late toxicity of patients with inflammatory bowel disease undergoing irradiation for abdominal and pelvic neoplasms. Int J Radiat Oncol Biol Phys 2000; 46:995-998.

66. Willins J, Wallner KE. Time-dependent changes in CT-based dosimetry of I-125 prostate brachytherapy. Radiat Oncol Invest 1998; 6:157-160.

67. Wong WW, Schild SE, Sawyer TE, Shaw EG. Analysis of outcome in patients reirradiated for brain metastases. Int J Radiat Oncol Biol Phys 1996; 34:585-590.

68. Yap J, Wallner K, Gray G. Cystourethroscopic findings and long-term urinary function after prostate brachytherapy. Journal of Brachytherapy International 2001;

13

Postimplant Cancer Assessment

Evaluating treatment efficacy for early-stage prostate cancer is hampered by the cancer's long natural history and by imprecise methods of assessing tumor control. Ideally, *survival* should be the endpoint by which efficacy is judged. However, survival analysis requires long follow-up, because most men with early stage disease aren't at risk for cancer-related death until ten years or more have passed.(ADOLFSSON) So in the shorter term, we've come to rely on digital rectal exam, repeat biopsies, and PSA to assess the effect of treatment. Unfortunately, all three measures are fraught with interpretive pitfalls, partly due to peculiarities in the postbrachytherapy setting. As brachytherapy becomes more widely practiced, it is important that physicians be aware of potential interpretive pitfalls. This is

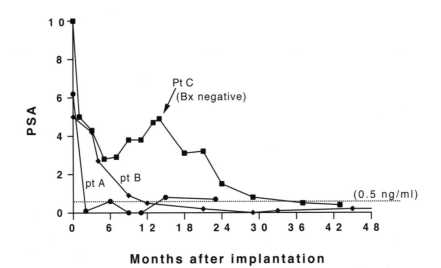

Figure 13-1. Typical postimplant PSA changes. There is striking variability in the rate of PSA decline. Patients A and B dropped below 1.0 ng/ml at one and nine months, respectively. Patient C took three years to reach nadir. He was biopsied at two years because of postimplant PSA rise near the one-year mark (negative), and eventually fell below 0.5 ng/ml.

especially true for physicians who perform brachytherapy as only a small part of their practice and who may be less familiar with the subtle interpretive nuances that are only now being described in the literature.(SMATHERS) Failing to do so places patients at risk for errors, ranging from needless worry to unnecessary salvage therapy. In fact, it is important that physicians *and* patients be made aware of the potential interpretive pitfalls, because so many patients track their own PSA closely and may become overly alarmed at certain PSA changes.

DIGITAL RECTAL EXAM
Until PSA was introduced, the digital rectal exam (DRE) was the most commonly used method to evaluate treatment results, with local control assessment based on regression of palpable tumor. Reliance on palpability is complicated by the subjectivity of the DRE and the fact that most tumors diagnosed in the PSA era are not palpable even prior to therapy (Stage T1c). Even for palpable tumors, the correlation between tumor regression on rectal exam and local or distant recurrence is tenuous. Perez and colleagues, for instance, showed that patients with Stage C disease did poorly, despite a high degree of tumor regression by DRE.(PEREZ)

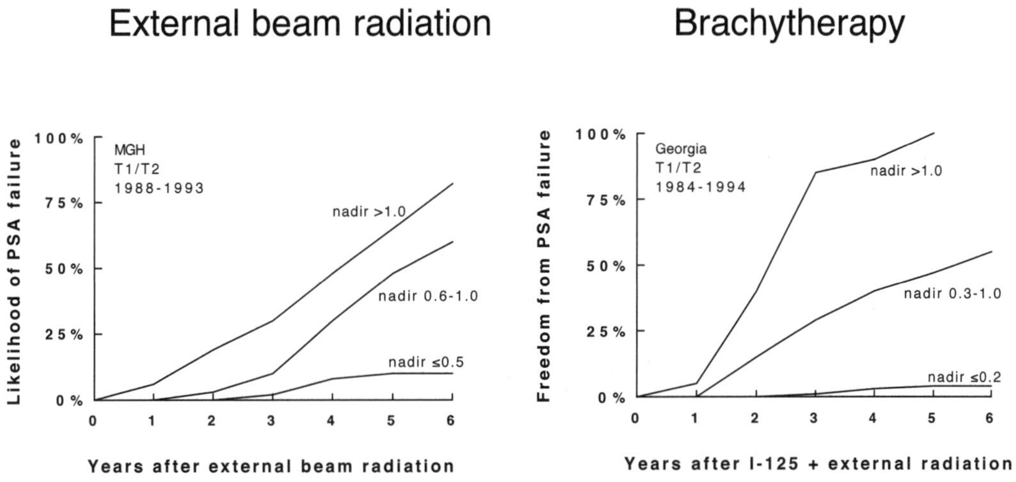

External beam radiation   Brachytherapy

Figure 13-2. Likelihood of subsequent biochemical failure, based on the PSA nadir. While the chance for recurrence decreases with decreasing nadirs, there is no nadir below which recurrences don't occur.(ZIETMAN, CRITZ)

PSA has rendered routine follow-up DRE nearly obsolete. In the absence of a rising PSA, repeat prostatic biopsies rarely show residual cancers, and a DRE is presumably even less likely to detect disease persistence.(ZELEFSKY) Similarly, after prostatectomy, a palpable tumor recurrence in the absence of a rising PSA is virtually unknown.(OBEK, POUND)

PROSTATE SPECIFIC ANTIGEN (PSA)
PSA is a much more sensitive and objective measure of residual cancer than DRE. It has dramatically decreased the time to detect cancer persistence. Following external beam radiation or brachytherapy, patients' PSAs typically decline markedly, reflective of local tumor regression. The rate of decline is highly variable and has not, in itself, been correlated with prognosis (**Figure 13-1**).(RITTER, KAVADI). In the postbrachytherapy setting, any relation between the rate of decline and prognosis is made especially murky by the occurrence of temporary PSA rises (see below).

Although the rate of PSA decline appears to have no significance, the *nadir* PSA appears to correlate with the likelihood of cure. The relationship between PSA nadir levels and disease-free status is a continuum down to low levels (**Figure 13-2**). However, there is no single nadir PSA value that guarantees against late bio-

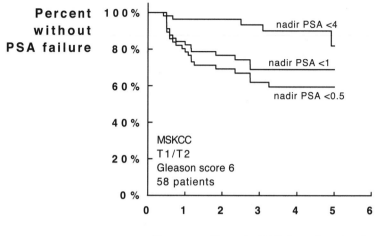

Figure 13-3. PSA-based cancer-free rates using biochemical cancer control criteria of PSA <4, <1 or <0.5 ng/ml. The lower the nadir PSA required to be considered cancer-free, the lower the apparent cure rate.

chemical failure. Additionally, because of the great variability in the rate and consistency of PSA declines after brachytherapy, the optimal time to allow for nadiring to occur is unknown—some patients nadir at six months, while others take six years. Using nadir values to determine disease-free status also requires wrestling with declining PSAs and PSA spikes (see below).

The simplest way to classify patients as to whether their disease has been eradicated is to use an absolute PSA criteria. The more stringent the criteria, the lower the cure rates will appear (**Figure 13-3**). While an absolute criteria of 1.0 was most popular during the 1990s, there is an increasing tendency to use 0.5 ng/ml as the cutoff for disease eradication.(CRITZ 00) Unfortunately, no matter how low the nadir value, an individual patient is not guaranteed a cure. And while low posttreatment PSA values are associated with a low likelihood of cancer recurrence, even some patients with undetectable postimplant PSA will ultimately develop late biochemical failure.

As an alternative to using nadir or absolute values to assess posttreatment cancer status, an ASTRO consensus panel recommended using three consecutive PSA

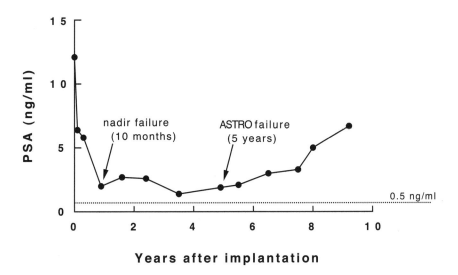

Figure 13-4. The major difference between using an absolute nadir value versus a rising PSA as a marker of disease status is that patients are scored as having failed much sooner with a nadir parameter. We now know that a high nadir value is almost certainly indicative of residual cancer, but it may take several years for residual cancer to begin to grow and to cause the PSA to rise.

rises as the marker for disease recurrence.(ASTRO) The conceptual appeal of using a *rising* value as the criteria for cancer recurrence is that some PSA nadirs, while not below 1.0 ng/ml, may remain stable for many years. In practice, the ASTRO consensus criteria make the disease-free curve look better in the short term, because many patients who would be considered to have failed, based on a high nadir PSA will, in fact, require several years to show a clear PSA rise. In other words, the ASTRO criteria delay the bad news (**Figure 13-4**). Debate over the preferability of the ASTRO criteria versus use of nadir values to score patients' cancer status will continue. With longer follow-up, however, the criteria used becomes less important because almost all cancer recurrences eventually declare themselves by a rising PSA, regardless of the nadir value.(VICINI, HANLON)

Whatever criteria are used to define biochemical failure, there will always be some ambiguous cases, probably the most common of which is the patient whose last PSA is slightly higher than previous values, but still below an arbitrary nadir criteria for tumor control. Ambiguous cases usually account for only a small fraction

13.5

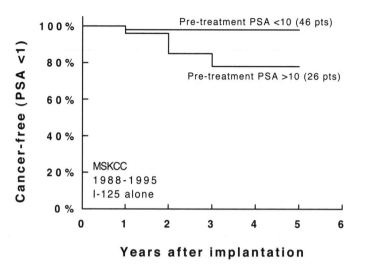

Figure 13-5. Freedom from biochemical failure in patients with nadir below 1.0 ng/ml is still influenced by the pretreatment PSA. Looking only at patients with a nadir below 1.0 ng/ml, those with a pretreatment PSA above 10 ng/ml had a higher failure rate than those with PSA below 10 ng/ml.

of the total and they should not have a substantial statistical effect on the reported cancer-free rates. Additionally, with longer follow-up, these ambiguous cases become less frequent.

PRETREATMENT PSA HOLDS ITS VALUE
Even among patients with posttreatment PSA nadir below 1.0 ng/ml following external beam radiation, the pretreatment PSA holds substantial prognostic significance.(KAVADI) In a preliminary look at brachytherapy patients treated at Memorial Sloan-Kettering Cancer Center (MSKCC), those with a nadir below 1.0 ng/ml and a pretreatment PSA below 10 ng/ml had fewer late biochemical failures than those with nadir below 1.0 ng/ml and pretreatment PSA above 10 ng/ml (**Figure 13-5**).

TEMPORARY PSA RISES
While the prognostic importance of nadir values applies to both external beam radiation and brachytherapy, there are some peculiar aspects of post-treatment PSAs that seem specific to brachytherapy. *Temporary PSA rises*, also referred to as *PSA bumps* or *PSA spikes*, occur commonly between 12 and 36 months after

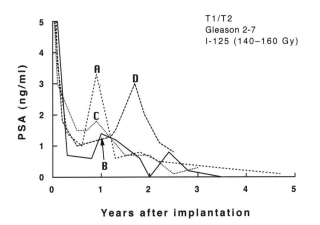

Figure 13-6. Typical examples of temporary PSA rises following brachytherapy.

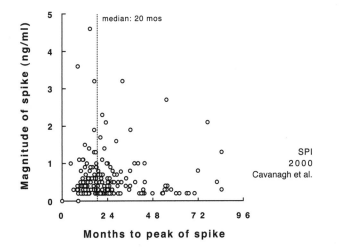

Figure 13-7. Magnitude of PSA spike peak versus time after brachytherapy. (CAVANAGH)

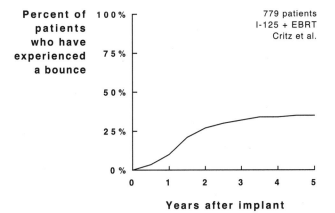

Figure 13-8. The incidence of a temporary PSA rise is greatest between one and two years postimplant.(CRITZ 00)

13.7

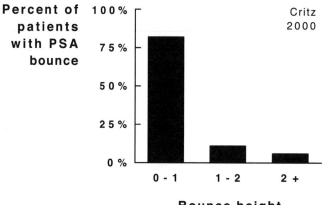

Figure 13-9. Of patients who experience a temporary PSA rise, 82% were a magnitude of 1.0 ng/ml or less, and only 6% were greater than 2.0 ng/ml.(CRITZ 00)

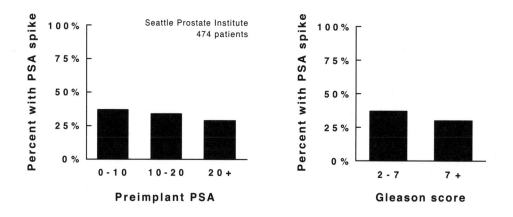

Figure 13-10. The likelihood of a patient demonstrating a temporary PSA rise is independent of pretreatment PSA or Gleason score.(CAVANAGH)

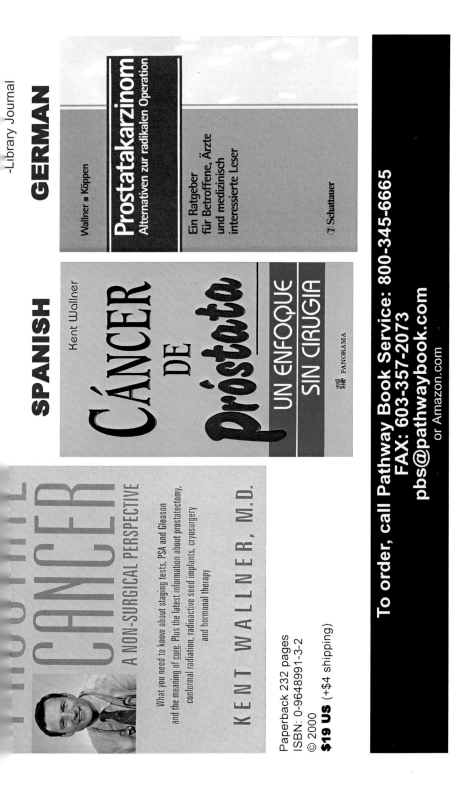

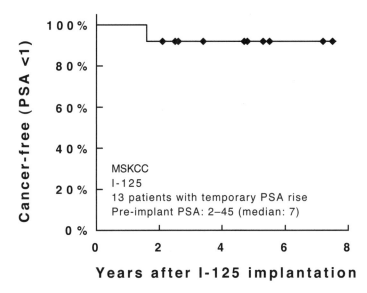

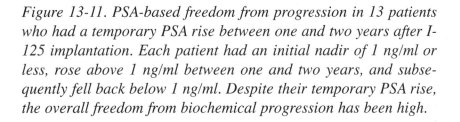

Figure 13-11. PSA-based freedom from progression in 13 patients who had a temporary PSA rise between one and two years after I-125 implantation. Each patient had an initial nadir of 1 ng/ml or less, rose above 1 ng/ml between one and two years, and subsequently fell back below 1 ng/ml. Despite their temporary PSA rise, the overall freedom from biochemical progression has been high.

implantation (**Figures 13-6, 13-7 & 13-8**). The magnitude of most temporary rises is less than 2.0 ng/ml, but rises as high as 16 ng/ml have been reported (**Figure 13-9**).(CRITZ 00, CAVANAGH) The incidence of temporary rises depends partly on how often PSAs are taken, and what magnitude of rise is considered a *rise*. If PSAs are taken at the typical 4 to 6 months intervals and *any* increase is considered, then about one-third of patients will experience a spike or bump.(**Figures 13-7 & 10**). The likelihood of a temporary rise is independent of pretreatment PSA, Gleason score, isotope, or use of supplemental external beam radiation (**Figure 13-11**). While they make for a lot of patient and physician anxiety, the long-term prognosis for PSA spike patients appears similar to patients without a spike (**Figure 13-10**).(CAVANAGH, CRITZ 00) Temporary posttreatment rises seem to correspond to late recurrence of radiation-related urinary symptoms. And spikes are apparently much less common after external beam radiation.

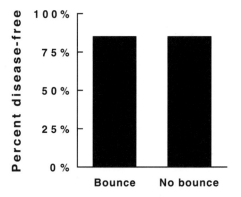

Figure 13-12. Likelihood of biochemical disease-free survival in patients with or without a temporary postimplant PSA rise.(CRITZ 00)

While there is currently no clear explanation for the occurrence of temporary rises, it's important to be aware of them because of the tendency of physicians and patients to panic with any PSA rise. To minimize the degree of panic, it's a good idea to warn patients in advance of the possibility of temporary PSA rises.

An appreciation of the frequent occurrence of temporary PSA rises is especially crucial in patients for whom a salvage prostatectomy would be considered. To the uninitiated, it seems commonsensical that a rising PSA in the first three post-implant years would be an indication for salvage prostatectomy. Not so fast. Any consideration of a salvage procedure during that time should be approached with great reluctance. In fact, for patients with a pretreatment PSA less than 20 ng/ml, a posttreatment PSA rise is far more likely to be temporary as opposed to a true indication of cancer persistence. The clinical dilemma of a rising PSA in the first three postimplant years is made doubly confusing when a postimplant biopsy in the same period is positive, because biopsies also may take two years or more to revert to negative (see below).(PRESTIDGE) The common occurrence of temporary PSA rises is further impetus to insist that investigators use longer follow-up times before reporting PSA-based cancer control rates.(SHIPLEY)

ACTUARIAL VERSUS "RAW" STATISTICS
Until the 1980s, cure rates were generally reported as *straight, raw,* or *crude* percentage of patients free of detectable disease at a point in time, with no consideration for the length of time they were followed. Using straight percentages, cure

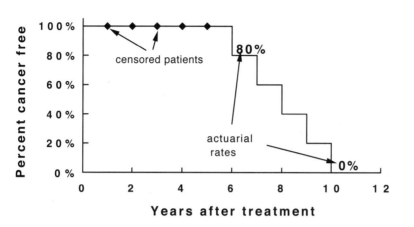

Figure 13-13. Example of freedom from biochemical failure, using crude versus actuarial calculations. In this example, five of ten patients have failed, all after the first five years of treatment. The crude freedom from failure is 50%. By actuarial calculation, the cure rate is 0%, because all patients followed beyond five years have failed.

rates appear falsely high because patients with shorter follow-up have not had sufficient time to manifest their disease recurrence, although they contribute to the denominator equally with longer-followed patients.

In contrast to straight percentages, *actuarial* calculations adjust the denominator over time, dropping patients out of the calculation as they reach their maximum follow-up time, a process called *censoring*. Censored patients are usually indicated on graphs by x's or dots, to give a visual estimate of their follow-up times (**Figure 13-13**). During the last twenty years, actuarial calculations have become the generally accepted method of reporting cancer-free rates, allowing for inclusion of patients with shorter follow-up times without favorably biasing longer-term results.

There are variations of actuarial calculation rates, the most common being Berkson-Gage (*life table*) and Kaplan-Meier (*product-limit method*). Kaplan-Meier is the most widely used in cancer research. It calculates changes in the cancer-free status whenever an event (failure) occurs, rather than at regular intervals

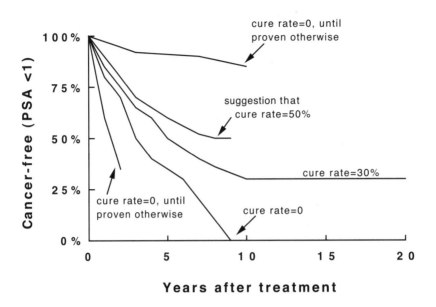

Figure 13-14. Cure rates are determined by where the freedom-from-cancer curve plateaus. If there is no plateau, no estimate of a cure rate can be made.

as is done for the Berkson-Gage calculation. Differences between the actuarial calculation methods are usually slight.

The statistical difference between curves can be calculated in several ways, the most common being the log-rank and the generalized Wilcoxin tests. Log-rank analysis is more reflective of differences in the late portion of the curves, and is probably preferable for slow-recurring cancers such as prostate cancer.

In contrast to temporary PSA rises, a persistently rising posttreatment PSA is highly likely to be followed by clinically evident failure, with a lag time of several years. With up to four years follow-up after external beam radiation, approximately 50% of patients with a rising PSA develop clinically evident local or distant recurrence.(KAPLAN, RITTER) With longer follow-up, probably all patients with a rising PSA would ultimately develop clinical failure. And nearly all patients who develop symptomatic cancer recurrence have a rising PSA several years prior to developing clinically detectable disease recurrence. To date, most data regarding PSA versus clinical cancer recurrence have come from external beam series, but brachytherapy series are likely to show similar trends.

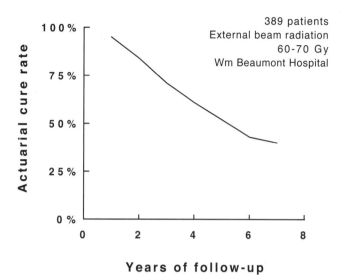

Figure 13-15. Due to the time required for posttreatment PSAs to start rising in patients with residual cancer, calculated cure rates are typically lower with longer follow-up.(VICINI)

CURE RATES

When tracking groups of patients at risk of cancer recurrence, there is no universally accepted definition of *cure*. With nearly all types of cancer, there is an initial rapid failure rate, followed by a leveling off of the curves, as the percent of the remaining patients with persistent cancer falls. Ideally, the time at which no further patients fail should be taken as the cure rate (**Figure 13-14**). With prostate cancer, there is probably no time, with any treatment modality, after which *no* more failures will occur—there is usually a small but persistent late failure rate. Some late failures could be due to second malignancies within the prostate, but differentiating late recurrences from second primaries is not currently practical. From a practical standpoint, that point at which the failure rate decelerates to near zero is generally taken as the *cure rate*. It would more appropriately be referred to as the *apparent* or *approximate* cure rate.

While actuarial statistics are a much more realistic statistical method than straight percentages, they can still favorably bias the data, especially with short follow-up times. Patients with short follow-up may make the initial portion of the curve look more favorable, simply because there has not been sufficient time to manifest clinical or biochemical failure, especially if the ASTRO requirement for three succes-

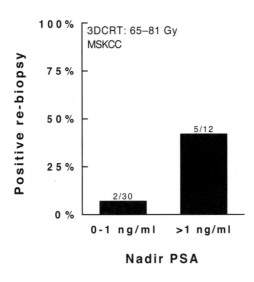

Figure 13-16. Likelihood of a positive rebiopsy after external beam radiation in patients with a nonrising nadir PSA below or above 1.0 ng/ml.(ZELEFSKY)

sive rises is used (**Figure 13-15**).(VICINI) Favorable statistical bias with short follow-up has rightly lead some investigators to call for exclusion of patients with less than 2.5 years follow-up.(SHIPLEY) Unfortunately, in the race to publish, common sense often goes out the window.

LOCAL VERSUS DISTANT FAILURE

A rising PSA is a general marker of disease progression—it does not in itself distinguish between local and distant failure. However, the rate of PSA rise helps distinguish between local and distant failures. After external beam radiation, patients with rapidly rising PSA (doubling time less than 12 months) are more likely to have distant metastases.(LEE, RITTER, SARTOR, POLLACK) However, the rate of rise is not a very specific criteria for local versus distant failure, because there is a large amount of overlap between the groups. To date, there are limited data specific to brachytherapy regarding the rate of PSA rise and the site of failure.

POSTTREATMENT BIOPSIES

Posttreatment biopsy has been used sporadically to assess intraprostatic tumor eradication. Compared to digital rectal exam, posttreatment prostatic biopsies always show a higher incidence of residual tumor. And in nearly all reported series, patients with histologically viable tumor have a greater likelihood of developing local recurrence and distant metastases.(KUBAN, SCARDINO) Some authors have argued that histologically viable tumor is irrelevant—wishful thinking. The

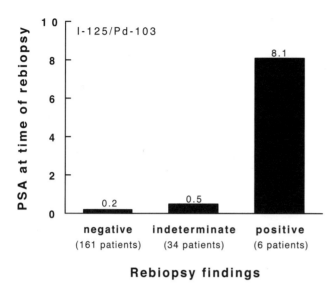

Figure 13-17. PSA at time of repeat biopsy versus biopsy results.(PRESTIDGE)

only series that failed to show worse outcomes in patients with positive follow-up biopsies was that by Cox and Kline.(COX) Their results were clouded, however, by the fact that some patients received hormonal ablation and that the biopsies were done under digital rather than TRUS guidance.

Postimplant biopsies are conceptually appealing, but their routine use is limited by ambiguity in interpretation of biopsy samples and the fact that biopsies are almost always negative in patients with a low PSA at the time of biopsy (**Figures 13-16 & 13-17**).(PRESTIDGE, ZELEFSKY) Immunostains have not been of much use so far, but they have the potential to help distinguish between a true biochemical failure versus a temporary PSA rise.(CROOK, BRAWER)

The majority of biopsies are clearly negative or positive. However, a small percent show residual cancer with radiation effect, and have been termed *indeterminate* (**Figure 13-18**). With time, most indeterminate samples become negative, suggesting that substantial radiation effect is indicative of tumorcidal damage, which simply needs more time to become histologically evident (**Figure 13-19**). (PRESTIDGE) Positive or indeterminate biopsies are especially vexing in the doubly confusing situation of a temporary PSA rise in the first three postimplant years (**Figures 13-20, 13-21, & 13-22**).(SMATHERS) Unfortunately, there's no way at pre-

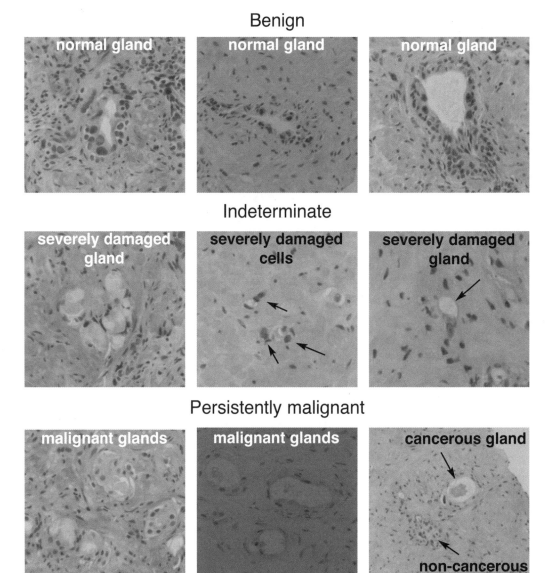

Figure 13-18. Findings on postimplant prostate biopsy range from irradiated noncancerous glands (top panels), to highly radiation-damaged glands of uncertain biologic potential for growth (middle panels), to what appear to be still viable irradiated cancer glands (bottom panels) (courtesy of Dr. Lawrence True).

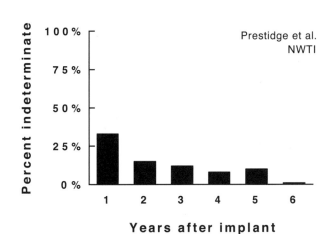

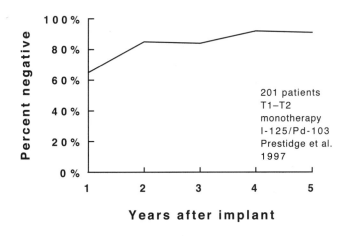

Figure 13-19. The percent of indeterminate biopsies decreases (top panel) and the percent of negative biopsies increases (lower panel) with greater time after implantation.(PRESTIDGE)

sent to be sure whether one is dealing with a true cancer recurrence or two transient phenomena.

While post-treatment biopsy results following external beam radiation have been less than stellar, anastomotic biopsies following prostatectomy aren't much better: Foster and Abi-Aad showed that anastamotic biopsies in the setting of an elevated post-prostatectomy PSA were positive in approximately 50% of patients.(FOSTER, ABI-AAD) Urologists who perseverate on postradiation biopsy studies need to be constantly reminded of this work.

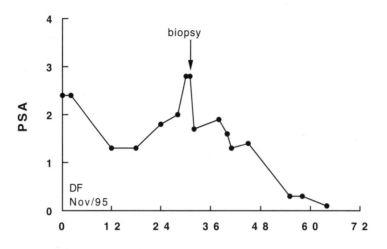

Months after I-125

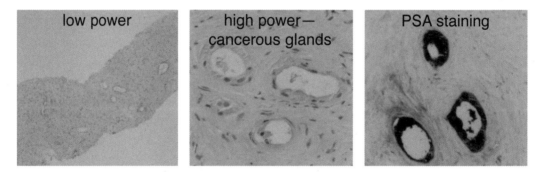

Figure 13-20. Postimplant PSA patterns and corresponding repeat biopsies can be doubly confusing. In this patient, a PSA rise two years after treatment for Gleason 3+3 cancer prompted a repeat biopsy, showing a single focus of histologically viable cancer. PSA staining was positive for cancer. In conjunction with the rising PSA, the patient's urologist strongly urged him to have a salvage prostatectomy. At K. Wallner's urging, the patient waited and his PSA subsequently fell to below 0.5 ng/ml. While further follow-up is needed, the point here is that even an apparently "positive" biopsy and a rising PSA are insufficient to make a definitive diagnosis of cancer persistence.

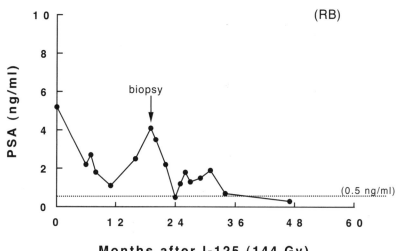

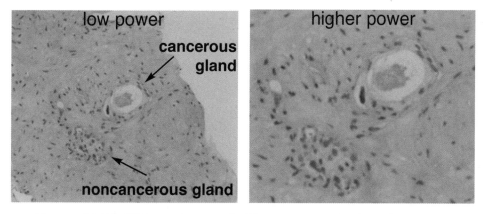

Figure 13-21. This patient, with Gleason score 3+3 and pretreatment PSA of 5.2 ng/ml, underwent I-125 implantation (144 Gy) at age 61. Eight months after implantation he developed a rising PSA, which fell concomitantly with antibiotic administration (top panel). A second PSA rise between 18 and 24 months after implantation prompted a repeat biopsy, which showed a single cancerous gland. He declined the advice to have a salvage prostatectomy. Subsequently, his PSA fell to below 1.0 ng/ml, 38 months after brachytherapy.(SMATHERS)

13.19

What would you do?

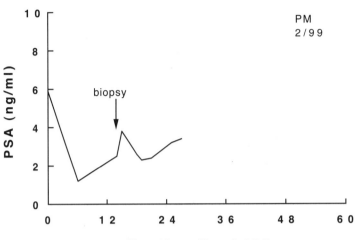

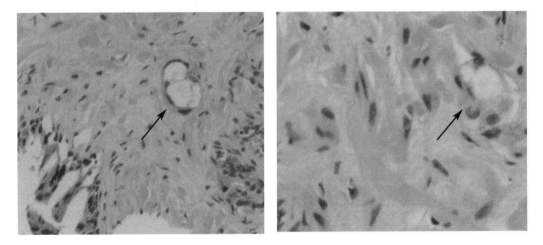

Figure 13-22. This 44-year-old patient had a I-125 (144 Gy) implant for a T1c cancer, with a pretreatment PSA of 5.9 and Gleason score 3+3. His PSA fell to 1.2, and then rose to 3.8 at 13 months postimplant. A repeat biopsy shows residual cancer glands with radiation effect (arrows) and he was strongly urged by his urologist to have a salvage prostatectomy. Instead, the patient has elected to wait... What would you advise? (See 3rd edition of Prostate Brachytherapy Made Complicated for the outcome.)

BONE SCANS

Routine follow-up bone scans in the absence of a rising PSA are not warranted. At initial diagnosis, bone scans are rarely positive with a PSA of less than 20 ng/ml. After prostatectomy, it has been clearly established that follow-up bone scans are not necessary in the absence of biochemical failure.(CHER) The same probably holds true for brachytherapy. Routine repeat bone scan, as part of follow-up, should be performed only if the PSA is greater than 10 ng/ml (or higher?) or if there is clinical suspicion of bone metastases.

IS BIOCHEMICAL FAILURE RELEVANT?

PSA has emerged as the most sensitive indicator of residual disease, making routine postimplant digital rectal exams or repeat biopsies almost obsolete.(TRALINS) But while a high nadir PSA or a rising PSA are statistically associated with a high likelihood of subsequent clinically evident failure, many patients with a rising posttreatment PSA will remain symptom-free for many years.(POUND 99, KUPELIAN) It has been argued that we're getting too concerned about a biochemical parameter that often has little practical relevance. Some would go so far as to argue that a posttreatment rising PSA is therefore not an indication of failed therapy. Whoa. Only partly true—patients who remain asymptomatic for many years in the face of a slowly rising posttreatment PSA probably are the ones who didn't need treatment in the first place!(ADOLFSSON)

REFERENCES

1. Abi-Aad AS, Macfarlane MT, Stein A, deKernion JB. Detection of local recurrence after radical prostatectomy by prostate specific antigen and transrectal ultrasound. J Urol 1992; 147:952-955.

2. Adolfsson J, Carstensen J, Lowhagen T. Deferred treatment in clinically localised prostatic carcinoma. Br J Urol 1992; 69:183-187.

3. ASTRO . Guidelines for PSA following radiation therapy. Int J Rad Oncol Biol Phys 1997; 37:1035-1041.

4. Brawer MK, Nagle RB, Pitts W, Freiha F, Gamble SL. Keratin immuoreactivity as an aid to the diagnosis of persistent adenocarcinoma in irradiated human prostates. Cancer 1989; 63:454-460.

5. Cavanagh W, Blasko JC, Grimm PD, Sylvester JE. Transient elevation of serum prostate-specific antigen following I-125/Pd-103 brachytherapy for localized prostate cancer. Sem in Urol Oncol 2000; 18:160-165.

6. Cher ML, Bianco FJ, Lam JS, et al . Limited role of radionuclide bone scintigraphy in patients with prostate specific antigen elevations after radical prostatectomy. J Urol 1998; 160:1387-1391.

7. Cox JD, Kline RW. Do prostatic biopsies 12 months or more after external irradiation for adenocarcinoma, Stage III, predict long-term survival? Int J Radiat Oncol Biol Phys 1983; 9:299-303.

8. Critz FA, Williams H, Holladay CT, Levinson AK, et al . Post-treatment PSA ≤0.2 ng/ml defines disease freedom after radiotherapy for prostate cancer using modern techniques. Urol 1999; 54:968-971.

9. Critz FA, Williams WH, Benton JB, Levinson AK, Holladay CT, Holladay DA. Prostate specific anitgen bounce after radioactive seed implantation followed by external beam radiation for prostate cancer. J Urol 2000; 163:1085-1089.

10. Critz FA, Williams WH, Levinson AK, Benton JB, Holladay CT, Schnell FJ. Simultaneous irradiation for prostate cancer: intermediate results with modern techniques. J Urol 2000; 164:738-743.

11. Crook J, Malone S, Perry G, Bahadur Y, Robertson S, Abdolell M. Postradiotherapy prostate biopsies: What do they really mean? Results for 498 patients. Int J Rad Oncol Biol Phys 2000; 48:355-367.

12. Foster LS, Jajodia P, Fournier G, Shinohara K, et al . The value of prostate specific antigen and transrectal guided biopsy in detecting prostatic fossa recurrences following radical prosatectomy. J Urol 1993; 149:1024-1028.

13. Hanlon AL, Hanks GE. Scrutiny of the ASTRO consensus definition of biochemical failure in irradiated prostate cancer patients demonstrates its usefulness and robustness. Int J Rad Oncol Biol Phys 2000; 46:559-566.

14. Kaplan I, Prestidge BR, Cox RS. Prostate Specific Antigen after Irradiation for Prostatic Carcinoma. J Urol 1990; 144:1172-1176.

15. Kavadi VS, Zagars GK, Pollack A. Serum prostate-specific antigen after radiation therapy for clonically localized prostate cancer: prognostic implications. Int J Rad Oncol Biol Phys 1994; 30:279-287.

16. Kuban DA, El-Mahdi AM, Schellhammer P. The significance of post-irradiation prostate biopsy with long- term follow-up. Int J Radiat Oncol Biol Phys 1992; 24:409-414.

17. Kupelian P, Katcher J, Levin H, Zippe C, Klein E. Correlation of clinical and pathologic factors with rising prostate-specific antigen profiles after radical prostatectomy alone for clinically locallized prostate cancer. Urol 1996; 48:249-260.

18. Lee WR, Hanks GE, Hanlon A. Increasing prostate-specific antigen profile following definitive radiation therapy for localized prostate cancer: Clinical observations. J Clin Oncol 1997; 15:230-238.

19. Obek C, Neulander E, Sadek S, Soloway MS. Is there a role for digital rectal examination in the follow-up of patients after radical prostatectomy? J Urol 1999; 162:762-764.

20. Perez CA, Pilepich MV, Zivnuska F. Tumor control in definitive irradiation of localized carcinoma of the prostate. Int J Radiat Oncol Biol Phys 1986; 12:523-531.

21. Pollack A, Zagars GK, Kavadi VS. Prostate specific antigen doubling time and disease relapse after radiotherapy for prostate cancer. Cancer 1994; 74:670-678.

22. Pound CR, Christens-Barry OW, Gurganus RT, Partin AW, Walsh PC. Digital rectal examination and imaging studies are unnecessary in men with undetectable prostate specific anitgen following radical prostatectomy. J Urol 1999; 162:1337-1340.

23. Pound CR, Partin AW, Eisenberger MA, Chan DW, Pearson JD, Walsh PC. Natural history of progression after PSA elevation following radical prostatectomy. JAMA 1999; 281:1591-1597.

24. Prestidge BR, Hoak DC, Grimm PD, Ragde H, Cavanagh W, Blasko JC. Posttreatment biopsy results following interstitial brachytherapy in early-stage prostate cancer. Int J Radiat Oncol Biol Phys 1997; 37:31.

25. Ritter MA, Messing EM, Shanahan TG, Potts S, Chappell RJ, Kinsella TJ. Prostate-specific antigen as a predictor of radiotherapy response and patterns of failure in localized prostate cancer. J Clin Oncol 1992; 10:1208-1217.

26. Sartor CI, Strawderman MH, Lin X, Kish KE, McLaughlin PW, Sandler HM. Rate of PSA rise predicts metastatic versus local recurrence after definitive radiotherapy. Int J Rad Oncol Biol Phys 1997; 38:941-947.

27. Scardino PT, Wheeler TM. Prostatic biopsy after irradiation therapy for prostatic cancer. Urol 1985; 25:39-46.

28. Shipley WU. PSA following irradiation for prostate cancer: The upcoming ASTRO symposium. Int J Radiat Oncol Biol Phys 1996; 35:1115.

29. Smathers S, Wallner K, Sprouse J, True L. Temporary PSA rises and repeat prostate biopsies after brachytherapy. Int J Rad Oncol Biol Phys 2001;

30. Tralins K, Wallner KE. Follow-up costs after external beam irradiation for low risk prostate cancer. Int J Rad Oncol Biol Phys 1999; 44:323-326.

31. Vicini FA, Kestin LL, Martinez AA. The importance of adequate follow-up in defining treatment success after external beam irradiation for prostate cancer. Int J Rad Oncol Biol Phys 1999; 45:553-561.

32. Zelefsky MJ, Leibel SA, Gaudin PB, et al . Dose escalation with three-dimensional conformal radation therapy affects the outcome in prostate cancer. Int J Rad Oncol Biol Phys 1998; 41:491-500.

33. Zietman AL, Tibbs MK, Dallow KC, et al . Use of PSA nadir to predict subsequent biochemical outcome following external beam radiation therapy for T1-2 adenocarcinoma of the prostate. Radiother and Oncol 1996; 40:159-162.

14

Cure rates

With the widespread adoption of prostate brachytherapy during the last five years, the body of literature regarding tumor control rates has grown rapidly.(BRACHMAN, CRITZ, GRADO, POLASCIK, POTTERS, RAGDE, RAMOS, STOKES, STOREY) Rather than present a detailed compilation of all published series, we'll summarize a few longer-term ones (good and bad!) that have received the most attention. We'll start with an update of the personal series from M. Dattoli—the unique feature of which is that all patients' biopsies have been reviewed by a single, highly regarded uropathologist (Dr. Lawrence True), making analysis of the role of Gleason scores more reliable. Then we'll summarize a half dozen much-quoted series. And finally, we'll take a look at one of the worst series ever published for *any* treatment modality, and ponder why some cancer specialists don't get it right.

PD-103 + BEAM RADIATION
Dattoli and colleagues have long experience with Pd-103 and supplemental beam radiation, treating patients with at least one adverse risk factor: a pretreatment PSA ≥10 or Gleason score of 7 or higher (**Figure 14-1**).(DATTOLI) From 1992 through 1995, 142 consecutive patients were treated, with ages ranging from 49 to 88 years (median: 71 years). Enzymatic acid phosphatase was determined by the method of Roy and colleagues.(ROY)

Due to concern regarding interobserver variability in grading, the original biopsy slides for 129 of the 142 patients were retrieved and re-reviewed by a single pathologist (L. True) at the University of Washington. Patients whose biopsy slides could not be reviewed were not included in the statistical analysis of Gleason score. Only one patient had a staging pelvic lymphadenectomy.

Patients received 41 Gy external beam radiation to a limited pelvic field, followed two to four weeks later by a Pd-103 boost (80 Gy, pre-NIST-99). A median of 89 mCi Pd-103 was implanted with a range of 52–144 mCi. The median source strength was 1.4 mCi (range:1.0–1.6 mCi/source) and the median number of sources was 64 (range: 37–100). Freedom from biochemical failure was defined as a serum PSA less than 1.0 ng/ml at last follow-up. Patients were censored at last follow-up if their serum PSA was still decreasing. Patients whose serum PSA plateaued at a value greater than 1.0 were scored as failures at the time at which their PSA plateaued. The follow-up period for nonfailing patients ranged from four to eight years (median: six years). Freedom-from failure curves were calculated by the method of Kaplan-Meier. Differences among groups were determined by the log-rank method.

Twenty-five patients developed biochemical failure. The overall actuarial freedom from biochemical progression at five years is 82%, with 81 patients followed beyond that time, particularly encouraging for patients with higher pretreatment PSAs or Gleason scores (**Figure 14-1**). No clinically evident local failures occurred. Thirty-five patients received a short course (2 months) of pretreatment androgen ablation.

Progressively more elevated pretreatment PSA, Gleason score, or PAP were each associated with a progressively higher failure rate (**Figure 14-2**). Gleason score of

Pretreatment parameters

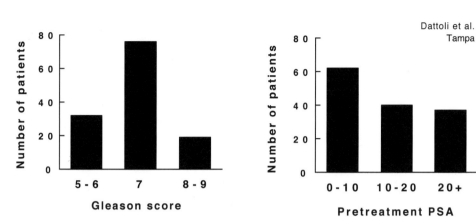

Cancer-free status

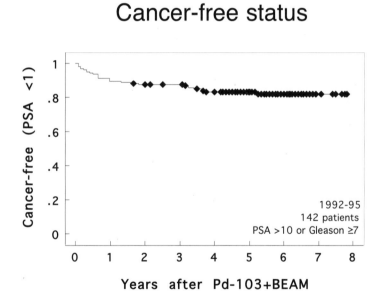

Years after Pd-103+BEAM

Figure 14-1. Patient characteristics (top panels) and freedom from biochemical progression for 142 patients with PSA >10 or Gleason score ≥7 treated with Pd-103 plus 41 Gy beam radiation. The curves level off at 82%, suggesting that a large percentage of patients with high risk features may be cured.

Pre-treatment PSA

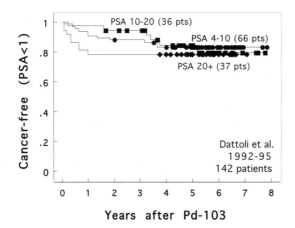

Gleason

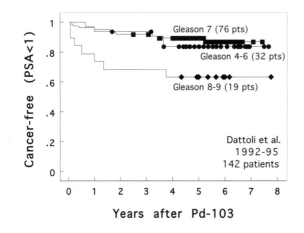

PAP

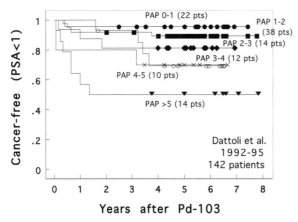

Figure 14-2. Freedom from biochemical failure for patients treated with Pd-103 + beam radiation, stratified by PSA, Gleason score, or PAP.

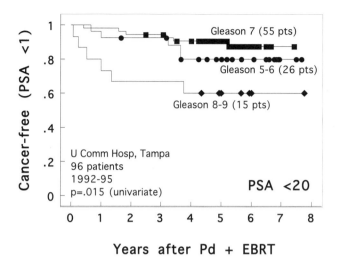

Figure 14-3. Freedom from biochemical failure for patients with pretreatment PSA less than 10, stratified by Gleason score.

8 or higher was predictive of biochemical failure in patients with a pretreatment PSA below 20 (**Figure 14-3**).

In Cox proportional hazard multivariate analysis, considering each factor as a continuous variable, the strongest predictor of failure was elevated acid phosphatase (p=.02), followed by Gleason score (p=.1) and PSA (p=.14). There was little correlation among pretreatment PSA, Gleason score, or PAP (**Figure 14-4**), as reported by other investigators.(STAMEY, MOUL)

FOLLOW-UP BIOPSIES
There is a growing body of postimplant biopsy data, showing remarkably high rates of cancer elimination. Approximately half the patients treated at Northwest Tumor Institute (NWTI) with I-125 or Pd-103 alone had follow-up biopsies at one year or more.(PRESTIDGE) Of 201 patients biopsied, only 3% showed residual, apparently viable cancer on their last biopsy. An additional 17% were read as *indeterminate*, or residual cancer with profound radiation changes that could be consistent with dying cancer. With longer follow-up, most indeterminate biopsies were negative when repeated (**Figure 14-5**). Not all patients were biopsied. Those with a rising PSA or abnormal digital rectal exam were more likely to agree to a second biopsy, likely biasing the results negatively.

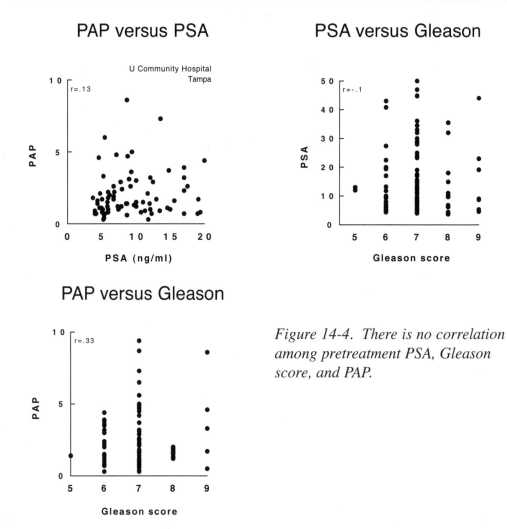

Figure 14-4. There is no correlation among pretreatment PSA, Gleason score, and PAP.

Sharkey and colleagues obtained follow-up biopsy on 86% of 288 patients with two years follow-up after Pd-103. The negative biopsy rate was 84% and 87%, respectively, for patients with or without adjuvant hormonal therapy. The repeat biopsies were nearly always negative, regardless of pretreatment PSA (**Figure 14-6**).(SHARKEY)

The likelihood of a positive posttreatment biopsy has historically been very high following conventional dose beam radiation, but in more recent series the positive biopsy rates have been lower.(CROOK) While the lower rate of positive biopsy after contemporary series is encouraging, we should pause before opening the champagne. Since introduction of PSA, cancers are being diagnosed at a far earlier stage, presumably with a much lower tumor burden than in earlier series. In fact,

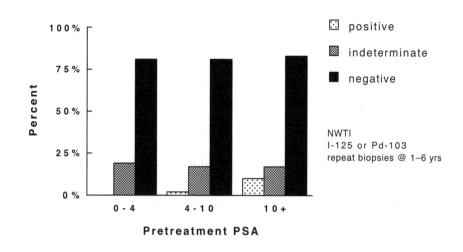

Figure 14-5. *Percent of patients with negative, indeterminate, or positive biopsies after I-125 or Pd-103 implant for early-stage cancer.*

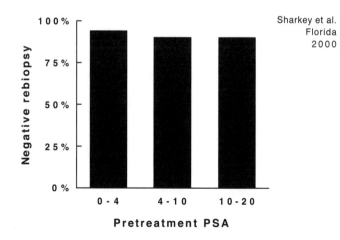

Figure 14-6. *Percent of patients with negative biopsies after Pd-103 implantation, with or without adjuvant hormonal therapy.*(SHARKEY)

14.7

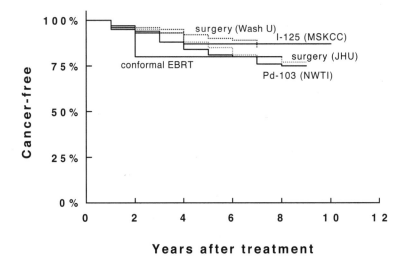

PSA 0-10

Figure 14-7. Freedom from failure after prostatectomy, external radiation, or brachytherapy for patients with pretreatment PSA less than 10 ng/ml, as reported from leading specialty centers with a reputation for excellence in their modality.(SHIPLEY, BLASKO, POUND, ZELEFSKY, CATALONA) The most striking findings are the apparent leveling off of the curves for all modalities used against small-volume cancers (PSA below 10).

repeat biopsies in patients with prior positive biopsies, are frequently negative even in the absence of therapy—the tumor burden is frequently so low in PSA-screened patients that it is difficult to find cancer even in the untreated patient!(SVETEC, STROUMBAKIS)

COMPARING MODALITIES

No modern controlled trials comparing surgery, external beam radiation, or brachytherapy have been performed, so we're left with retrospective uncontrolled comparisons—but things could be worse. Before PSA, retrospective comparisons were nearly worthless, because patients grouped by clinical stage alone are so heterogeneous. With the advent of PSA, there is remarkable prognostic agreement among institutions, within similar PSA categories, using the same modalities.(ZIETMAN, ZAGARS) Accordingly, comparing outcome with different modalities for the same PSA groupings likely gives a reasonably good idea of each modality's effectiveness.

14.8

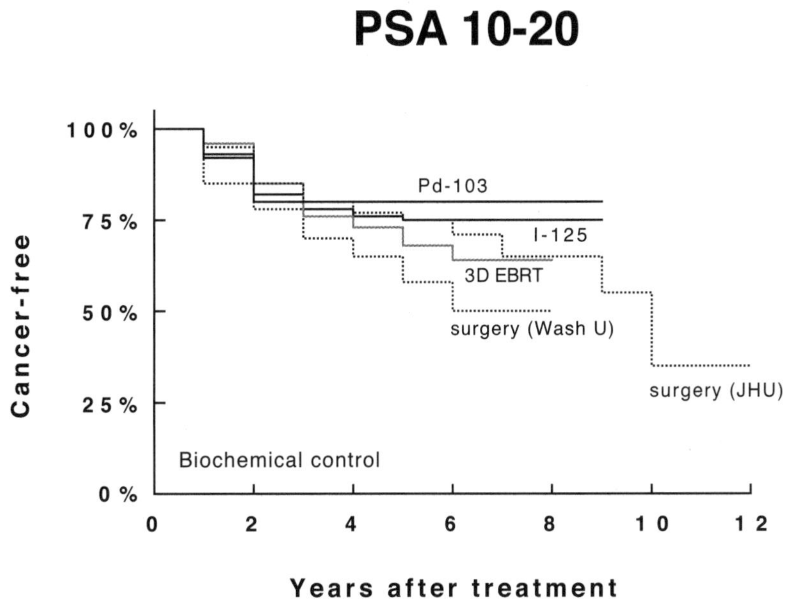

PSA 10-20

Figure 14-8. Freedom from failure after prostatectomy, external radiation, or brachytherapy for patients with pretreatment PSA between 10 and 20 ng/ml, as reported from leading specialty centers with a reputation for excellence in their modality.(SHIPLEY, BLASKO, POUND, ZELEFSKY, CATALONA) *The most striking finding is the lack of a plateau in prostatectomy patients with a pretreatment PSA above 10. These results, by renowned surgeons, suggest that radical prostatectomy is purely palliative for men with a PSA above 10.*

In comparing brachytherapy with surgery, two concepts have been remarkably consistent. First, patients with low tumor burden (low PSA) do well with either modality, when treated by capable physicians. With follow-up of approximately 10 years, each modality appears to eradicate cancer in 80% to 90% of such patients (**Figure 14-7**). If there is a cure rate advantage to any of the modalities, it's not apparent within the first ten years follow-up. This makes sense—if the cancer burden is small it can probably be eradicated with either therapy.

The second consistent finding in contemporary series is that patients with higher tumor burden (PSA >10) have a high risk of early biochemical failure, regardless of treatment modality. It is in the higher-risk patients that results with beam radi-

D'Amico and colleagues

prostatectomy:

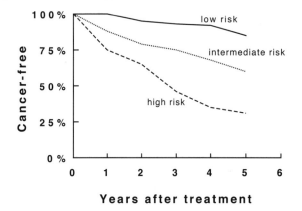

Figure 14-9. PSA-based cure rates for each modality in patients treated at the Joint Radiation Center in Boston or the University of Pennsylvania. The most striking thing about these results is that few of the cancer-free curves level off with any modality, suggesting that the ultimate cure rates may be very low no matter what treatment is employed.(D'AMICO) *(low risk=PSA <10 and Gleason score 2–6; intermediate risk=PSA 10–20 or Gleason score 7; high risk=PSA >20 or Gleason score ≥8.)*

external beam radiation:

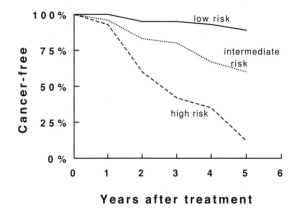

brachytherapy:

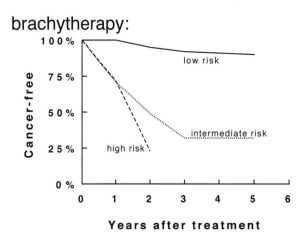

Table 14-1. Reasons why some brachytherapists results could be vastly inferior to others.

- early experience, still learning
- lack of adequate treatment margins (see Chapter 6)
- ?

ation alone or prostatectomy deteriorate so markedly (**Figure 14-8**). In the absence of controlled trials, the best that can be said is that patients with PSA above 10 appear to do better with brachytherapy-based therapy, but this needs to be confirmed in many centers, and preferably in controlled studies.

While the previous paragraph may elicit howls of protest from some of our colleagues, it shouldn't. The idea of using brachytherapy to maximize radiation-induced tumor eradication is not some weird new idea from Mars. Brachytherapy is widely used to enhance local control of advanced solid tumors in other sites, including the cervix, endometrium, and base of tongue. That brachytherapy would add to the cure of patients with more advanced prostate cancers should come as no great surprise.

EXCEPTIONALLY POOR RESULTS
While outcomes reported by brachytherapy enthusiasts have generally compared favorably with those of surgery or external beam radiation, there are reports of remarkably poor brachytherapy results. Probably the most widely quoted are from D'Amico and colleagues, who have published extensively their low cure rates after all forms of prostate cancer therapy, including brachytherapy (**Figure 14-9**).(D'AMICO) It's always tough to reconcile favorable reports from leading physicians with poor results by others. There are a number of plausible explanations—you be the judge in this case (**Table 14-1**).

The first important lesson to be learned from occasional poor outcome reports are that all forms of therapy require good quality implementation to be effective. The second lesson is that isolated poor outcome reports more likely reflect misuse of a technique, rather than that the technique is inherently flawed.

MORE
The growing number of PSA-based follow-up reports is still dominated by a few select brachytherapists. Like the situation for nerve-sparing prostatectomy and conformal external beam radiation, the vast majority of published brachytherapy

data come from a handful of subspecialist physicians, and may not be representative of the overall brachytherapy experience. In the next few years, more reports should emerge as other brachytherapy teams accumulate longer follow-up, making it clear just how generalizable the favorable results are.

REFERENCES
1. Blasko JC, Grimm PD, Sylvester JE, Badiozamani KR, Hoak D, Cavanagh W. Palladium-103 brachytherapy for prostate carcinoma. Int J Rad Oncol Biol Phys 2000; 46:839-850.

2. Brachman DG, Thomas T, Hilbe J, Beyer DC. Failure-free survival following brachytherapy alone or external beam irradiation alone for T1-2 prostate tumors in 2222 patients: results from a single practice. Int J Rad Oncol Biol Phys 2000; 48:111-117.

3. Catalona WJ, Smith DS. Cancer recurrence and survival rates after anatomic radical retropubic prostatectomy for prostate cancer: intermediate-term results. J Urol 1998; 160:2428-2434.

4. Critz FA, Levinson AK, Williams WH, Holladay CT, Griffin VD, Holladay DA. Simultaneous radiotherapy for prostate cancer: 125-prostate implant followed by external-beam radiation. Ca J Sci Am 1998; 4:359-363.

5. Critz FA, Williams WH, Levinson AK, Benton JB, Holladay CT, Schnell FJ. Simultaneous irradiation for prostate cancer: intermediate results with modern techniques. J Urol 2000; 164:738-743.

6. Crook J, Malone S, Perry G, Bahadur Y, Robertson S, Abdolell M. Postradiotherapy prostate biopsies: What do they really mean? Results for 498 patients. Int J Rad Oncol Biol Phys 2000; 48:355-367.

7. D'Amico AV, Whittington R, Malkowicz SB, et al . Biochemical outcome after radical prostatectomy, external beam radiation therapy, or interstitial radiation therapy for clinically localized prostate cancer. JAMA 1998; 280:969-974.

8. Dattoli M, Wallner K, True L, Sorace R, Koval J, et al . Prognostic role of serum prostatic acid phosphatase for 103-Pd-based radiation for prostatic carcinoma. Int J Rad Oncol Biol Phys 1999; 45:853-856.

9. Grado GL, Larson TR, Balch CS, et al . Actuarial disease-free survival after prostate cancer brachytherapy using interactive techniques with biplane ultrasound and fluoroscopic guidance. Int J Rad Oncol Biol Phys 1998; 42:289-298.

10. Moul JW, Connelly RR, Perahia B, McLeod DG. The contemporary value of pretreatment prostatic acid phosphatase to predict pathological stage and recurrence in radical prostatectomy cases. J Urol 1998; 159:935-940.

11. Polascik TJ, Pound CR, DeWeese TL, Walsh PC. Comparison of radical prostatectomy and iodine 125 interstitial radiotherapy for the treatment of clinically localized prostate cancer: A 7-year biochemical (PSA) progression analysis. Urol 1998; 51:884-890.

12. Potters L. Permanent prostate brachytherapy: Lessons learned, lessons to be learned. Oncology 2000; 14:981-991.

13. Pound CR, Partin AW, Epstein JI, Walsh PC. Prostate-specific antigen after anatomic radical retropubic prostatectomy. Urol Clin N Am 1997; 24:395-406.

14. Prestidge BR, Hoak DC, Grimm PD, Ragde H, Cavanagh W, Blasko JC. Posttreatment biopsy results following interstitial brachytherapy in early-stage prostate cancer. Int J Radiat Oncol Biol Phys 1997; 37:31.

15. Ragde H, Elgamal A, Snow P, et al . Ten-year disease free survival after transperineal sonography-guided iodine-125 brachytherapy with or without 45-Gray external beam irradiation in the treatment of patients with clinically localized, low to high Gleason grade prostate carcinoma. Cancer 1998; 83:989-1001.

16. Ramos CG, Carvalhal GF, Smith DS, Mager DE, Catalona WJ. Retrospective comparison of radical retropubic prostatectomy and 125-Iodine brachytherapy for localized prostate cancer. J Urol 1999; 161:1212-1215.

17. Roy AV, Brower ME, Hayden JE. Sodium thymolphthalein monophosphate: a new acid phosphatase substrate with greater specificity for the prostatic enzyme in serum. Clin Chem 1998; 17:1093-1102.

18. Sharkey J, Chovnick SD, Behar RJ, et al . Evolution of techniques for ultrasound-guided palladium 103 brachytherapy in 950 patients with prostate cancer. Tech Urol 2000; 6:128-134.

19. Sharkey J, Chovnick SD, Behar RJ, Perez R, et al . Minimally invasive treatment for localized adenocarcinoma of the prostate: Review of 1048 patients treated with ultrasound-guided palladium-103 brachytherapy. J Endourol 2000; 14:343-350.

20. Shipley WU, Thames HD, Sandler HM, Hanks GE, Zietman AL, Perez CA, Kuban DA, Hancock SL, Smith CD. Radiation therapy for clinically localized prostate cancer. A multi-institutional pooled analysis. JAMA 1999; 281:1598-1604.

21. Stamey TA, Kabalin JN, McNeal JE, Johnstone IM, Freiha F, Redwine EA, Yang N. Prostate specific antigen in the diagnosis and treatment of adenocarcinoma of the prostate. II. Radical prostatectomy treated patients. J Urol 1989; 141:1076-1083.

22. Stokes SH. Comparison of biochemical disease-free survival of patients with localized carcinoma of the prostate undergoing radical prostatectomy, transperineal ultrasound-guided radioactive seed implantation, or definitive external beam irradiation. Int J Rad Oncol Biol Phys 2000; 47:129-136.

23. Storey MR, Landgren RC, Cottone JL, et al . Transperineal 125-iodine implantation for treatment of clinically localized prostate cancer: 5-year tumor control and morbidity. Int J Radiat Oncol Biol Phys 1999; 43:565-570.

24. Stroumbakis N, Cookson MS, Reuter VE, Fair WR. Clinical significance of repeat sextant biopsies in prostate cancer patients. Urol 1997; 49(S 3A):113-118.

25. Svetec D, McCabe K, Peretsman S, Klein E, Levin H, Optenberg S, Thompson I. Prostate rebiopsy is a poor surrogate of treatment efficacy in localized prostate cancer. J Urol 1998; 159:1606-1608.

26. Zagars GK. Prostate specific antigen as an outcome variable for T1 and T2 prostate cancer treated by radiation therapy. J Urol 1994; 152:1786.

27. Zelefsky MJ, Hollister T, Raben A, Matthews SM, Wallner KE. Five-year biochemical outcome and toxicity with transperineal CT-planned permanent I-125 prostate implantation for patients with localized prostate cancer. Int J Rad Oncol Biol Phys 2000; 47:1261-1266.

28. Zietman AL, Coen JJ, Dallow KC, Shipley WU. The treatment of prostate cancer by conventional radiation therapy: An analysis of long-term outcome. Int J Radiat Oncol Biol Phys 1995; 32:287-292.

15

Morbidity

Many physicians and prospective patients have a false perception that prostate brachytherapy has fewer side effects and complications than external beam radiation, a perception derived in part from the seemingly logical assumption that the more localized radiation of an implant should lead to fewer problems. Wrong. Brachytherapy typically causes *more* marked and *more* prolonged radiation-related urinary symptoms, at least in the first six to twelve postimplant months. Fortunately, nearly all implant-related problems resolve spontaneously.

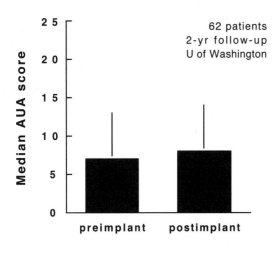

Figure 15-1. Pre- and postimplant AUA scores in 62 patients, followed for two years.

URINARY MORBIDITY

Nearly all patients experience varying degrees of radiation-related prostatitis. If given the choice, approximately half the patients use medication (alpha-blockers) for several months or longer following their implant.(WALLNER 96) Fortunately, radiation prostatitis is rarely incapacitating and typically resolves spontaneously within six to twelve months (see chapter 10).(KLEINBERG, MERRICK 00) Most patients return to their baseline AUA scores (**Figure 15-1**). Somewhat surprisingly, long-term AUA scores are not influenced by such pretreatment parameters as prostate volume, age, preimplant AUA scores, or urinary flow parameters (**Figure 15-2**).(LANDIS) Although spontaneous resolution of radiation prostatitis is the norm, there is some chance of more serious complications, including superficial urethral necrosis and incontinence.

Superficial urethral necrosis

Superficial urethral necrosis (SUN), associated with severe dysuria and urinary incontinence, was reported to occur in up to 4% of patients treated by Blasko and colleagues in the late 1980s and early 1990s (**Figure 15-3**).(BLASKO) Its occurrence among patients treated in the early TRUS experience probably reflected astronomical urethral doses from homogeneous seed placement patterns typically used at that time. With the peripheral loading patterns typical of today, urethral necrosis is very uncommon.(STONE)

Urinary Incontinence

Reports regarding the incidence of postimplant urinary incontinence are mixed. With short-term follow-up, none of 184 Northwest Tumor Institute (NWTI)

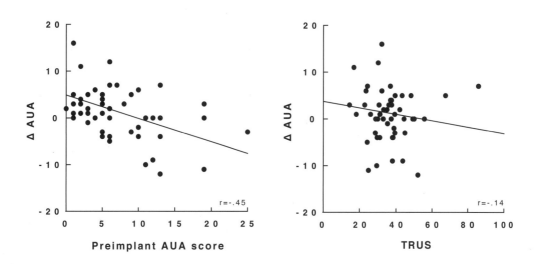

Figure 15-2. Change in AUA score at two years following brachytherapy in 62 patients treated at the University of Washington in 1998. There was no correlation between preimplant AUA scores or preimplant TRUS volume and AUA scores two years after therapy.(LANDIS)

patients without TURP developed incontinence (**Figure 15-4**). However, incontinence was more common in patients who had a TURP before or after implantation. There was no obvious difference in the risk of incontinence in patients treated with implant alone versus those treated with implant and supplemental external beam radiation.

The homogeneous source loading pattern that led to an increased incidence of SUN in some early patients likewise resulted in an increased risk of long-term incontinence. With longer follow-up of the early NWTI patients, a relatively high rate of incontinence was seen even in patients without a prior TURP, likely secondary to excessive urethral doses from homogeneous source loading patterns used at the time.(TALCOTT)

In contrast to the excessive morbidity reported in some early series, more recent experience has been that urinary incontinence is unusual when peripheral source loading patterns are used.(MERRICK 00) Only 2 of 91 patients implanted at MSKCC without a prior TURP developed urinary incontinence requiring use of pads

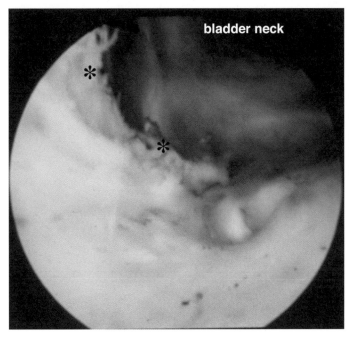

bladder neck

Figure 15-3. Cystoscopic view of superficial urethral necrosis with sloughing tissue (*). SUN is rarely seen since peripheral source placement has been widely adopted.

(**Figure 15-5**). Six patients described minimal urgency or stress incontinence not requiring use of pads.

The current trend is to quantify urinary incontinence with survey instruments far more detailed than previously published scales, such as those of the Radiation Therapy Oncology Group (RTOG).(LAWTON, LEE) More detailed quality of life (QOL) instruments attempt to make lifestyle effects more uniformly reported, in part so that different modalities can be compared. While admirable in their intent, such efforts culminate in such scores as *urinary bother* or *functional well-being* or *EPIC scores*, indices so nebulous that they are almost meaningless.(KRUPSKI, BRANDEIS, LIM, WEI)

BRACHYTHERAPY AFTER A TURP
There are conflicting reports regarding the risk of urinary incontinence in patients with prior TURP (see chapter 12). Both TURP and radiation can impair urinary continence and their combination may have additive adverse effects. TURP may predispose patients to radiation-related incontinence by compromising the urinary sphincters or by denuding the urethral lining. Blasko, Grimm, and Ragde were the first to draw attention to the higher risk of incontinence in men with prior TURP (**Figure 15-4**).(BLASKO) Of 90 patients with pre- or postimplant TURP, there was a 17% likelihood of incontinence, usually associated with superficial urethral

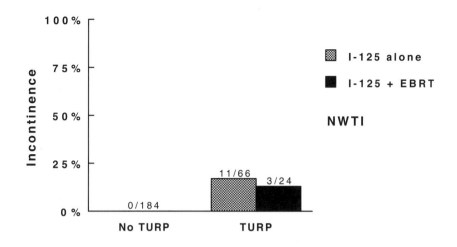

Figure 15-4. Incidence of urinary incontinence in patients treated at NWTI with I-125 alone or I-125 combined with external beam radiation. Patients who had a preimplant TURP had a higher likelihood of developing postimplant incontinence.(BLASKO)

necrosis. And the likelihood of incontinence increased with longer follow-up (unpublished data).

Fortunately, the early brachytherapy experience in patients with prior TURP has not been representative of later series. In a more recent report, only two of twenty-four patients developed postimplant urine incontinence (one mild and one severe), with the lower incidence attributable to a more peripheral source placement pattern (see chapter 6).(WALLNER 97) Since adopting a more peripheral source loading as of 1994, Blasko and colleagues have also noted a lower incidence of urinary incontinence (unpublished data). Other investigators have confirmed a low incidence of incontinence in patients with a prior TURP, provided that a peripheral source loading pattern is used.(STONE)

TURP AFTER BRACHYTHERAPY
Patients who undergo TURP to relieve refractory urinary retention after implantation are probably at increased risk of developing urinary incontinence. Hu and Wallner reviewed ten patients who underwent TURP or TUIP (transurethral incision of the prostate) to relieve urinary obstruction unrelated to local tumor recurrence, from 1 to 22 months following brachytherapy.(HU 98) Seven of the ten patients developed some degree of permanent urinary incontinence. Three have

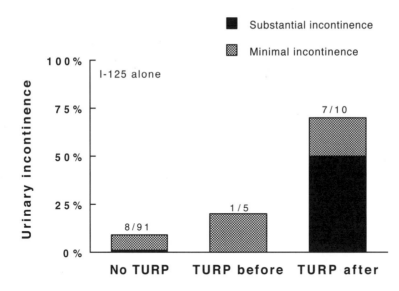

Figure 15-5. Incidence of urinary incontinence in patients treated with I-125 alone by Wallner and colleagues. The six patients who developed incontinence without having had a TURP before or after implant described urgency, that would occasionally lead to slight leakage if they could not get to a bathroom, symptoms that would not be considered incontinent by the LENT scoring system.(LEE, LAWTON)

minimal stress incontinence and four developed severe incontinence. There was no obvious relationship between the extent of the surgical procedure (TURP versus TUIP) and the likelihood of incontinence. Equally perplexing, there was no obvious relationship between the development of incontinence and the amount of tissue resected at the time of TURP or between the time from implant to TURP.

In five of the patients for whom urethral dose calculations were done, the maximal dose exceeded the prescription dose by 2.5-fold, the level at which the risk of urinary morbidity may rise.(WALLNER 95) The high incidence of incontinence in postimplant TURP patients reported by Hu and Wallner is likely higher than would be expected in today's patients, because more effort is being taken to keep the urethral doses within acceptable levels. However, because of the risk of incontinence, patients with refractory postimplant urinary retention should be managed conservatively, with prolonged self-catheterization if necessary. Postimplant resections

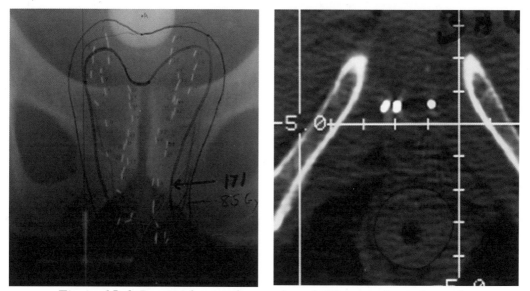

Figure 15-6. Postimplant radiograph and CT scan of a patient who developed an apical urethral stricture 18 months after I-125 implant. An excessive number of sources were placed at prostatic apex, probably contributing to late stricture formation.

should be postponed much longer, if not indefinitely, to allow spontaneous resolution of urinary obstruction (see chapter 11).

Urethral stricture

Urethral stricture is an uncommon complication of modern brachytherapy, probably related to excessive apical radiation doses.(MERRICK 02) One of the few cases the authors identified was associated with excessive sources placed at the prostatic apex (**Figure 15-6**), one reason to avoid excessive apical margins (see chapter 6). When stricture does occur, it typically is successfully managed with one or more urethral dilations.

PROCTITIS

Some degree of postimplant radiation proctitis is almost inevitable, given the proximity of the prostate to the rectum. Patients commonly develop more frequent bowel movements, but not diarrhea. They may also experience an urge to defecate when urinating—some will actually sit down to urinate, out of concern that they may also pass stool. Although radiation-related rectal symptoms are common, rectal incontinence is unusual. Proctitis symptoms usually resolve within a few

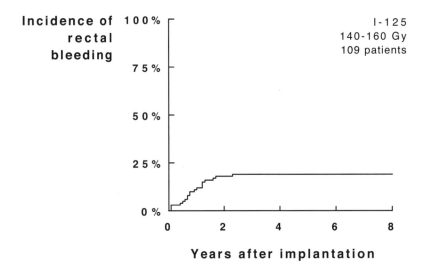

Incidence of rectal bleeding

I-125
140-160 Gy
109 patients

Years after implantation

Figure 15-7. Incidence of rectal bleeding over time—nearly all cases manifest in the first six to twenty-four postimplant months.(HU 98)

months, and nearly all patients' rectal function returns to the preimplant level by one to two years.(MERRICK 99)

Rectal bleeding
Radiation proctopathy with bleeding occurs in 2% to 10% of patients, and nearly always manifests between 6 and 18 months of implantation (**Figures 15-7 & 15-8**).(GELBLUM, HAN, MERRICK 99) Endoscopy typically reveals a circumscribed area of intense erythema, telangiectasias, and friability on the anterior rectal wall, overlying the prostate (**Figure 15-9**). Blood loss is typically minimal, rarely requiring transfusions. Fortunately, rectal ulceration is far less common that proctitis (**Figure 15-10**).(HAN) Rectal bleeding from radiation proctitis is typically painless. When pain does occur, it may indicate involvement of the sphincter muscles. Pain itself does not appear to portend a worse outcome.(HU 98)

In some cases of proctitis, misplaced sources are obvious on postimplant CT scan (**Figure 15-11**). Most of the time, however, errors are not obvious and rectal doses are only mildly higher than in patients without clinically apparent proctitis (see chapter 9). The loose correlation between dosimetry and rectal complications might be explained by a predisposition of some patients to rectal complications

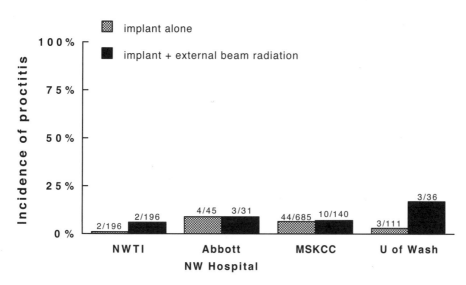

Figure 15-8. Incidence of implant-related rectal bleeding after brachytherapy, with or without supplemental external beam radiation.(BLASKO, KAYE, GELBLUM, HAN)

due to inherent radiation sensitivity, diabetes, or microvascular damage from other causes.

Reports regarding the effects of supplemental external beam radiation on rectal morbidity are mixed. Iversen and colleagues treated patients with a full dose (160 Gy) I-125 implant followed by 47 Gy whole-pelvic irradiation at 220 cGy/day.(IVERSEN) Severe late complications, including rectal ulceration, colostomy, and severe radiation cystitis, were reported in 14 of 33 patients. This toxicity would be unacceptable by any standard, and likely resulted from their use of whole pelvic irradiation at high daily fractions, preceded by a full dose implant. Combining full doses of brachytherapy and supplemental external beam radiation is unwise. Although the report by Iversen and colleagues was frightening, the incidence of significant proctitis with combined implant plus external beam radiation is low with current techniques.(HAN) In most series, the addition of supplemental beam radiation has increased the likelihood of rectal bleeding, but has not clearly been associated with more severe complications, such as ulceration or fistula (**Figure 15-8**).(HOWARD) Some authors report higher rates of severe rectal complications with supplemental beam radation performed *after* brachytherapy, but this issue is unsettled.(ZEITLIN, PATEL)

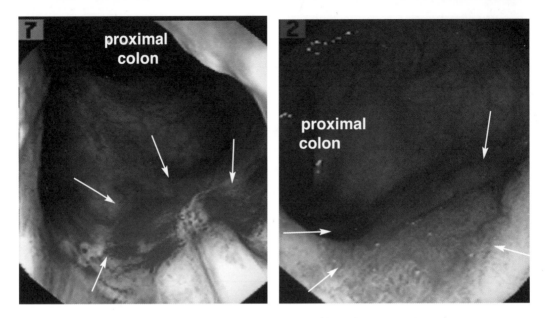

Figure 15-9. Postimplant proctitis with telangiectasias (arrows) in patients who developed painless rectal bleeding. The erythema is well localized to the anterior rectal wall.

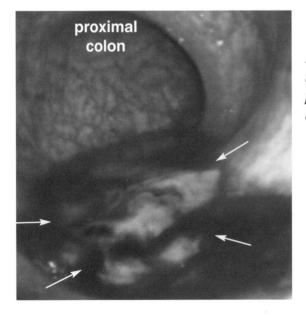

Figure 15-10. Postimplant rectal ulceration (arrows) overlying the prostate, a much less common occurrence.

15.10

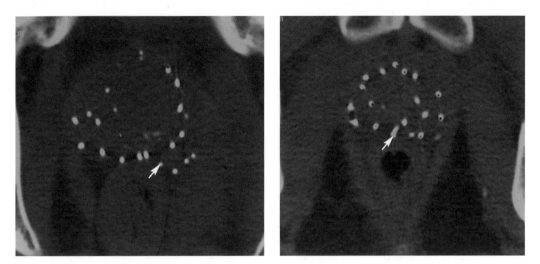

Figure 15-11. These patients with postimplant rectal bleeding have a few errant sources (arrows) in their rectal wall. But in most cases of postimplant proctitis, even these minor placement errors are not seen.

Management

The need for intervention in the case of implant-related rectal bleeding is unclear. Most patients who develop bleeding after external beam radiation or brachytherapy do not progress to rectal fistula. Given enough time, most will heal spontaneously.(CROOK, SHIPLEY, TESHIMA, HU) However, healing is typically slow, sometimes requiring many years. While slow, spontaneous healing is likely, persistent bleeding can be a substantial nuisance for patients—repeated soiling of the underwear is especially distressing. Medical therapies, including meselamine or steroid enemas, are commonly prescribed, with mixed results.(BABB, KOCHBAR) Nonetheless, such therapies are seldom harmful and a therapeutic trial seems reasonable, with discontinuation if no benefit is seen. Of eighteen I-125 patients reported by Hu and Wallner, nine were treated with steroid enemas, three had laser coagulation, and six had no intervention. Although the series was retrospective and with no set criteria for the choice of one therapy over another, there was no obvious difference in the resolution rate between treatment groups.(HU)

In contrast to medical therapies, more invasive therapies with electrocoagulation, laser, argon plasma coagulation (APC), or topical formalin have been highly effective therapy for bleeding from radiation proctitis, with what appears to be a low likelihood of complications (**Figure 15-12**).(VIGGIANO, KAASSIS, ROCHE, BISWAL) The limitation of most reports is that they mix patients with proctitis from varied

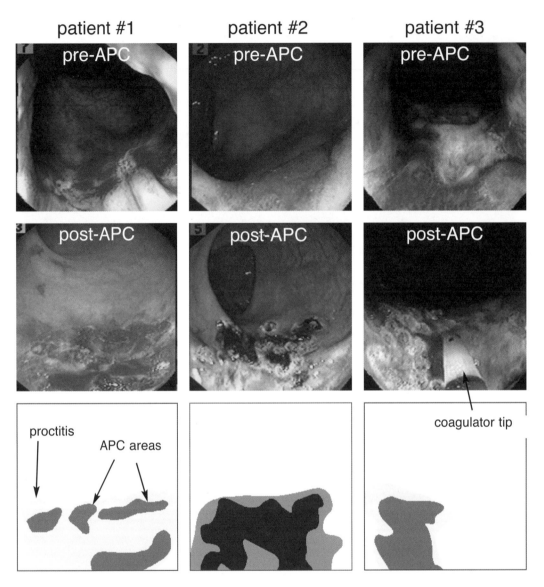

Figure 15-12. Examples of extent of argon plasma coagulated (APC) areas in patients treated by Dr. Jason Dominitz at the Puget Sound Health Care System VA Hospital.(SMITH)

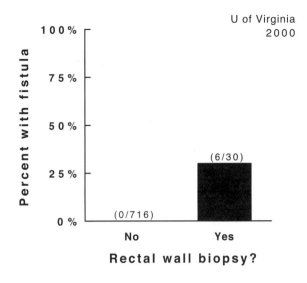

Figure 15-13. Incidence of rectal fistula formation by whether or not a post-implant rectal wall biopsy had been performed. (THEODORESCU)

types of radiation, without attention specifically to prostate brachytherapy. At the Puget Sound Health Care System VA hospital, patients with radiation-related proctitis have generally responded well to one or more treatment sessions with argon plasma laser coagulation.(SMITH) However, we are aware of cases where laser therapy may have exacerbated bleeding, followed by fistualization, so that such therapy should be undertaken cautiously.

One of the more controversial areas in the management of implant-related proctitis has been the inclination of gastroenterologists to biopsy the rectal wall to rule out the possibility of carcinoma. While there are rare reports of postimplant rectal cancers, such a finding is much less likely than a simple case of radiation proctitis.(HU) In a large series from the University of Virginia, patients who underwent rectal wall biopsy in the course of evaluation for implant-related proctitis were clearly at higher risk of fistula formation.(THEODORESCU) In fairness, however, it should be pointed out that the majority of patients in the Virginia series, and all three in the series by Howard and colleagues, did *not* have a biopsy prior to developing a fistula (**Figure 15-13**). Accordingly, it seems that while biopsy may predispose patients to further damage, most cases of fistualization are due to the implant rather than subsequent procedures.

Proper management of the tiny fraction of patients who progress to fistula or clinically significant blood loss is unclear (**Figures 15-14 & 15-15**). Cases of spontaneous healing after suprapubic catheterization, diverting colostomy, or both have

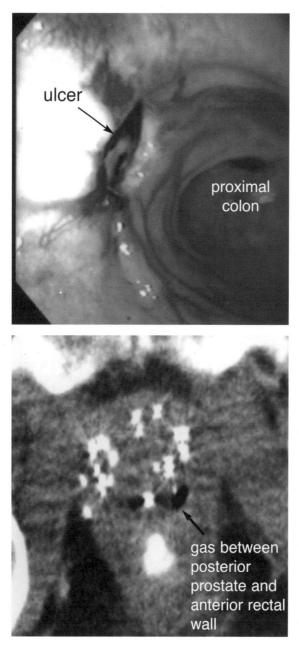

Figure 15-14. Endoscopic view of 62-year-old patient who developed a rectal ulcer and then fistula (arrows) 18 months after 144 Gy I-125 implant. The ulcer measured about 10 mm across. CT scan (below) shows gas between the outer rectal wall and the posterior prostate, leaking through the fistula. In this case, no gross necrosis of the prostate is evident on CT, but the patient may progress to more tissue destruction. He is currently undergoing hyperbaric oxygen therapy. As with most cases of an implant-related fistula, perusal of the postimplant dosimetry failed to show an obvious cause for this severe complication (opposite page). The lateral view did not show excessive posterior sources, and only a small portion of the rectum was included in the high-dose region, and the prostate V100, V200, and V300 were in the typical range (opposite page, bottom graphs).

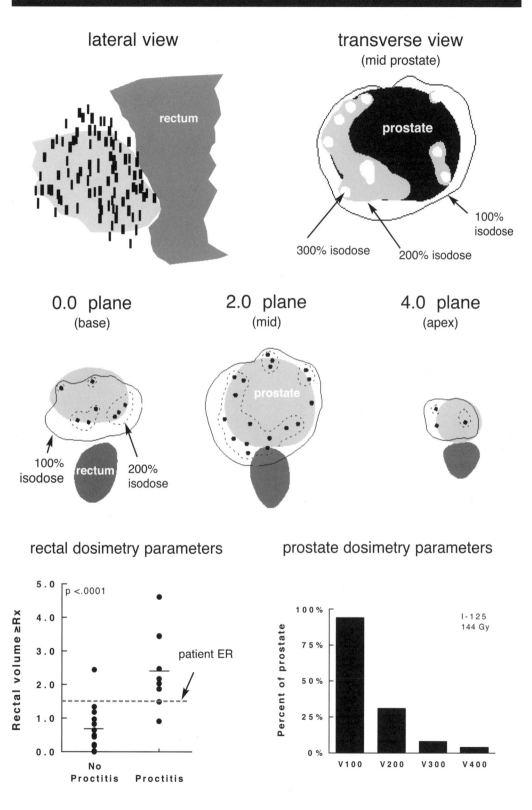

lateral view

transverse view
(mid prostate)

rectum

prostate

100% isodose

300% isodose   200% isodose

0.0 plane
(base)

2.0 plane
(mid)

4.0 plane
(apex)

prostate

100% isodose   rectum   200% isodose

rectal dosimetry parameters

prostate dosimetry parameters

p <.0001

Rectal volume ≥Rx

patient ER

No Proctitis   Proctitis

Percent of prostate

I-125
144 Gy

V100   V200   V300   V400

15.15

day 1

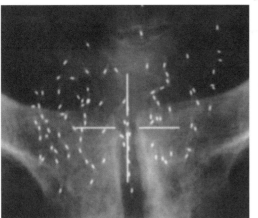
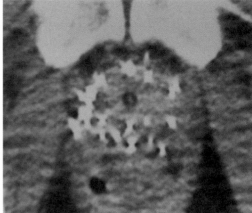

14 months

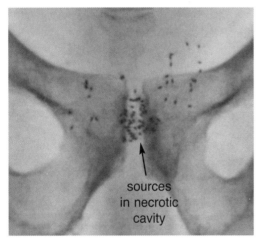

sources
in necrotic
cavity

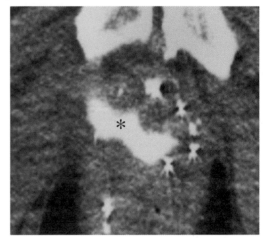

*

postplan dosimetry
(midprostate)

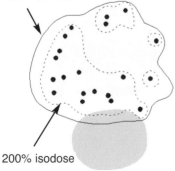

100% isodose

200% isodose

Figure 15-15. Day 1 AP film (top) and CT of patient who developed diffuse prostatic necrosis one year after a 115 Gy Pd-103 implant. The middle photos show diffuse source loss and clumping within a central necrotic cavity (*). The preplan and postplan were not unusually hot (bottom, left). To date, complications like this have been rare. But adding larger and larger treatment margins to the planning images could lead to more such cases (see chapter 6).

been reported.(HOWARD, THEODORESCU) From the limited data available, it appears that spontaneous healing of fistulas is unlikely, even with a diverting colostomy. To date, there are limited data regarding the surgical repair of rectal fistulas.(JORDAN, THEODORESCU) Colo-anal anastomosis might be an alternative to more elaborate repair procedures.

> ***Special note from K. Wallner***
> We need more information regarding the proper management of the rare patient with a prostato-rectal fistula. If you have one or more such patients, please contact me. I'm keeping a list of them with the hope of getting enough cases to figure out how best to treat them.

WE'VE PROBABLY SEEN THE WORST

Modern prostate brachytherapy, using TRUS and CT guidance, has been widely practiced only for ten years. The first few years' experience, on which most of the published morbidity data is based, almost certainly indicates a higher complication rate than should currently be expected, given what we have learned about radiation tolerance and the technical experience that has been gained. The substantial short-term and long-term morbidity in the early experiences of Wallner, Blasko, and others in the early 1990s is not representative of current implants. Morbidity in more recently treated patients, whose urethral and rectal doses were better controlled, has been much lower.(MERRICK 99, BROWN, HAN) In experienced hands, serious complications are now surprisingly infrequent. One note of caution is that late complications may surface with longer follow-up, possibly related to very high urethral doses that can occur. But we doubt it.

REFERENCES

1. Babb RR. Radiation proctitis: A review. Am J Gastro 2000; 91:1309-1311.

2. Biswal BM, Lal P, Rath GK, Shukla NK, Mohanti BK, Deo S. Intrarectal formalin application, an effective treatment for grade III haemorrhagic radiation proctitis. Radiother Oncol 1995; 35:212-215.

3. Blasko JC, Ragde H, Grimm PD. Transperineal Ultrasound-Guided Implantation of the Prostate: Morbidity and Complications. Scand J Urol Nephrol Suppl 1991; 137:113-118.

4. Brandeis JM, Litwin MS, Burnison CM, Reiter RE. Quality of life outcomes after brachytherapy for early stage prostate cancer. J Urol 2000; 163:851-857.

5. Brown D, Colonias A, Miller R, Benoit R, et al . Urinary morbidity with a modified peripheral loading technique of transperienal 125-I prostate implantation. Int J Radiat Oncol Biolo Phys 2000; 47:353-360.

6. Crook J, Esche B, Futter N. Effect of pelvic radiotherapy for prostate cancer on bowel, bladder, and sexual function: The patient's perspective. Urology 1996; 47:387-394.

7. Gelblum DY, Potters L. Rectal complications asociated with transperineal interstitial brachytherapy for prostate cancer. Int J Rad Oncol Biol Phys 2000; 48:119-124.

8. Han B, Wallner K. Dosimetric and radiographic correlates to prostate brachytherapy-related rectal complications. (submitted) 2002;

9. Howard A, Wallner K, Han B, Schneider B, et al . Rectal fistulas after prostate brachytherapy. Journal of Brachytherapy International 2001; (in press):

10. Hu K, Wallner K. Clinical course of rectal complications following I-125 prostate brachytherapy. Int J Rad Oncol Biol Phys 1998; 41:263-265.

11. Hu K, Wallner KE. Urinary incontinence in patients who have a TURP/TUIP following prostate brachytherapy. Int J Radiat Oncol Biol Phys 1998; 40:783-786.

12. Iversen P, Nielsen L, Bak M, Rasmussen F, Juul N, Torp-Pederson S, Laursen F, Holm HH, von der Maase H. Ultrasonically guided 125Iodine seed implantation with external radiation in management of localized prostatic carcinoma. Urol 1989; 34:181-186.

13. Jordan GH, Lynch DF, Warden SS, McGraw JD, Hoffman GC, Schellhammer PF. Major pelvic complications following interstitial implantation of Iodine-125 for carcinoma of the prostate. J Urol 1985; 134:1212-1214.

14. Kaassis M, Oberti F, Burtin P, Boyer J. Argon plasma coagulation for the treatment of hemorrhagic radiation proctitis. Endoscopy 2000; 32:673-676.

15. Kaye KW, Olson DJ, Payne JT. Detailed preliminary analysis of 125 iodine implantation for localized prostate cancer using percutaneous approach. J Urol 1995; 153:1020.

16. Kleinberg L, Wallner K, Roy J, Zelefsky M, Arterbery VE, Fuks Z, Harrison L. Treatment-related symptoms during the first year following transperineal I-125 prostate implantation. Int J Radiat Oncol Biol Phys 1994; 28:985.

17. Kochbar R, Patel F, Dhar A, Sharma SC, Ayyagari S, Aggarwal R, Goenka MK, Gupta BD, Mehta SK. Radiation-induced proctosigmoiditis: Prospective, randomized, double-blind controlled trial of oral sulfasalazine plus rectal steroids versus rectal sucralfate. Digestive dis sci 2000; 36:103-107.

18. Krupski T, Petroni GR, Bissonette EA, Theodorescu D. Quality-of-life comparison of radical prostatectomy and interstitial brachytherapy in the treatment of clinically localized prostate cancer. Urol 2000; 55:736-742.

19. Landis D, Wallner K, Locke J, Ellis W, Russell K, Cavanuagh W, Blasko J. Late urinary morbidity after prostate brachytherapy. (submitted) 2002;

20. Lawton CA, Won M, Pilepich MV. Long-term Treatment Sequelae Following External Beam Irradiation for Adenocarcinoma of the Prostate: Analysis of RTOG Studies 7506 and 7706. Int J Radiat Oncol Biol Phys 1991; 21:935-939.

21. Lee WR, Schultheiss TE, Hanlon AL, Hanks GE. Urinary incontinence following external beam radiotherapy for clinically localized prostate cancer. Urol 1996; 48:95-99.

22. Lim AJ, Brandon AH, Fiedler J, Brickman AL, et al . Quality of life: radical prostatectomy versus radiation therapy for prostate cancer. J Urol 1995; 154:1420-1425.

23. Merrick GS, Butler WM, Dorsey AT, Galbreath RW, Blatt H, Lief JH. Rectal function following prostate brachytherapy. Int J Rad Oncol Biol Phys 2000; 48:667-674.

24. Merrick GS, Butler WM, Dorsey AT, Lief JH, Walbert HL, Blatt HJ. Rectal dosimetric analysis following prostate brachytherapy. Int J Rad Oncol Biol Phys 1999; 43:1021-1027.

25. Merrick GS, Butler WM, Lief JH, Dorsey AT. Temporal resolution of urinary morbidity following prostate brachytherapy. Int J Radiat Oncol Biolo Phys 2000; 47:121-128.

26. Merrick GS, Butler WM, Tollenaar BG, Galbreath RW, Lief JH. The dosimetry of prostate brachytherapy-induced urethral strictures. (submitted) 2002;

27. Patel J, Worthen R, Abadir R, Weaver DJ, Weinstein S, Ross G. Late results of combined Iodine-125 and external beam radiotherapy in carcinoma of prostate. Urol 1990; 36:27-30.

28. Roche B, Chautems R, Marti MC. Application of formaldehyde for treatment of hemorrhagic radiation-induced proctitits. World J Surg 1996; 20:1092-1095.

29. Shipley WU, Zietman AL, Hanks GE, Coen JJ, Caplan RJ, Won M, Zagars GK, Asbell SO. Treatment related sequelae following external beam radiation for prostate cancer: A review with an update in patients with Stages T1 and T2 tumor. J Urol 1994; 152:1799-1805.

30. Smith S, Wallner K, Han B, Sutlief S, Blasko J, Dominitz J, Billingsley K. Argon plasma coagulation for rectal bleeding following prostate brachytherapy . (submitted) 2000;

31. Stone NN, Ratnow ER, Stock RG. Prior transurethral resection does not increase morbidity following real-time ultrasound-guided prostate seed implantation. Tech Urol 2000; 6:123-127.

32. Syed AM, Puthawala A, Austin P, Cherlow J. Temporary iridium-192 implant in the management of carcinoma of the prostate. Cancer 1992; 69:2515-2524.

33. Talcott JA, Clark JC, Stark P, Nadir B, Ragde H. Long-term treatment-related complications of brachytherapy for early prostate cancer: A survey of treated patients. Proc ASCO 1999; 18:311a.

34. Teshima T, Hanks GE, Hanlon AL, Peter RS, Schultheiss TE. Rectal bleeding after conformal 3D treatment of prostate cancer: Time to occurrence, response to treatment and duration of morbidity. Int J Radiat Oncol Biol Phys 1997; 39:77-83.

35. Theodorescu D, Gillenwater JY, Koutrouvelis PG. Prostatourethral-rectal fistula after prostate brachytherapy: Incidence and risk factors. Cancer 2000; 89:2085-2091.

36. Viggiano TR, Zighelboim J, Ahlquist DA, Gostout CJ, Wang KK, Larson MV. Endoscopic Nd:YAG laser coagulation of bleeding from radiation proctopathy. Gastrointest endosc 2000; 39:513-517.

37. Wallner K, Lee H, Wasserman S, Dattoli M. Low risk of urinary incontinence following prostate brachytherapy in patients with a prior TURP. Int J Radiat Oncol Biol Phys 1997; 37:565-569.

38. Wallner KE, Roy J, Harrison L. Dosimetry guidelines to minimize urethral and rectal morbidity following transperineal I-125 prostate brachytherapy. Int J Radiat Oncol Biol Phys 1995; 32:465-471.

39. Wallner KE, Roy J, Harrison L. Tumor control and morbidity following transperineal I-125 implantation for Stage T1/T2 prostatic carcinoma. J Clin Oncol 1996; 14:449-453.

40. Wei JT, Dunn RL, Litwin MS, Sandler HM, Sanda MG. Development and validation of the expanded prostate cancer index composite (EPIC) for comprehensive assessment of health-related quality of life in men with prostate cancer. Urol 2000; 56:899-905.

41. Zeitlin SI, Sherman J, Raboy A, Lederman G, Albert P. High dose combination radiotherapy for the treatment of localized prostate cancer. J Urol 1998; 160:91-96.

16

Potency

Potency loss is the most common, permanent sequela of treatment for early-stage prostate cancer. Brachytherapy is generally believed to offer some advantage over surgery or external radiation in regards to potency preservation, but the true magnitude of its advantage is still unclear.

DEFINITION

Quantification of treatment effects requires a working definition of sexual potency. The one used typically in mainstream surgical literature is *the ability to maintain an erection sufficient for intercourse.* The most widely quoted potency figures, by the most widely known surgeons, are based on this simple, practical

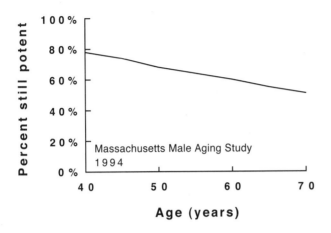

Figure 16-1. Sexual potency versus age in the general population. Data are based on personal interviews.(FELDMAN)

definition.(CATALONA, QUINLAN) Unfortunately, this definition leaves considerable room for interpretation on the part of the patient and the investigator. Critics of the current state of affairs have called for more detailed criteria.(ZINREICH, BANKER) Quality-of-life experts are using increasingly sophisticated measures of sexual function—quantifiers such as "sexual bother" or "SFIQ scores" are becoming commonplace.(KRUPSKI, BRANDEIS) The problem with these more sophisticated but more nebulous measures is that they make it difficult for physicians and patients to relate to the findings, an effect that prostatectomy proponents probably find appealing.

SPONTANEOUS POTENCY LOSS
Analysis of the effect of treatment on potency is clouded by the fact that prostate cancer occurs in an age group for which there is a substantial incidence of impotence prior to treatment. As much as 50% of men are already impotent by the time they are diagnosed with prostatic carcinoma.(ZINREICH) The Massachusetts Male Aging Study summarized the incidence of impotence versus age in normal men.(FELDMAN) Based on personal interviews, men between the ages of 40 and 80 spontaneously lose potency at a rate of approximately 1.5% per year (**Figure 16-1**). In the short term, gradual, "natural" potency loss should not substantially affect treatment-related potency changes. However, with increasing follow-up time, age-related potency changes need to be taken into consideration.

COLLECTING POTENCY INFORMATION
Collecting potency data is frequently an exercise in frustration. Patients sometimes are surprisingly inconsistent in their responses, for a variety of reasons. Many are simply not sexually active at this time of their life and others are reluctant to admit

potency loss. Most vexing are the substantial fluctuations in sexual function in the first few years after brachytherapy, probably related to development and resolution of radiation-related inflammation.

Another common assumption regarding analysis of potency status is that spouses should be interviewed separately, because patients may not be realistic or honest in reporting their erectile capacity. On the contrary, patients and spouses generally report similar function.(ZINREICH, CHINN) Another commonly raised concern has been that potency data should be verified with physiologic testing, in order to be more objective. But considering that patients and spouses are generally consistent in their answers when interviewed separately, the necessity of physiologic testing is questionable.

CAUSES

The mechanism of radiation-related impotence is not known. An early report of radiation-induced arterial occlusion of the internal iliac, internal pudendal, and penile arteries, based on only two patients, has never been confirmed.(GOLDSTEIN) Pelvic neural testing after external beam radiation has been unremarkable, not surprising considering that peripheral nerves readily tolerate high doses in the course of radiation for extremity sarcomas and other pelvic tumors.(GOLDSTEIN) Radiation-induced impotence generally responds to intracavernosal papaverine or PGE1 injection or to Viagra™.(PIERCE, MERRICK 99, ZELEFSKY 99) The relationship between a response to pharmacologic agents and the mechanism(s) of impotence is unclear. Whether impotence is due to arterial, venous, neural, or some other type of damage, pharmacologic agents may work simply by virtue of bolstering a multicompromised system. It is likely that radiation-related impotence will turn out to be multifactorial, with radiation damage to the neurovascular bundles and to the penile venous system being the most obvious candidates for the blame.(ZELEFSKY 98)

Neurovascular bundles

Walsh and colleagues have attributed postprostatectomy impotence to neurovascular bundle (NVB) trauma.(LEPOR, WALSH) Similarly, excessive radiation doses to vascular or neural components of the NVBs might account for brachytherapy-related impotence. The typical onset of radiation-related impotence, months or years after treatment, is more consistent with delayed radiation damage as the cause of impotence, rather than to needle trauma.

To investigate the role of NVB radiation doses in brachytherapy-related impotence, DiBiase and colleagues estimated the doses in brachytherapy patients

CT   TRUS   MR

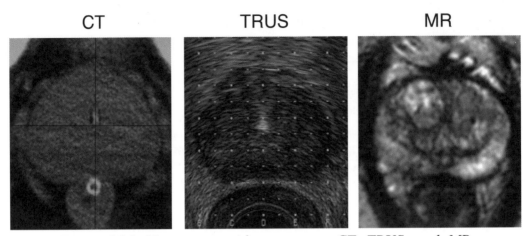

Figure 16-2. Transverse mid-prostate on CT, TRUS, and MR. Contrary to some claims in the literature, the NVBs are not typically well visualized with any modality. Published studies of NVB doses have instead relied on arbitrary NVB location estimates.(DIB-IASE, MERRICK 01)

treated at the University of Washington and the Puget Sound VA. Because the NVBs cannot be visualized consistently on CT, TRUS or MR (**Figure 16-2**), calculation points were taken posterior-laterally, 2.0 mm from the prostatic capsule, according to the anatomic description of Lepor and colleagues (**Figure 16-3 & 16-4**).(LEPOR)

In contrast to popular perception, NVB doses were usually far higher than the prescription dose, because of the typical 3–6 mm treatment margins that typically lie beyond the NVBs (see chapter 6). Doses varied widely between the right and left side of the same patient and among patients (**Figures 16-5 and 16-6**). Average NVB doses along the course of the NVB ranged from 150% to 200% of the prescription dose and are similar for Pd-103 and I-125 (**Figure 16-7**).

Merrick and colleagues did not find a relationship between NVB doses and impotence among patients followed up to four years postimplantation (**Figure 16-8**).(MERRICK 00) The lack of an effect of NVB radiation doses is consistent with growing evidence that NVBs are not as crucial to potency as alleged by investigators at Johns Hopkins University Hospitals.(KIM) Also keep in mind that the two classic reports regarding NVB location were each based on a single autopsy study, and that more sophisticated intraoperative investigations are raising considerable doubt about the location and function of the NVBs.(WALSH, LEPOR, MICHL)

posterior view   cross-section

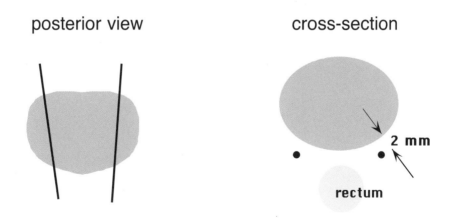

Figure 16-3. The neurovascular bundles are allegedly located approximately 2 millimeters from the posterior prostatic capsule.(LEPOR) The problem with using this description is that it is based on only two cases.(WALSH, LEPOR) There is remarkably little other published information regarding the typical location of the NVBs.

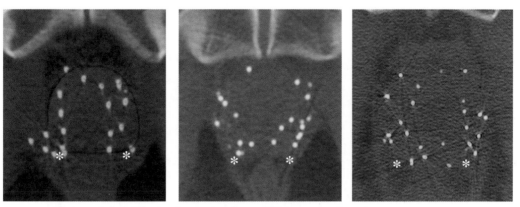

Figure 16-4. Typical postimplant CT images showing sources near or even behind the neurovascular bundles (*). Typical postimplant images like these have lead us to question the assertion by Stock and colleagues that brachytherapy is a NVB-sparing therapy. (STOCK 96)

16.5

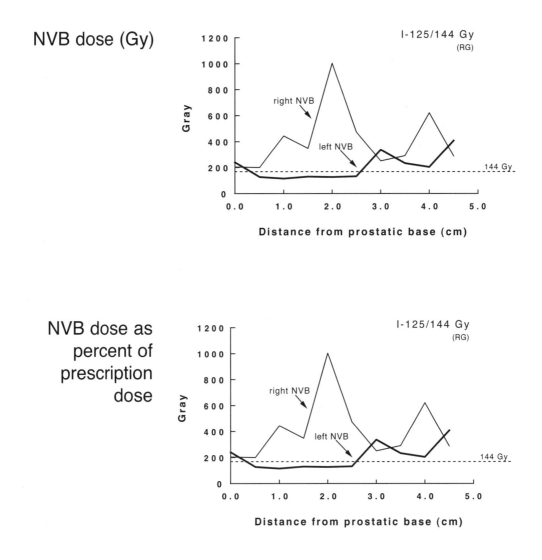

Figure 16-5. NVB doses from base to apex of the prostate expressed in Gy (top panel) or as the percentage of the prescription dose (lower panel). Note the substantial difference from one side to the next, a typical finding among patients.

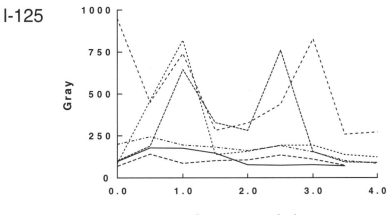

I-125

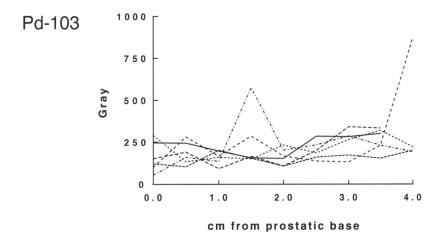

Pd-103

Figure 16-6. Composite NVB doses from three unselected I-125 (top) and Pd-103 (lower panel) patients. Note the remarkable variability among patients.

16.7

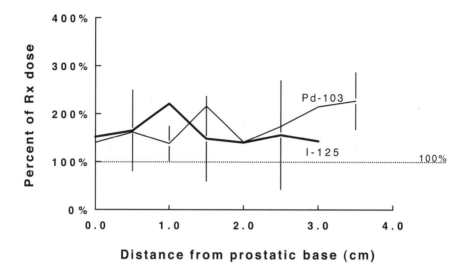

Figure 16-7. Average NVB doses expressed as the percentage of the prescription dose from base to apex of the prostate for full dose I-125 or Pd-103 implants. Note the similarities in the averages between the two isotopes.(DIBIASE)

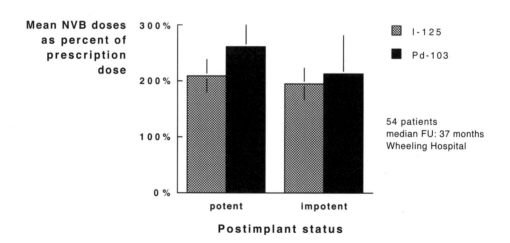

Figure 16-8. NVB doses among patients with or without post-implant impotence.(MERRICK 00)

16.8

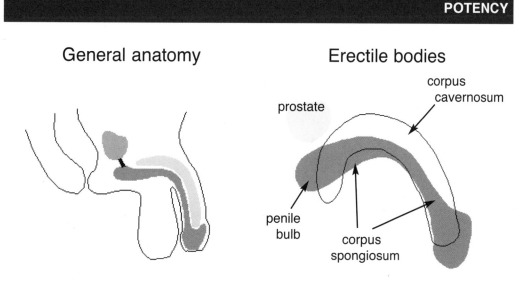

Figure 16-9 .General anatomy and erectile bodies of the penis.

However, because the onset of impotence is often delayed by several years, longer follow-up may show some relationship between dose and treatment-related sexual dysfunction. In the next few years, the role that NVB doses have on potency impairment should be clarified, by correlating NVB dose calculations with larger numbers of patients with longer follow-up.

PENILE BULB
A second possible cause of radiation-induced impotence is venous insufficiency from damage to the proximal corpus spongiosum, or *bulb,* of the penis (**Figure 16-9**). Separated from the prostate by the striated urethral sphincter, the bulb typically lies 0.5–1.0 cm below the prostatic apex and is fairly well visualized on CT, TRUS, or MR (**Figures 16-10 & 16-11**). It typically has a volume of 5–7 cc and usually receives a maximal radiation dose of about 50% of the brachytherapy prescription dose (**Figure 16-12 & 16-13**).

Venous leakage is increasingly being considered as a mechanism of postradiation impotence. Pickett, Roach, and colleagues have shown that bulb doses from external beam radiation correlate well with posttherapy impotence (**Figure 16-14**).(PICKETT, ROACH)

Brachytherapy doses to the penile bulb depend on the distance between the prostatic apex and bulb, as well as the magnitude of the planning treatment margins. Because of the proximity of the bulb to the prostatic apex and the tendency to use

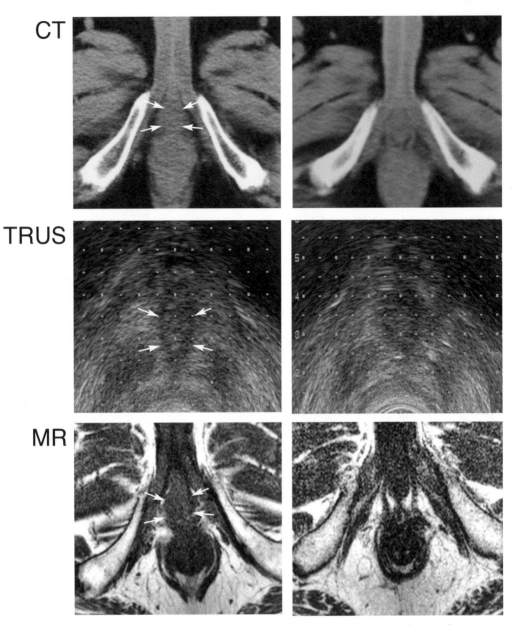

Figure 16-10. Typical CT, TRUS, or MR images through the mid-bulb (arrows). The bulb shows up surprisingly well on preimplant scans, but not as clearly in the postimplant setting (see Figures 16-12 and 16-13).

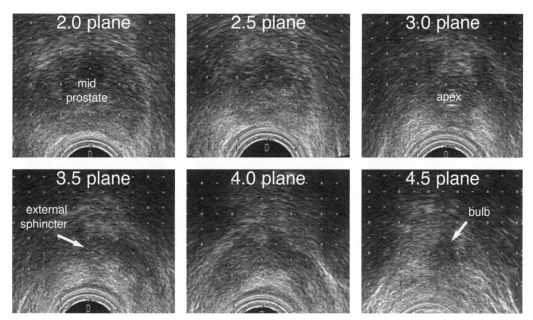

Figure 16-11. The bulbous spongiosum is typically separated from the prostatic apex by 5–10 mm of the striated external sphincter/pelvic floor. In this series of TRUS images, the prostatic apex ends at the 3.0 plane, and the top of the bulb is seen at the 4.5 plane.

generous treatment margins at the the apex, it is fairly common that sources are adjacent or even inside of the bulb (**Figures 16-12 & 13**). Cases of excessive peribulbar sources are not difficult to find (**Figures 16-15 & 16-16**).

Using post-implant CT to identify the bulb, Merrick and colleagues showed a strong correlation between bulb doses and postimplant impotence (**Figure 16-17**).(MERRICK 01) While this work is highly suggestive that bulb doses are important, postbrachytherapy potency frequently fluctuates in the years following implantation, so that longer-term follow-up is needed to determine their precise role in permanent impotence. In the future, it is likely that NVB and penile bulb dose parameters will be incorporated into dosimetry guidelines to maximize tumor control and minimize treatment-related morbidity.

BRACHYTHERAPY-RELATED SEXUAL DYSFUNCTION
While most reports of treatment-related dysfunction have focused exclusively on erectile function, there are a variety of subtle and not-so-subtle changes in sexual function following brachytherapy, most of which are just now being

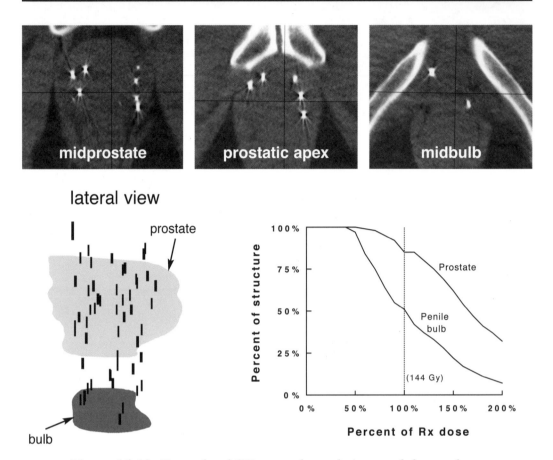

Figure 16-12. Example of CT scans, lateral view, and dose volume histogram of prostate and penile bulb doses from a 144 Gy I-125 implant. Note that in this patient, several sources were placed distal to the prostatic apex, resulting in higher-than-average bulb doses. 51% of the 6 cc bulb received a dose in excess of the prescription, which is high even by external beam radiation standards.

16.12

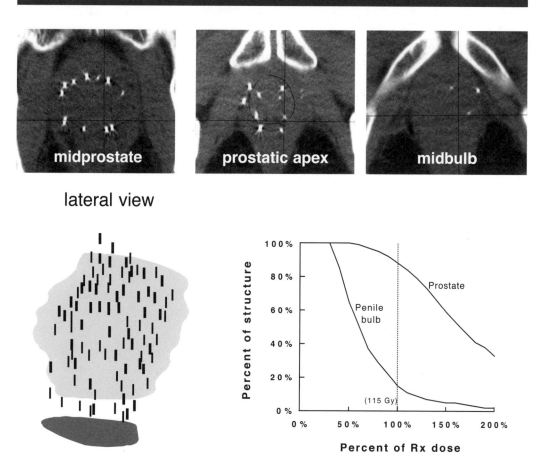

Figure 16-13. Example of CT scans, lateral view, and dose volume histogram of prostate and penile bulb doses from a 115 Gy Pd-103 implant. In this patient, fewer sources were near the bulb, with only 15% of the 4.9 cc bulb volume receiving in excess of the prescription dose.

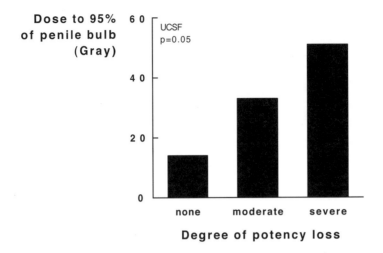

Figure 16-14. Bulb doses from external beam radiation correlate with posttreatment impotence.(PICKETT)

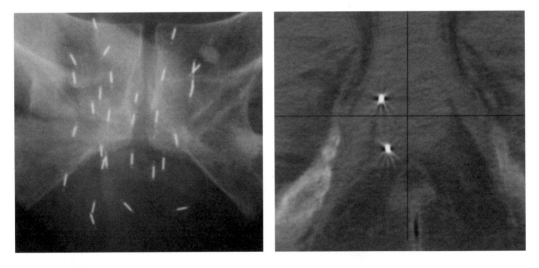

Figure 16-15. One cause of excessive penile bulb brachytherapy doses is that sources are pulled too far inferiorly. In this example, several sources were deposited too distal. Mistakes like this probably contribute to brachytherapy-related impotence. As we learn more about where not to place sources, it should be possible to decrease the adverse potency effects of brachytherapy.

16.14

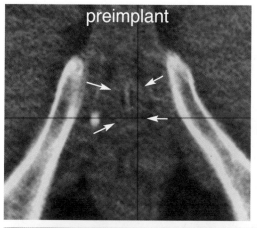
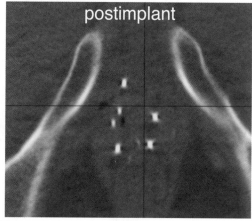

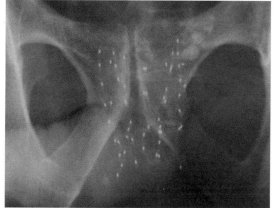

Figure 16-16. Another example of excessive sources around the penile bulb (arrows), a result of overly generous treatment planning margins at the prostatic apex. Notice how low the implant extends on the anterior view (left).

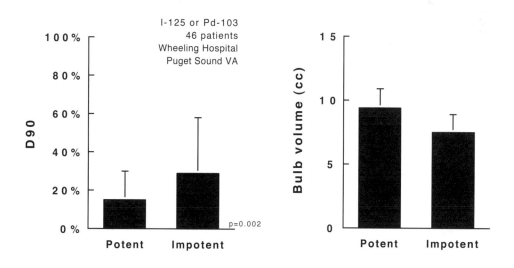

Figure 16-17. Mean penile bulb doses (left) and volumes (right) in patients with or without postimplant impotence.(MERRICK 01)

16.15

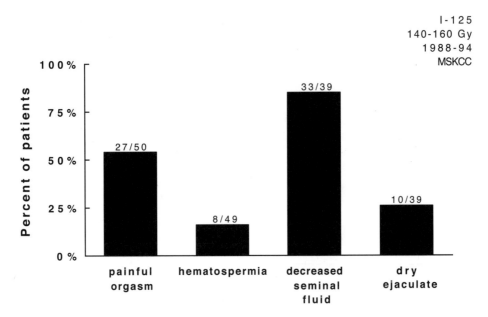

Figure 16-18. Incidence of painful ejaculation, bloody seminal fluid, or dry ejaculate in patients treated with I-125 implant at MSKCC.

described.(MERRICK 02) None of the popular quality of life scales adequately addresses brachytherapy-related symptoms.

Acute sexual sequelae
Patients commonly experience burning with orgasm (orgalmasia) in their first six to twelve postimplant months, probably related to inflammation of the terminal portion of the ejaculatory ducts and the urethra. In retrospective surveys, approximately one-third to one-half of patients report painful ejaculation for several months or longer, necessitating temporary abstinence (**Figure 16-18 & 6-19**).(MERRICK 02) Bloody ejaculate is very common in the first several weeks after implantation, without apparent significance. Patients commonly report a diminished amount of ejaculate fluid and a change in its consistency in the first few years following brachytherapy. Dry ejaculate occurs in approximately one-fourth of patients. Similarly, intermittent bloody semen (hematospermia) occurs commonly, as both an early and late phenomenon. It is probably due to radiation-induced capillary fragility and seems to be of no clinical significance.

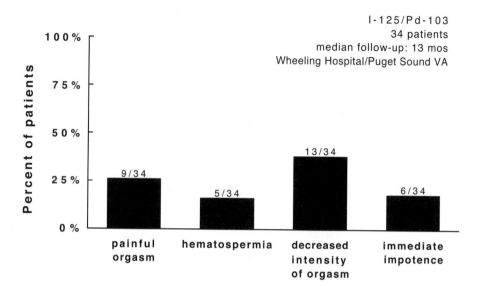

Figure 16-19. Sexual symptomatology among patients randomized to I-125 or Pd-103.(MERRICK 02)

Some patients develop impotence immediately after their implant procedure, presumably due to needle trauma to the neurovascular bundles or venous bodies (**Figure 16-19**). Patients with acute postimplant impotence often spontaneously improve over time, but the likelihood of recovery has not yet been well documented.

Erectile dysfunction

There has been wide discrepancy among investigators regarding the likelihood of potency preservation after brachytherapy, for several reasons. First, it is becoming increasingly apparent that potency rates are highly dependent on how much time has passed from the implant date. Favorable reports of high potency rates after brachytherapy were almost uniformly based on short-term follow-up of 1–3 years. Unfortunately, the likelihood of impotence increases in the 10 years after radiation, a phenomenon first revealed by Bagshaw and colleagues in the 1980s but conveniently ignored by advocates of both external beam and implant radiation.(BAGSHAW)

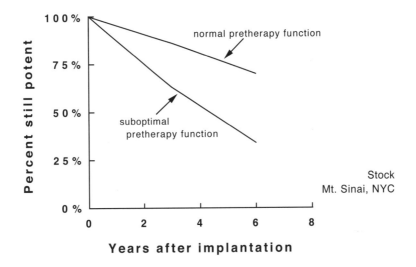

Figure 16-20. Increased potency loss in patients with diminished preimplant function.(STOCK 01)

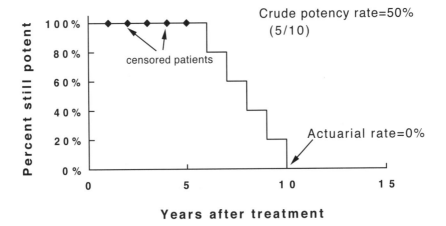

Figure 16-21. Example of crude versus actuarial potency rates. Assume that one patient is treated per year from 1985 through 1995 and that the first five patients become impotent in 1995, the year that the potency rate is calculated. Actuarial calculation gives a potency rate of 0% at 10 years, while the crude rate is 5 of 10, or 50%!

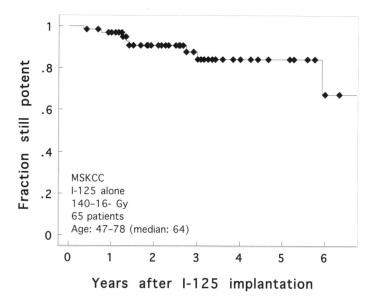

Figure 16-22. Potency preservation following I-125 implantation at MSKCC, based on the potency definition of ability to have an erection sufficient for intercourse. Data was collected from personal interview (K. Wallner). This graph shows the worst case scenario, in that patients who voiced concern about the quality of their erections or erectile time were considered impotent, even if they were able to achieve vaginal penetration. The data would look better with less strict interpretation of the patients' potency perception.

A second reason for the discrepancy regarding postimplant potency preservation is that rates may vary depending on the degree of compromise prior to therapy. Stock and colleagues have shown that patients with substantially compromised preimplant erectile function are at higher risk of complete impotence than are patients with full potency (**Figure 16-20**). This variability in potency with the level of pretherapy functioning is exacerbated by frequent potency fluctuation over time in the postimplant period, a phenomenon that hasn't been adequately addressed to date.

A third reason for discrepancies in postimplant potency rates has been the (mis)use of statistical methods—the use of crude percentages can grossly inflate the potency preservation rates. Because potency rates decline over time, actuarial statistics, which account for length of time patients have been followed since treat-

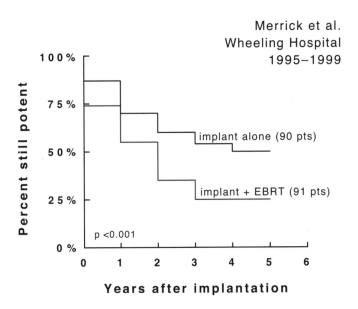

Figure 16-23. Potency preservation following implantation with or without supplemental beam radiation (manuscript in preparation).

ment, give a much more realistic potency rate calculation (**Figure 16-21**). Surprisingly, most published series from mainstream academicians have used crude rates and short follow-up times.

At Memorial Sloan-Kettering Cancer Center (MSKCC), the actuarial potency rate at five years following I-125 implantation in fully potent patients was 79% (**Figure 16-22**). The potency rate continued to fall over time, but only a small percent of patients have been followed beyond five years. Merrick and colleagues have shown greater potency loss in patients who receive supplemental external beam radiation (**Figure 16-23**). In some series, younger patients do better than older ones (**Figure 16-24**). However, in multivariate analysis of patients treated to 70–80 Gy with conformal external beam radiation or brachytherapy at MSKCC, antiandrogen use and patient age were not associated with diminished potency preservation. (ZELEFSKY 99)

COMPARING MODALITIES

Despite the huge number of patients treated with external beam radiation during the last thirty years, long-term reports regarding potency preservation are amazingly few, a red flag that outcomes are much worse than commonly acknowledged. The largest series regarding the effect of external beam radiation on potency is

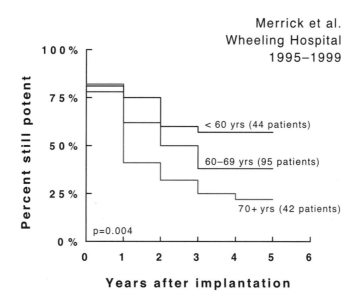

Merrick et al.
Wheeling Hospital
1995–1999

16-24. Potency preservation by age group (manuscript in preparation).

from Stanford, based on a questionnaire mailed to patients.(BAGSHAW) Potency was preserved in 86% of patients at fifteen months after treatment, but only in 50% at 5 years (**Figure 16-25**). The loss of potency decelerated at 30%, approximately ten years after treatment. Drs. Bagshaw, Cox and Ray should be congratulated on their early interest and statistical prowess but their results should be interpreted cautiously, because they are based on an anonymous survey of a small percent of patients treated, and with no mention of how potency was defined. More recently, Zelefsky and colleagues reported longer-term actuarial potency preservation rates following 3D conformal external beam radiation, with their rates being somewhat better than those reported by Bagshaw (**Figure 16-25**). The relationship between potency loss and radiation volume, patient age, field size, or radiation dose has not been rigorously examined.

In the early 1980s, Walsh and colleagues alleged that potency could often be preserved after radical prostatectomy if the pelvic splanchnic nerves were identified and preserved.(WALSH) In the most favorable report by Dr. Walsh at Johns Hopkins University, maintenance of potency was achieved in approximately 60% of patients, with markedly better results in younger patients. Patients younger than 60 years of age had a 68% likelihood of maintaining potency, versus 55% in patients 60 years or older.(QUINLAN)

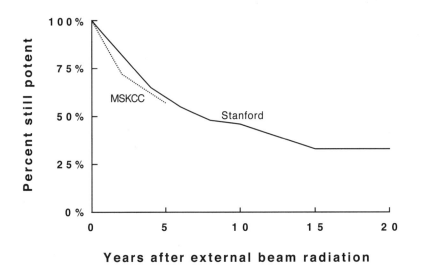

Figure 16-25. Longer-term potency preservation in external beam patients treated at Stanford with conventional external beam radiation or at Memorial Sloan-Kettering (MSKCC) with conformal radiation.(BAGSHAW, ZELEFSKY 99)

While the potential for potency-sparing surgery was quickly parroted by urologists around the world, giddy reports by surgeons at Johns Hopkins should be viewed skeptically, at best—they have not been widely reproduced by other surgeons and their favorable data have never been verified by an independent observer. Most disturbing is that potency rates by other experienced surgeons have typically been far, far lower (**Figures 16-26 & 16-27**). And like most external radiation series, no surgical series has included actuarial calculations, which would probably substantially decrease the stated rates of potency preservation. Furthermore, no investigator has ever reported longer-term follow-up of post-nerve-sparing prostatectomy potency preservation, numbers that would seem to be of prime interest given the frequent recommendation that "young patients should be treated by prostatectomy rather than radiation" (**Figure 16-28**).

TREATMENT
Patients who develop radiation-related impotence generally respond to corrective measures. Treatment with vasoactive agents after external beam radiation is usually successful.(PIERCE) Patients with treatment-related impotence after surgery or any form of radiation are likely to respond favorably to Viagra™/sildenafil (**Figure

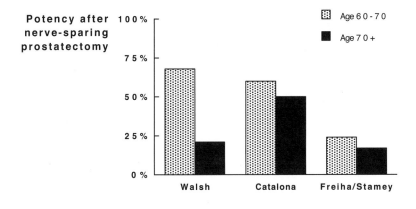

Figure 16-26. More examples of the tremendous variability in reported potency preservation rates following nerve-sparing prostatectomy.(QUINLAN, GEARY, CATALONA)

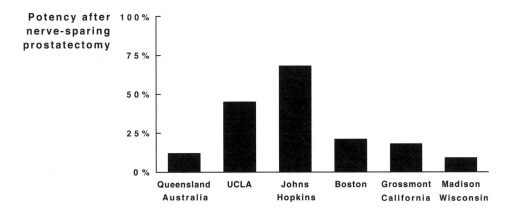

Figure 16-27. There is a large, perplexing variation in reported potency preservation rates following nerve-sparing prostatectomy.(TALCOTT, RITCHIE, QUINLAN, HEATHCOTE, GAYLIS, JONLER) *Either some surgeons are an awfully lot better than others, or some are particularly adept at massaging their data. Chances are, both factors are at work!*

16.23

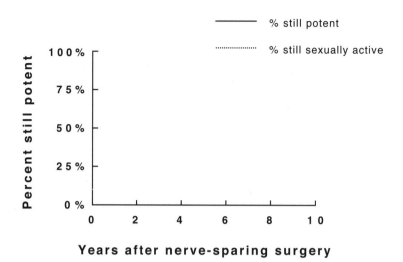

—————— % still potent

················· % still sexually active

Figure 16-28. Compilation of long-term potency follow-up reports after nerve-sparing prostatectomy. (No mistake here—there are none!)

16-29). There is no clear correlation with clinical or implant parameters and the response to Viagra.(MERRICK 99)

Penile implants typically are highly effective and well tolerated in radiation patients.(DUBOCQ) However, considering that brachytherapy patients commonly recover some erectile function with time, mechanical implants should be recommended cautiously, because their placement usually destroys any remaining erectile function.

While the success of therapies for brachytherapy-related impotence has been a pleasant surprise, enthusiasm for corrective measures should be tempered by reports of high attrition rates for potency therapies in general.(MULHALL, VARDI)

WHOM SHOULD WE BELIEVE?
The precise effect that different treatment modalities have on potency is still far from clear. In general, reported potency rates following brachytherapy have been higher than those following prostatectomy or external beam radiation. However, comparisons between modalities should be made with caution and qualification, considering the dearth of good quality actuarial long-term data for any modality. In the meantime, judging from the available data from disparate sources to date,

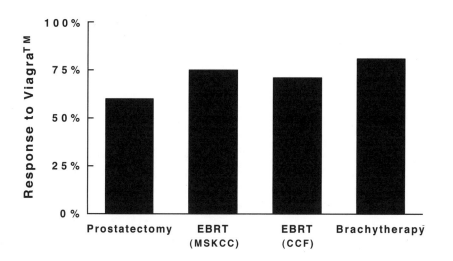

Figure 16-29. Approximate response to Viagra/sildenafil after prostatectomy, external beam radiation (EBRT), or brachytherapy. (LOWENTRITT, ZELEFSKY 99, KEDIA, MERRICK 99)

brachytherapy probably offers less potency preservation advantage than once believed.

REFERENCES

1. Bagshaw MA, Cox RS, Ray GR. Status of Radiation of Prostate Cancer at Stanford University. NCI Monogr 1988; 7:47-60.

2. Banker RL. The preservation of potency after external beam irradiation for prostate cancer. Int J Radiat Oncol Biol Phys 1988; 15:219-220.

3. Brandeis JM, Litwin MS, Burnison CM, Reiter RE. Quality of life outcomes after brachytherapy for early stage prostate cancer. J Urol 2000; 163:851-857.

4. Catalona WJ, Basler JW. Return of erections and urinary continence following nerve sparing radical retropubic prostatectomy. J Urol 1993; 150:905-907.

5. Chinn DM, Holland J, Crownover RL, Roach M. Potency following high-dose three-dimensional conformal radiotherapy and the impact of prior major urologic surgical procedures in patients treated for prostate cancer. Int J Radiat Oncol Biol Phys 1995; 33:15-22.

6. DeLaney TF, Shipley WU, O'Leary MP, Biggs PJ, Prout GR. Preoperative irradiation and 125-Iodine implantation for patients with localized carcinoma of the prostate. Int J Radiat Oncol Biol Phys 1986; 12:1779-1785.

7. DiBiase SJ, Wallner KE, Tralins K, Sutlief S. Brachytherapy radiation doses to the neurovascular bundles. Int J Rad Oncol Biol Phys 2000; 46:1301-1307.

8. Dubocq FM, Bianco FJ, Maralani SJ, Forman JD, Dhabuwala CB. Outcome analysis of penile implant surgery after external beam radiation for prostate cancer. J Urol 1997; 158:1787-1790.

9. Feldman HA, Goldstein I, Hatzichristou DG, et al . Impotence and its medical and psychosocial correlates: Results of the Massachusetts Male Aging Study. J Urol 1994; 151:54-61.

10. Fisch BM, Pickett B, Weinberg V, Roach M. Dose of radiation received by the bulb of the penis correlates with risk of impotence after three-dimensional conformal radiotherapy for prostate cancer. Urol 2001; 57:955-959.

11. Fowler JE, Barzell W, Hilaris BS, Whitmore WF. Complications of 125-Iodine Implantation and Pelvic Lymphadenectomy in the Treatment of Prostatic Cancer. J Urol 1979; 121:447-451.

12. Gaylis FD, Friedel WE, Armas OA. Radical retropubic prostatectomy outcomes at a community hospital. J Urol 1998; 159:167-171.

13. Geary ES, Dendinger TE, Freiha FS, Stamey TA. Nerve sparing radical prostatectomy: A different view. J Urol 1995; 154:145-149.

14. Goldstein I, Feldman MI, Deckers PJ, et al . Radiation-associated impotence: A clinical study of its mechanism. JAMA 1984; 251:903-910.

15. Heathcote PS, Mactaggart PN, Boston RJ, James AN, Thompson LC, Nicol DL. Health-related quality of life in Australian men remaining disease-free after radical prostatectomy. MJA 2001; 168:483-486.

16. Jonler M, Messing EM, Rhodes PR, Bruskewitz RC. Sequelae of radical prostatectomy. Br J Urol 1994; 74:352-358.

17. Kedia S, Zippe CD, Agarwal A, Nelson DR, Lakin MM. Treatment of erectile dysfunction with sildenafil citrate (Viagra) after radiation therapy for prostate cancer. Urol 1999; 54:308-312.

18. Kim HL, Stoffel DS, Mhoon DA, Brandler CB. A positive CaverMap response poorly predicts recovery of potency after radical prostatectomy. Urol 2000; 56:561-564.

19. Krupski T, Petroni GR, Bissonette EA, Theodorescu D. Quality-of-life comparison of radical prostatectomy and interstitial brachytherapy in the treatment of clinically localized prostate cancer. Urol 2000; 55:736-742.

20. Lepor H, Gregerman M, Crosby R, et al . Precise localization of the autonomic nerves from the pelvic plexus to the corpora cavernosa: A detailed anatomical study of the adult male pelvis. J Urol 1985; 133:207-212.

21. Lowentritt BH, Scardino PT, Miles BJ, Orejuela FJ, Schatte EC, Slawin KM, Elliott SP, Kim ED. Sildenafil citrate after radical retropubic prostatectomy. J Urol 1999; 162:1614-1617.

22. Mantz CA, Song P, Farhangi E, et al . Potency probability following conformal megavoltage radiotherapy using conventional doses for localized prostate cancer. Int J Radiat Oncol Biol Phys 1997; 37:551-557.

23. Merrick GS, Butler WM, Dorsey AT, Lief JH, Donzella JG. A comparison of radiation dose to the neurovascular bundles in men with and without prostate brachytherapy induced erectile dysfunction. Int J Rad Oncol Biol Phys 2000; 48:1065-1070.

24. Merrick GS, Butler WM, Lief JH, Stipetich RL, Abel LJ, Dorsey AT. Efficacy of sildenafil citrate in prostate brachytherapy patients with erectile dysfunction. Urol 1999; 53:1112-1116.

25. Merrick GS, Wallner K, Butler WM, Galbreath RW, Lief JH, Benson ML. A comparison of radiation dose to the bulb of the penis in men with and without prostate brachytherapy induced erectile dysfunction. Int J Rad Oncol Biol Phys 2001; (in press):

26. Merrick GS, Wallner KE, Butler WM, Lief JH, Sutlief S. Sexual function after prostate brachytherapy. (submitted) 2002;

27. Michl U, Dietz R, Huland H. Is intraoperative electrostimulation of erectile nerves possible? J Urol 1999; 162:1610-1613.

28. Mulhall JP, Jahoda AE, Cairney M, et al . The causes of patient dropout from penile self-injection therapy for impotence. J Urol 1999; 162:1291-1294.

29. Pickett B, Fisch BM, Weinberg V, Roach M. Dose to the bulb of the penis is associated with the risk of impotence following radiotherapy for prostate cancer. Int J Rad Oncol Biol Phys 1999; 45(supp):263.

30. Pierce LJ, Whittington R, Hanno PM, et al . Pharmacologic erection with intra-cavernosal injection for men with sexual dysfunction following irradiation: A preliminary report. Int J Radiat Oncol Biol Phys 1991; 21:1311-1314.

31. Quinlan DM, Epstein JI, Carter BS, Walsh PC. Sexual Function Following Radical Prostatectomy: Influence of Preservation of Neurovascular Bundles. J Urol 1991; 145:998-1002.

32. Reddy EK, Mebust WK, Weigel JW, Krishnan L. Iodine-125 Implantation in Localized Prostatic Cancer. Endo/Hypertherm Oncol 1990; 6:239-244.

33. Ritchie AWS, James K, deKiernion JB. Early post-operative morbidity of total prostatectomy. Br J Urol 1989; 64:511-515.

34. Roach M, Winter K, Michalski J, Bosch W, Lin X. Mean dose to the bulb of the penis correlates with risk of impotence at 24 months: preliminary analysis of Radiation Therapy Group (RTOG) phase I/II dose escalation trial 9406. Int J Rad Oncol Biol Phys 2000; 48:#2104.

35. Stock RG, Kao JK, Stone NN. Penile erectile function after permanent radioactive seed implantation for the treatment of prostate cancer. J Urol 2001; 165:436-439.

36. Stock RG, Stone NN, Iannuzzi C. Sexual potency following interactive ultrasound-guided brachytherapy for prostate cancer. Int J Radiat Oncol Biol Phys 1996; 35:267-272.

37. Talcott JA, Rieker P, Propert KJ, Clark JA, et al . Patient-reported impotence and incontinence after nerve-sparing radical prostatectomy. J Natl Ca Inst 1997; 89:1117-1123.

38. Vardi Y, Sprecher E, Gruenwald I. Logistic regression and survival analysis of 450 impotent patients treated with injection therapy: long-term dropout parameters. J Urol 2000; 163:467-470.

39. Wallner KE, Roy J, Harrison L. Dosimetry guidelines to minimize urethral and rectal morbidity following transperineal I-125 prostate brachytherapy. Int J Radiat Oncol Biol Phys 1995; 32:465-471.

40. Walsh PC, Donker PJ. Impotence following radical prostatectomy: Insight into etiology and prevention. J Urol 1982; 128:492-497.

41. Zelefsky MJ, Eid JF. Elucidating the etiology of erectile dysfunction after definitive therapy for prostatic cancer. Int J Rad Oncol Biol Phys 1998; 40:129-133.

42. Zelefsky MJ, McKee AB, Lee H, Leibel SA. Efficacy of oral sildenafil in patients with erectile dysfunction after radiotherapy for carcinoma of the prostate. Urol 1999; 53:775-778.

43. Zelefsky MJ, Wallner KE, Ling CC, Raben A, et al . Comparison of the 5-year outcome and morbidity of three-dimensional conformal radiotherapy versus transperineal permanent iodine-125 implantation for earl-stage prostatic cancer. J Clin Oncol 1999; 17:517-522.

44. Zinreich ES, Derogatis LR, Herpst J, Auvil G, Piantadosi S, Order SE. Pre and posttreatment evaluation of sexual function in patients with adenocarcinoma of the prostate. Int J Radiat Biol Phys 1990; 19:729-732.

17

Salvage Therapy

There are two aspects with regard to salvage therapy and brachytherapy—the use of implants as salvage, and salvage for a failed implant. Data regarding either situation are limited.

IMPLANTS AS SALVAGE THERAPY

The biggest potential use for brachytherapy as salvage is for patients with local tumor persistence after external beam irradiation. With conventional dose external beam radiation, the likelihood of persistent intraprostatic cancer has been high in most series, and the number of patients who might be considered for brachytherapy salvage is huge—approximately 20% of the 40,000 patients treated with exter-

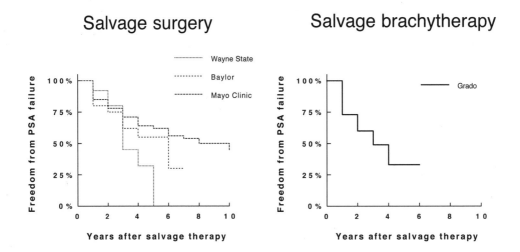

Figure 17-1. Overall freedom from second biochemical failure after salvage prostatectomy or salvage brachytherapy for locally recurrent cancer after external beam radiation failure.(AMLING, ROGERS, TEFILLI, BEYER, GRADO)

nal beam radiation annually in the United States. The biggest question regarding salvage of external beam failures is how many are really salvageable with *any* local therapy. Some patients already have micrometastatic disease by the time intraprostatic tumor persistence is demonstrated, and local therapy is unlikely to have an impact on their survival or improve their quality of life.

The limited number of salvage prostatectomy series published to date are unanimous in showing that the surgical salvage rates are low, at best (**Figure 17-1, left**). While the biochemical control rates are acceptable in the first couple of postsalvage years, the number of second failures continues to climb with longer follow-up, so that the ultimate salvage rates appear very low.

Two investigators have reported results with salvage brachytherapy for failed external beam patients. Grado reported on 49 patients salvaged with either I-125 or Pd-103 between 1990 and 1996.(GRADO) At five years, the biochemical freedom from failure in salvaged patients was 33%, similar to that reported in surgical salvage series (**Figure 17-1, right**). Six percent of patients developed urinary incontinence and one patient required a colostomy for rectal bleeding.

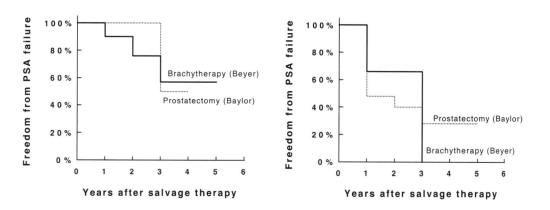

Figure 17-2. Freedom from second biochemical failure after salvage brachytherapy or salvage prostatectomy for locally recurrent cancer after external beam radiation (the Beyer series line for PSA less than 10 ng/ml excludes patients with a PSA of 0–4).(BEYER, ROGERS)

Beyer reported 17 patients treated with reduced dose I-125 or Pd-103 salvage implants.(BEYER) At five years, the overall freedom from second relapse was 53%, with 24% of patients developing urinary incontinence.

The chance for successful salvage brachytherapy could be predicted in part by the pretreatment PSA. For patients with a PSA below 10 there appears to be a leveling off of the biochemical freedom-from-failure curves at about 50% after salvage surgery or brachytherapy, suggesting that a substantial percentage of such patients might still be cured. Patients with a PSA above 10 at the time of salvage fare poorly (**Figure 17-2**).

In contrast to salvage prostatectomy, the risk of incontinence has been relatively low after salvage brachytherapy (**Figure 17-3**). However, it is possible that the incidence could rise with longer follow-up.

While these limited results are mildly encouraging, it should be remembered that they likely represent a highly selected patient group and may not be representative of what we'd see if salvage implants were done on a widespread basis. What is missing from the reports are the details of how the implants were actually done.

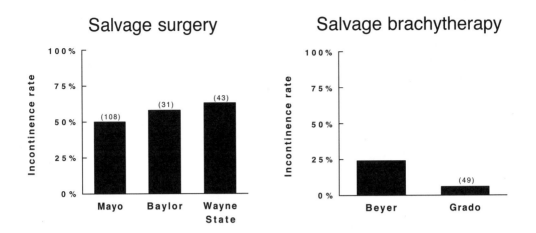

Figure 17-3. Urinary incontinence after salvage implant or salvage prostatectomy for locally recurrent cancer after external beam radiation.(AMLING, ROGERS, TEFILLI, BEYER, GRADO)

Implant doses used by Dr. Grado, for instance, varied during the study period. And it's likely that both Drs. Grado and Beyer varied their implant techniques during the study periods. Simply stating the prescription dose of a salvage implant does not tell enough about the implant technique to safely duplicate it at another center (see Chapter 6). The treatment margins used in the planning process, in particular, can have a substantial impact on the true dose to the prostate and adjacent normal tissues. For instance, Dr. Beyer was careful to avoid over-radiating the prostatic apex by ensuring that sources were not placed outside of the prostate apex, a limitation that he does not use for previously untreated patients (personal communication). More information on how salvage doses and treatment margins can affect the complication rates is needed.(BICE)

Keeping in mind the myriad caveats, both salvage brachytherapy reports suggest that it may be effective in a sizable percentage of failed external beam radiation patients. But more detailed scrutiny of the techniques used and the longer-term outcomes are called for before widespread adoption of salvage brachytherapy for beam radiation failures.

SALVAGE FOR FAILED IMPLANTS
While data regarding salvage implants for beam failures are slim, data for salvage of brachytherapy failures are even slimmer. Using external beam radiation to salvage failed implant patients is not practical—if an implant failed to eradicate a cancer, it seems highly unlikely that external beam radiation could. If the implant

was technically poor, a reimplant would probably be preferable to salvage external radiation.

To date, no series of salvage prostatectomy specifically for failed transperineal implants have been published. The Baylor report of salvage surgery included failed beam radiation patients and 26 failed retropubic implant patients, which likely have limited relevance to today's transperineal techniques. Data regarding salvage surgery for failed *transperineal* implants are anecdotal at this time. And as more reports of salvage surgery emerge, it will be important to interpret alleged salvage "cure" rates in light of the possibility that some surgical salvage patients will likely have undergone salvage for temporary PSA rises, rather than for true cancer persistence (see chapter 13).

REFERENCES
1. Amling CL, Lerner SE, Martin SK, et al . Deoxyribonucleic acid ploidy and serum prostate specific antigen predict outcome following salvage prostatectomy for radiation refractory prostate cancer. J Urol 1999; 161:857-863.

2. Beyer DC. Permanent brachytherapy as salvage treatment for recurrent prostate cancer. Urol 1999; 54:880-883.

3. Bice WS, Freeman JE, Russell LF, et al . Use of image coregistration in salvage prostate brachytherapy. Tech Urol 2000; 6:151-156.

4. Grado GL, Collins JM, Kriegshauser JS, et al . Salvage brachytherapy for localized prostate cancer after radiotherapy failure. Urol 1999; 53:2-10.

5. Rogers E, Ohori M, Kassabian VS, et al . Salvage radical prostatectomy: Outcome measured by serum prostate specific antigen levels. J Urol 1995; 153:104-110.

6. Tefilli MV, Gheiler EL, Tiguert R, et al . Salvage surgery or salvage radiotherapy for locally recurrent prostate cancer. Urol 1998; 52:224-229.

18

Really Bad Mistakes

Prostate brachytherapy has come a long way, thanks to good quality, easy-to-use TRUS equipment and sophisticated but user-friendly treatment planning systems. And we've learned, sometimes the hard way, what *not* to do to avoid complications. If you follow basic guidelines printed here and elsewhere, you should get good tumor control rates and acceptable complication rates. But you still have to pay attention to what you're doing, while you're doing it. Even though guidelines are fairly well worked out and should keep you out of serious trouble, there's always the possibility of making a really stupid mistake. And unfortunately, even the smartest, most conscientious people make one once in a while.

Mistake   Correction

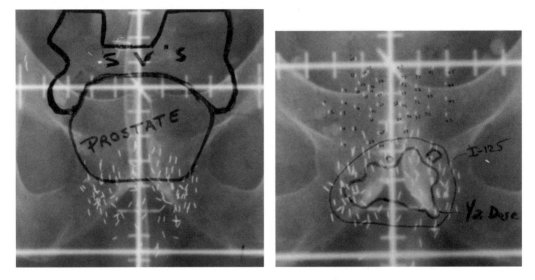

Figure 18-1. In this example, the brachytherapist somehow didn't visualize the prostate correctly, perhaps mistaking a backward view (sacrum) for the prostate, or believing that the external sphincter was prostatic tissue. We don't know exactly what went wrong in this case, but when consulted about the patient, Michael Dattoli elected to go back and implant the prostate as should have been done in the first place. The patient did well, and has not developed rectal complications in the two years after his "patch-up" implant.

Whatever the reason—you weren't feeling well, you were distracted, or you simply blew it—disasters *can* occur. And if you do enough procedures, one probably *will* occur at some point in your practice. Just to get you in the proper frame of mind to handle disaster, we've collected a number of them that we've seen over the years.

MISSING THE PROSTATE
One of the most embarrassing mistakes you could make is to miss the prostate (**Figure 18-1**). It happens—we know of several instances, probably related to misinterpreting the TRUS images at the time of initial setup. Unfortunately, you can't go back and remove the misplaced sources, short of resecting the wrongly implanted tissue in bulk.

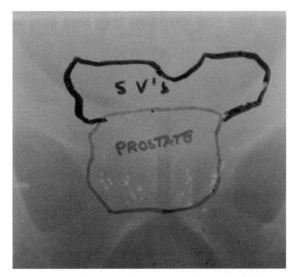

Figure 18-2. This is another miss-the-prostate mistake, apparently due to gross underplanning. It may have resulted from a faulty pre-implant volume study suggesting a prostate volume much smaller than it really was. When consulted about the patient after this implant, Michael Dattoli elected to go back and implant the prostate as should have been done in the first place. Like the patient in Figure 18-1, the patient has done well after his "patch-up" implant.

The prostate should appear obvious on TRUS. If you're setting up and not sure whether you're looking at the prostate, something is *very* wrong—stop and reposition the probe or take it out and start again. Either the probe setup is wrong (backward, looking at the sacrum, for instance) or you're not in far enough. A quick anterior fluoroscopic view with a catheter in place is the surest way to prevent mistakes like the one in **Figure 18-1**. If you *really* goof up and miss the prostate altogether, often the best remedy is to go back and reimplant (correctly), providing the patient isn't going to wind up with excessive rectal doses.

GROSS UNDERDOSE
More common than outright missing the prostate is grossly underdoing it. Mistakes like this probably result from a brachytherapy team *really* not knowing what they're doing. And we're talking about the *whole team* here. A gross undertreatment like the one shown in **Figure 18-2** can be avoided if even one member of the brachytherapy team has even an ounce of brains—the radiation oncologist should know from simple inspection of the planning images and treatment plan

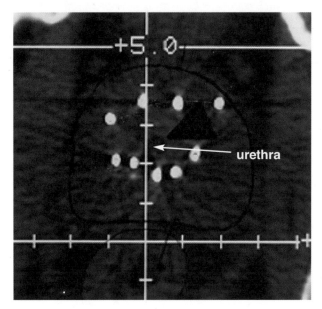

Figure 18-3. This mistake was committed in the early 1990s. For some reason, the posterior sources were too anterior, resulting in an excessive urethral dose and inadequate dose to the back of the prostate. If this occurred today, we'd probably go back and add a few sources in the posterior prostate, to make sure of an adequate cancercidal dose posteriorly, even if it meant overdosing the urethra—a problem from which patients nearly always recover spontaneously.

that something is wrong, the dosimetrist should know that the target is going to be grossly underdosed, and even the urologist, without formal training, should see that this kind of seed distribution could not *possibly* be adequate to treat a patient's prostate. The saving grace for blunders like this is that they are relatively easy to fix—it's pretty straightforward to run the postimplant dosimetry and go back and add sources to bring coverage of the prostate up to where it should be. The chance for complications (apart from severe embarrassment) should be minimal. Probably the worst thing to do with a mistake such as this is to ignore it—the patient will likely develop cancer recurrence and possibly die from your mistake (and the proof of your guilt is obvious to anyone taking even a cursory look at the films!).

OVERDOSE
The two really bad mistakes in Figures 18-1 and 18-2 were related to underdosing the prostate, the primary clinical result being a missed chance at cure. The other type of really bad mistake is *over*dosing. Overdosing the prostate itself is typically not the issue; the real problem is overdosing the urethra or rectum. And remember, there are overdoses, and there are *over*doses—the second type is the one we're talking about here.

With relatively consistent source loading patterns in current practice, there typically are only minor variations in the urethral and rectal doses being used. Extreme outliers are more likely due to a really bad placement error than to a faulty plan.

Gross urethral overdose

Following typical peripheral source placement patterns, urethral doses are easily kept below the recommended maximum of 2–2.5 times the prescription dose. Deviations from the peripheral pattern, however, can lead to huge urethral doses, a problem that could come from a faulty plan, source placement error, or a lack of appreciation of a markedly asymmetric urethra, leading to gross overdosage despite a peripheral loading pattern. The patient in **Figure 18-3** had several high activity I-125 sources placed too close to his urethra, resulting in excessive urethral doses and prolonged urinary morbidity. Fortunately, his symptoms resolved spontaneously with no long-term permanent complications of which we are aware.

Gross rectal overdose

While serious rectal complications are infrequent and not usually associated with *really* bad mistakes, it is possible to place several sources too posteriorly, resulting in grossly excessive rectal doses (**Figure 18-4**). There are two potential serious sequela from this kind of mistake. The first is that such patients are at high risk of rectal complications—ulceration or prostatic-rectal fistula. The second, equally serious problem is that such patients are at substantial risk of cancer progression, since many of the sources that were supposed to contribute to their prostatic radiation are instead contributing to their rectal dose.

WRONG SOURCE, WRONG PATIENT, WRONG PLAN, ETC.

Perhaps the most common really bad mistake is mixing up patients' intended therapy (**Figure 18-5**). Especially in a high-volume practice, it's not surprising that such errors occasionally occur. The best safeguard is to have a system of checks in place, whereby multiple people involved in the planning and implementation recheck that everything is consistent, from the prescription to the actual sources taken to the operating room. But if NASA researchers can use the wrong units in calculating the distance to Mars, you can be sure that a small brachytherapy team can get the wrong sources or wrong dose for an implant patient.

WHEN YOU DISCOVER A MISTAKE

Like we said earlier, no matter how smart you are, if you do enough procedures, you're likely to make a really bad mistake at some point, probably when you're most confident of the safeguards in your practice and when you least expect it. You may discover *your* bad mistake at any time in the implant process. Assuming the

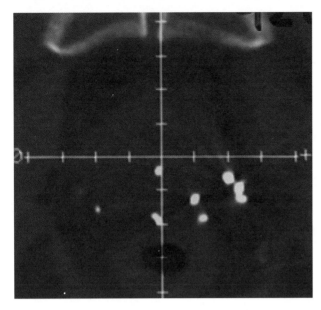

Figure 18-4. This error was committed in the early days of transperineal implants—we're not sure how it happened. The patient developed a severe rectal ulcer, but no fistula. His ulcer gradually healed spontaneously, but he developed local tumor progression.

It's tough to know what would have been the proper action at the time the error was detected. One reasonable option might have been to proceed with a prostatectomy, in the hope of curing him and preventing overradiation of the rectum. Another option, going back and implanting additional sources to achieve an adequate cancericidal dose to the prostate, might have pushed him over the edge, to a fistula.

mistake is discovered sometime after the sources have been placed, the most natural response to the kind of things shown here is to go into a frenzied panic, immediately counting the ways you'll get into big trouble with your patient, your hospital administration, and maybe a jury. But wait—like any crisis situation, it's important not to panic. Most of what you initially think are bad mistakes will likely turn out to be only *sort of bad* ones, or even within the range of accepted practice. For instance, if you mix up the sources between two patients, the target coverage could easily still be well within acceptable treatment guidelines. Take time to asses the situation before going to the patient and saying that something's wrong. First, do the dosimetry and assess whether your error makes any clinical difference. Remember, any corrective action likely won't be made immediately anyhow.

If you're in the middle of the implant when you discover the mistake, call other experts from your institution into the operating room to assess the mistake realtime and determine what, if anything, can be done intraoperatively to correct it. It may be that a mistake can be corrected, at least partially, on the spot. For instance,

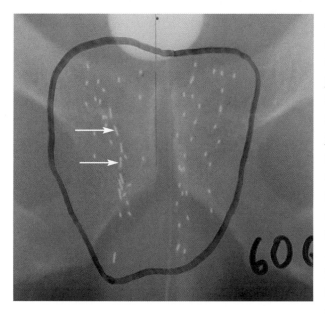

Figure 18-5. This is the best illustration that we could find of what is probably the most common mistake—mixing up sources. This patient's sources were mixed up with another's at the time of sterilization. The mistake was caught early on fluoroscopy when a few I-125 sources (thin arrows) were apparent instead of the intended Pd-103 sources. There are a variety of source mix-ups that can occur. So the first thing to do when you discover a source mix-up error is to make sure you're not about to make the reciprocal error in the next patient.

you mix up two plans, using that of a smaller prostate than the one you were supposed to do. You may be able to add sources ad hoc, with the patient still under anesthesia. Even if you implanted the smaller prostate with excess sources from another plan, it's likely that the TMs achieved won't be far out of the range typically used (see chapter 9). So even if you make a clear error in the case, the medical significance may be slight or insignificant. But determine the clinical significance before alarming the patient.

LAWSUITS
Finally, keep in mind that none of the really bad errors shown here have resulted in lawsuits (yet). The suits that the authors *have* been involved with to date have instead involved complications from technically acceptable implants. But like any other area of medicine, a small number of bad complications will occur in a small percent of patients, regardless of how well their treatment was delivered. So our advice is to assess the situation from the viewpoint of the actual dosimetry and its deviation from the fairly broad range of currently accepted practice. Once you've sized up the problem, then consider informing the patient as to how it occurred and what the corrective options are. And like any other potential medical malpractice

situation, make yourself readily available to answer questions. Honesty is (almost) always the best policy.

19

Cost

Treatment of prostate cancer is expensive. Of approximately 200,000 new cases diagnosed annually in the Unites States, 80% are clinically localized to the prostate. If all patients with localized disease are treated with definitive therapy, at an average charge of $12,000, the annual consumer cost of primary treatment alone would be almost $2 billion per year (**Table 19-1**). Treating all early-stage patients amounts to approximately 1% of the yearly Medicare budget (**Figure 19-1**). And the cost of palliative care for patients with more advanced cancers is probably considerably higher.(CARLSSON)

Table 19-1. Approximate annual cost of potentially curative treatment of clinically localized prostate cancer in the United States.	
New cases:	200,000
Clinically localized (80%):	160,000
Average cost per patient:	$12,000
Total cost, all patients:	$1,900,000,000

PRICES, CHARGES, AND COSTS

Prices, charges, and *costs* are relative terms, the proper choice of which depends on the context in which they are used. By definition, the *price* of a commodity is the market-based agreement between what the consumer is willing to pay and the provider is willing to accept. Thus, in a free-market system, price is arrived at efficiently. In contrast, the price of medical care is influenced by third-party payers (government, insurers, employers) who stand between the patient (consumer) and the medical industry (provider). Because they represent large numbers of patients,

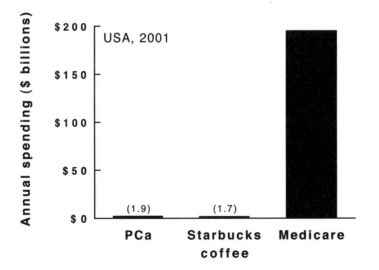

Figure 19-1. Approximate cost to provide primary, curative treatment to all U.S. patients with clinically localized prostate cancer, compared with the gross revenues from Starbucks coffee products or the annual Medicare budget. (*1999 annual financial report)

Table 19-2. Who pays the bills.

Type of payer	Source of money	Primary price-setter
Medicare	Federal tax	Health Care Financing Admin (HCFA)
Medicaid	Federal/state tax	HCFA/state agencies
Managed care	Employer/individual	Market
Fee-for-service	Employer/individual	Physician/hospital

third-party payers have a remarkable influence on the market-derived price. *Charges* are the fees that providers (physicians and hospitals) bill for their services. In the past, charges were similar to prices. But prices of medical services currently are typically substantially lower than the charges, because of discounting demanded by third parties. And the prices, charges, and costs of medical care in the United States are changing, as managed care gains market share and providers (physicians and hospitals) compete for patients.

The best way around the vagaries of prices and charges would be to analyze medical care in terms of its *production cost*. Unfortunately, the production cost of medical care is even harder to determine than current charges or prices, due in part to the complexity of separating out the production cost of a service from the myriad overlapping activities of physician time and hospital services. In fact, most institutions don't know their production cost for a complex procedure like prostate brachytherapy. And if they do, they're typically not interested in publishing it.(CIEZKI)

To make matters worse, the definition of *cost* varies. For instance, a hospital bill for open-heart surgery is viewed as a "charge" by the local dominant HMO, only a starting point for negotiations in the final price. But the same hospital bill is clearly a *cost* to a private patient, paying out-of-pocket and legally obligated to pay in full. Any discussion regarding the specifics of medical costs is fraught with opportunities to nitpick about how dollar figures are cited. So if you think you've found an inconsistency in the next few pages, keep it to yourself.

WHO PAYS THE BILLS
Analysis of medical costs is complicated by the plethora of payer types within U.S. health care. There are four general categories of payers in the U.S. health market: individuals, government programs (Medicare and Medicaid), private fee-for-ser-

Costs of cancer recurrence

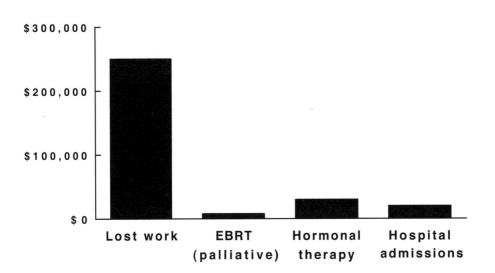

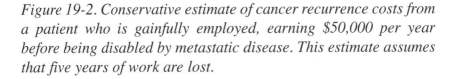

Figure 19-2. Conservative estimate of cancer recurrence costs from a patient who is gainfully employed, earning $50,000 per year before being disabled by metastatic disease. This estimate assumes that five years of work are lost.

vice (the "Blues" and other indemnity plans), and managed care (HMOs, PPOs, etc.) (**Table 19-2**). Medicare rates have a disproportionate effect on other pricing systems because they are used for guidance by nongovernmental parties when setting the price of medical care. The percent of patients in various payer categories has changed substantially, and the movement toward managed care probably will continue.

Of the four payer types, fee-for-service plans generally offer the highest reimbursements to providers, presumably the cost for patients to have their free choice of doctors and to be treated in the more prestigious institutions (perhaps) by the more prestigious doctors (perhaps). The cost of fee-for-service plans is inflated by cost-shifting, whereby fee-for-service patients are charged more because they are not organized to negotiate lower prices. Fee-for-service patients cannot negotiate down their costs, and are legally responsible for the amount billed by the hospital and physician. There have been sporadic attempts to control fee-for-service charges through government-mandated price controls, but such efforts have con-

Cost of recurrence versus therapy

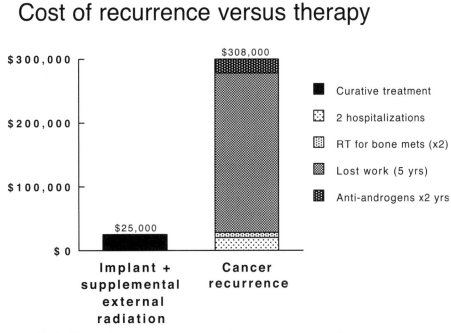

Figure 19-3. Even the most expensive therapy appears cheap compared to that of cancer recurrence.

sistently failed. Cost-shifting will continue to some extent, as long as there is some element of fee-for-service in the system. However, as the percent of patients enrolled in managed care climbs, cost-shifting will become an increasingly impractical way for physicians and hospitals to cover costs or boost income.

THE COST OF FAILURE

Before delving into the cost of therapy, it's important to emphasize that cancer therapy costs are dwarfed by the cost of recurrence. Patients who are not cured may require palliative therapy and long-term hormonal ablation, and suffer substantial loss of income. A patient who lives five years with recurrent, metastatic disease might lose five years of productive work time, valued at $250,000. He would typically receive five years of androgen ablation at an approximate total cost of $30,000. At the more advanced stage of metastatic disease, he might be hospitalized twice for pain control ($20,000) and two courses of palliative irradiation would total $8,000. These costs do not include extra imaging studies or other palliative therapies that are commonly used. A conservative estimate of the additional cost in this case would be $308,000, dwarfing the initial treatment charges

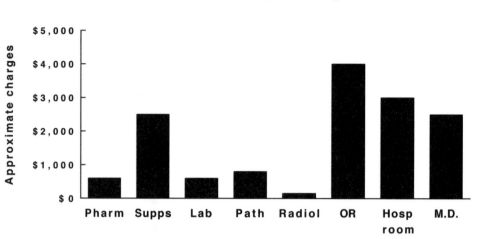

Figure 19-4. Breakdown of charges for radical prostatectomy.

of more than $25,000 for even the most costly therapy—combined implant plus supplemental external radiation (**Figures 19-2 & 19-3**). And the actual cost of cancer recurrence could rise to many times the $308,000 estimated in Figure 19-3, depending on whether salvage therapy is used and how much palliative care is required. For younger patients especially, the cost of lost wages could be far higher.

COMPARING MODALITIES
There is still surprisingly little written about the cost of prostate cancer treatment. Earlier studies comparing external radiation, prostatectomy, and brachytherapy are outdated due to substantial changes in the way treatments are delivered.(HANKS, COTTER)

Prostatectomy
Based on 1999 Medicare reimbursements, the total consumer cost of a prostatectomy is approximately $14,000, 80% of which represents hospital charges and 20% physician fees (**Figure 19-4**).(ONCOLOGY)

Since most of the surgical costs represent hospital charges, substantial savings can be achieved through early abdominal drain removal, early ambulation and oral feeding, early hospital discharge, and more judicious use of laboratory tests. These goals can be achieved through aggressive preoperative patient education and by continuous monitoring by a dedicated cost-control team. With a concerted

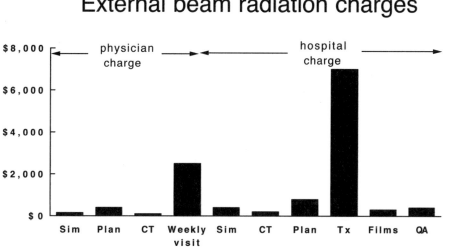

Figure 19-5. Approximate charges for conformal external radiation (75 Gy).

effort, substantial savings have been achieved. University of Chicago surgeons were able to decrease the average hospitalization from five days to two days, with total treatment cost cut by 34%.(PALMER) Such cost savings require constant vigilance to maintain.

External beam radiation

Based on current Medicare reimbursement, the cost of EBRT (70–75 Gy) is approximately $14,000, 80% of which is due to hospital charges and 20% to physician fees (**Figure 19-5**).

In past analyses, charges for external beam radiation have been lower than that of a prostatectomy.(HANKS, COTTER) However, the provider cost to deliver external radiation has risen with increasingly sophisticated treatment plans and delivery systems, such that private charges for high-dose conformal external radiation run between $20,000 and $35,000. While managed care plans currently may not reimburse at this charge level, if outcomes data show that better technical delivery and higher doses increase cure rates while decreasing complication rates, there will be upward price pressure. The figures quoted here are charges. Actual production cost figures are hard to come by. European investigators estimate external beam production costs at about $220 per dose, pooling all departmental costs and dividing

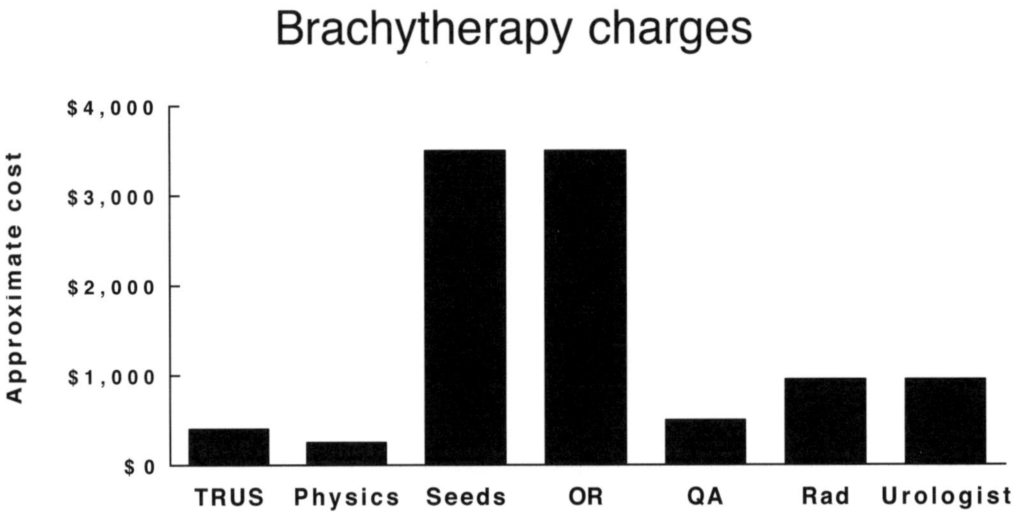

Brachytherapy charges

Figure 19-6. Approximate Medicare brachytherapy reimbursements.(QA=postimplant dosimetry, Rad=radiation oncologist)

by the number of patients treated.(WODINSKY) Keep in mind, though, that the cost of providing conformal therapy may be substantially higher.(HORWITZ)

Implant alone
Based on 1996 Medicare reimbursement rates, the charges for a permanent prostate radioactive implant totals approximately $12,000, 80% of which represents hospital charges and 20% physician charges (**Figure 19-6**).

The cost of the sources themselves is a substantial portion of the bill. The typical cost to the provider for I-125 or Pd-103 is about $2,500 to $5,000. Some hospitals mark up the source price, bringing the charges to $6,000 or more.

Implant + supplemental external radiation
Implant alone is a cost-competitive therapy relative to prostatectomy or external radiation. However, the addition of supplemental external beam radiation increases the cost substantially. The consumer cost of the supplemental radiation (40–50 Gy) is close to that of full-course radiation alone, since a simulation is still needed and the number of treatments is decreased by only 30%. The brachytherapy costs are decreased from those of a full-dose implant only by use of 30% fewer sources than would be used for a full implant. Based on current Medicare reimbursement, the consumer cost of an implant plus supplemental external radiation

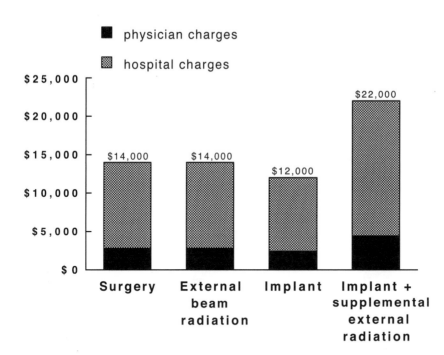

■ physician charges

▧ hospital charges

Figure 19-7. Approximate physician and hospital charges for prostatectomy, beam radiation, transperineal implant or implant+beam.

(45 Gy) is approximately $22,000, almost twice that of an implant alone and at least 50% greater than Medicare fees for 80 Gy 3D conformal external beam radiation.

If the high cure rates reported by some investigators are truly representative, then the high up front costs of implant plus supplemental external radiation could be a bargain in the long-term by avoiding the costs of cancer recurrence (**Figure 19-7**). But in the short term, it's very expensive therapy.

COMPARING MODALITIES

Several reports regarding the charges for brachytherapy versus radical prostatectomy have appeared. Disregarding the cost of the radioactive sources, brachytherapy is comparable to surgery, the primary cost components being operative room time and physician fees. But when the cost of the sources is included, brachytherapy charges are about 10-20% higher than surgery (**Figures 19-8, 19-9 & 19-10**).(WAGNER, KOHAN, CIEZKI) Published studies, to date, compared only *charges*, as opposed to actual provider's cost to deliver therapy. But either way, probably

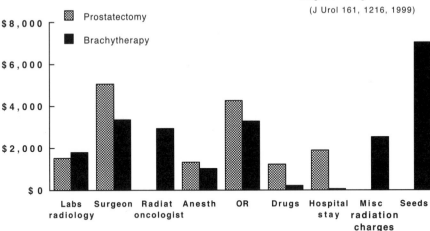

Ohio State University
33 patients
1996-7
Private charges
-Wagner, Young & Bahnson
(J Urol 161, 1216, 1999)

Figure 19-8. Breakdown comparison of private charges for prostatectomy versus brachytherapy at Ohio State University (above). Total charges for brachytherapy (left) were almost $6,000 higher, but included supplemental external beam radiation in some patients.(WAGNER)

the same conclusion would be reached—there is no clear cost advantage of one modality over the other.

DIRECT, INDIRECT, AND INTANGIBLES

Using Medicare or private charges is the most common way to compare the cost of medical therapies. But the total cost of a medical therapy is far more complicated than simply tabulating the initial charges for the treatment itself. First of all,

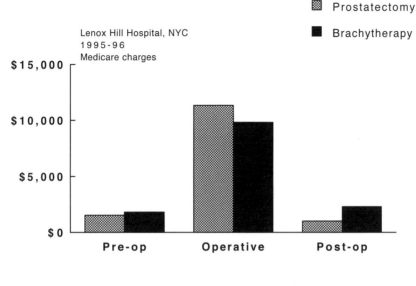

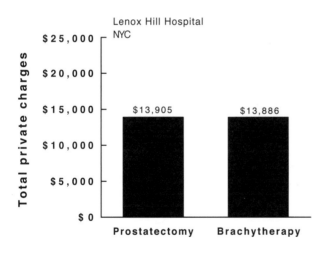

Figure 19-9. Breakdown comparison of private charges for prostatectomy versus brachytherapy at Lenox Hill Hospital (above). Total charges between modalities were almost identical (left).(KOHAN)

it is nearly impossible to calculate accurate production cost figures, which are difficult to separate from other services provided at a large medical center. Second, therapy charges quoted don't include the associated costs of treatment-related complications and accessory therapies. To get a more realistic cost estimate, medical costs can be divided into direct, indirect, and intangible costs (**Table 19-3**).(WALLNER)

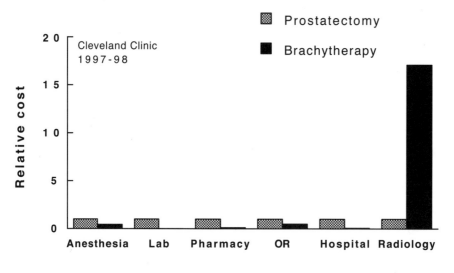

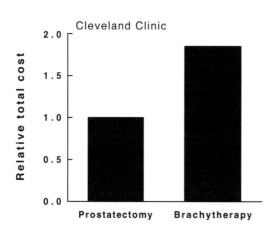

Figure 19-10. Alleged hospital costs to perform prostatectomy compared to brachytherapy. This study is the first to use actual costs rather than charges. However, due to propriety concerns of Cleveland Clinic Foundation, the figures were reported as relative to those of prostatectomy, rather than actual dollar figures, making it difficult to compare this to other hospitals. Unfortunately, actual costs are difficult to separate from those of a large, complex medical institution, and the figures should be viewed skeptically.(CIEZKI)

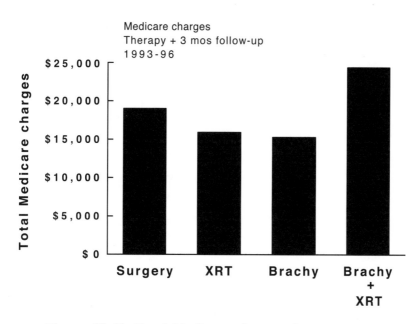

Figure 19-11. Total Medicare charges for prostatectomy, external beam radiation (XRT), outpatient transperineal implant, and implant+XRT.(BRANDEIS)

Direct costs

Direct costs include amounts paid to medical providers for medical goods and services. They can be divided into *primary* and *secondary* direct costs. Primary direct costs include those of the treatment itself: physician fees, operating room time, hospitalization, medication, laboratory fees, etc. These are the costs typically quoted by providers and typically used to calculate published comparisons between modalities.

Secondary direct costs are the insidious *extras*, including treatment-related complications, accessory treatments, and treatment for recurrent disease. Secondary direct costs can be referred to as *hidden* costs, because they are not easily anticipated and are often ignored in providers' price quotes. Identifying secondary direct costs is crucial to determining a realistic, total consumer cost.

Indirect costs

Traditionally, indirect medical costs are the personal costs that a patient incurs by receiving treatment, including such things as travel costs and child care. *Lost*

Table 19-3. Direct and indirect consumer medical costs.

<u>Category</u>	<u>Example</u>
Primary direct	hospitalization
	physician fees
	lab tests
Secondary direct	complications
	accessory treatments
	salvage therapy
Indirect	lost wages
(societal, personal)	

wages is the most easily quantified indirect cost and is the only one considered here.

Intangibles

As with most serious diseases and their treatments, there are substantial intangible costs to prostate cancer therapies, including physical discomfort, mental stress, and social disruptions. While clearly important, intangible medical costs are not easy to quantify and are not included in the cost considerations here. To date, indications are that relatively few major problems are associated with brachytherapy, and that it compares favorably to prostatectomy and external beam radiation.(BRANDEIS, HAN)

HIDDEN COSTS

Hidden costs make a big difference. Looking only at the primary direct costs of treating potentially curable prostate cancer, surgery and implants both compare favorably to external radiation. But when the hidden costs are added, external radiation and implants both compare more favorably to surgery (**Figures 19-12 to 19-15**).

While there is room to quibble about some of the calculations here, the important point is that substantial hidden costs exist and that they need to be recognized along with the primary direct costs in order to make a realistic estimate of the total consumer cost.

REDUCING THE COST OF IMPLANTATION
Several commonly used procedures of questionable benefit add to the cost of prostate brachytherapy. These procedures are not uniformly followed by all physicians, and those who do not use the procedures do not appear to have a higher likelihood of complications or a lesser cure rate. In the absence of data to support the use of such procedures, it seems prudent to discontinue them, both to save resources and to prevent complications, which can accompany any medical treatment (**Table 19-4**).

Hospitalization
Hospitalization is the single most expensive, unnecessary item that adds to the cost of implantation. A patient typically is charged $600 to $1,000 for overnight hospitalization. Some physicians and patients would prefer overnight hospitalization due to the 10% possibility of urinary retention or the remote possibility of postimplant bleeding. In fact, urinary retention is not an emergency, and can be managed on an outpatient basis. Significant postimplant bleeding is rare; it has never been reported in the literature and is not a reason for hospitalization.

There are occasional patients who require hospitalization following implantation. Probably the most common are those with significant cardiac problems who need to be closely observed postimplantation. Patients with serious general health problems would generally not be advised to have definitive treatment of early stage prostatic carcinoma, so that the number of people who *need* overnight hospitalization should be very small.(HAN)

Antibiotics
Prophylactic antibiotics are nearly universally given. While this policy may seem prudent, there is little or no data to support it (see chapter 7). The only retrospective studies that examined routine prophylactic antibiotics showed no benefit to their use. Avoiding the routine use of antibiotics can save $20 to $200/patient, depending on the drugs used.

Postimplant cystoscopy
Postimplant cystoscopy is commonly performed to remove sources left in the bladder or protruding into the urethra, or to remove blood clots in the bladder. While postimplant cystoscopy seems superficially logical, there is no data to support it as a routine procedure.(GRAY, YAP)

Prostatectomy: grand total

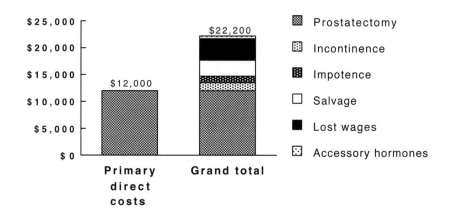

Figure 19-12. Primary direct cost of prostatectomy compared to the combined primary and secondary direct and indirect costs.

EBRT: grand total

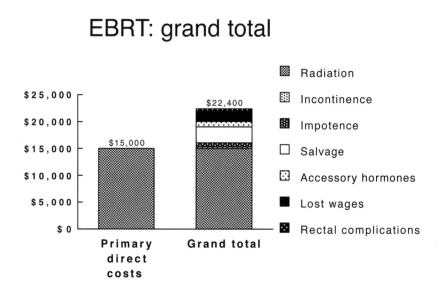

Figure 19-13. Primary direct cost of external beam radiation compared to the combined primary and secondary direct and indirect costs.

Implants: grand total

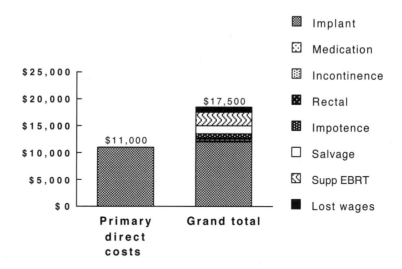

Legend:
- ▨ Implant
- ⊡ Medication
- ▦ Incontinence
- ▪ Rectal
- ▤ Impotence
- ☐ Salvage
- ⊠ Supp EBRT
- ■ Lost wages

Figure 19-14. Primary direct costs of implant alone, compared to their total costs, including secondary direct and indirect costs. (Supp EBRT=supplemental external radiation)

Comparing grand totals

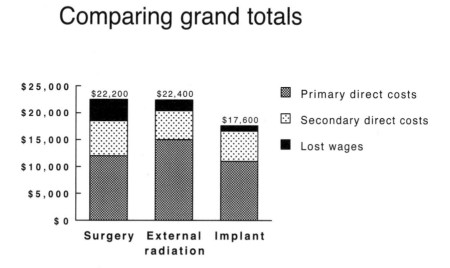

Legend:
- ▨ Primary direct costs
- ⊡ Secondary direct costs
- ■ Lost wages

Figure 19-15. Comparison of combined direct and indirect costs of prostatectomy, external radiation, or implants.

Table 19-4. Unnecessary procedures that could be omitted to contain costs.

Item	Cost to hospital	Cost to patient
Inpatient stay (1 day)	$200	$800
Antibiotics	50	100
Postimplant cysto	10	100
Postimplant CBC	2	15
Sterile drapes/gowns	11	22
General/spinal anesthesia	500	3,000

Because the postimplant cystoscopy charge has been bundled into the urology Medicare codes, its use seems to have declined. Ending the practice of postimplant cystoscopy saves time and resources, without affecting the quality of care.

Blood work
Routine pre- and postimplant lab tests are unnecessary, except what might be required by anesthesia. Similarly, routine chest Xrays are unnecessary.

Sterile supplies
Sterile drapes has never been proven to decrease the risk of infection in any type of surgery, and may actually make infection more likely in some circumstances (see chapter 7). Curtailing their use can eliminate $10 to $20 in hospital costs.

Local anesthesia
The biggest potential to cut the cost of brachytherapy is to move the procedure out of the operating room, and get away from the routine use of anesthesia (see chapter 7). Switching to local anesthesia, and moving the procedure to the radiation oncology department, eliminates approximately $3,000 in private charges. (Not only are resources saved; bypassing the operating room scheduling maze can cut down on much of the hassle factor in arranging procedures.)

LOST WAGES
Perhaps the largest cost of treatment is lifestyle effect. A full accounting of lifestyle cost has not been attempted for any treatment modality and is beyond the scope of this text. However, a relatively easily estimated factor is the time lost from work. On that basis, work days lost with implantation compares favorably

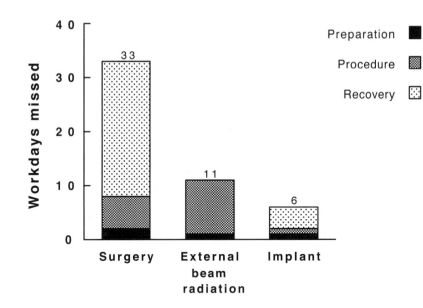

Figure 19-16. Work days missed with each modality. Numbers are estimations and could vary substantially, based on patient circumstances and physician policy regarding postoperative care.

with external beam radiation or prostatectomy (**Figure 19-16**). Work time missed with an implant includes an office visit for treatment planning volume study and preanesthesia testing. The treatment itself, performed on an outpatient basis, requires one day off work. The at-home recovery time typically would be 1 to 3 days.

Work time missed with a prostatectomy includes time spent donating autologous blood, estimated at one day. The hospital stay is typically 3 to 5 days, in the absence of serious complications. The recovery time at home is generally 3 to 6 weeks, although some of that time could be spent working at home, depending on the nature of the patient's occupation.

Work days missed with beam radiation include those for simulation and for daily treatments. If one assumes a half day missed for simulation and plan verification and two hours missed for each of 40 treatments, a total of approximately eleven days would be missed.

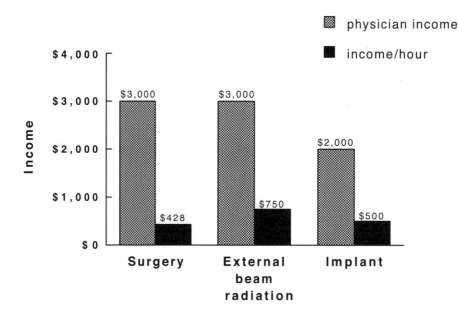

Figure 19-17. Approximate total and hourly physician income from each modality. Numbers are approximations, and will vary substantially, depending on geographic region and specific policies of the treating physician and institution.

PHYSICIANS' FINANCIAL INCENTIVES

There may be a marked disparity in physician compensation with different treatment options due to differences in charges, physician time required to perform each procedure, and the amount of uncompensated follow-up care required. To date, very little data are available from any source regarding physician compensation for specific treatment modalities.

Assuming physician reimbursement of $3,000, $3,000, and $2,000 for prostatectomy, beam radiation and implant, respectively, and total time of 7 hours, 4 hours, and 4 hours, respectively, the total physician income would be highest with prostatectomy and lowest with brachytherapy. However, the comparisons are radically different when income is calculated on an hourly basis (**Figure 19-17**). These reimbursement and time estimations could vary from region to region and from one physician to another. Additionally, financial incentives for the institution are far more complex to estimate and could differ markedly from those for the physician.

The physician's financial incentives are affected by the form of a patient's health insurance. Patients in capitated systems presumably would be discouraged from prostatectomy because they could be treated more quickly and cheaply with brachytherapy. In the absence of evidence that surgery is more effective, the financial considerations will likely encourage substitution of brachytherapy for surgery, at least when an implant is used without supplemental external radiation. Once managed care organizations better understand the overall cost savings of brachytherapy, it is not inconceivable that prostatectomy (the *fool's-gold standard*), would be allowed only if brachytherapy is first ruled out.

COST–THE ULTIMATE MEDICAL MYSTERY

Medial costs, incomes, and profits, especially from complex procedures, are difficult to quantify accurately. They vary by region and are constantly changing as the medical marketplace shifts increasingly toward managed care. The numbers given here are broad estimates. They are food for thought but suffer from substantial uncertainties. Assuming that brachytherapy cure rates are equal to those for surgery or external beam radiation, implant alone is probably the most cost-effective therapy, but not necessarily the most lucrative for the physician or the hospital. It is likely that future cost analyses will follow the example of Kent Wallner's *SmartMedicine: How to cut medical costs and cure cancer*, which offers a more complete picture of therapy costs than most out-the-door cost comparisons published to date.(WALLNER)

REFERENCES

1. Adolfsson J, Carstensen J, Lowhagen T. Deferred treatment in clinically localized prostatic carcinoma. Br J Urol 1992; 69:183-187.

2. Brandeis J, Pashos CL, Henning JM, Litwin MS. A nationwide charge comparison of the principal treatments for earlly stage prostat carcinoma. Cancer 2000; 89:1792-1799.

3. Carlsson P, Hjertberg H, Jonsson B, Varenhorst E. The cost of prostatic cancer in a defined population. Scand J Urol Nephrol Suppl 1989; 23:93-96.

4. Ciezki JP, Klein EA, Angermeier KW, Ulchaker J, Zippe CD, Wilkinson DA. Cost comparison of radical prostatectomy and transperineal brachytherapy for localized prostate cancer. Urol 2000; 55:68-72.

5. Cotter GW. Surgery or radiation therapy: A comparative cost analysis for early carcinoma of the prostate and breast. App Radiol 1990; January:25-28.

6. Gray G, Wallner K, Roof J, Corman J. Cystourethroscopic findings before and after prostate brachytherapy. Tech Urol 2000; 6:109-111.

7. Han BH, Demel KC, Wallner KE, Young L. Patient reported short-term complications after prostate brachytherapy. J Urol 2001; (in press):

8. Hanks GE, Dunlap K. A comparison of the cost of various treatment methods for early cancer of the prostate. Int J Radiat Oncol Biol Phys 1986; 12:1879-1881.

9. Kohan AD, Armenakas NA, Fracchia JA. The perioperative charge equilvalence of interstitial brachytherapy and radical prostatectomy with 1-year followup. J Urol 2000; 163:511-514.

10. Oncology . Prostate surgeries: Average charges throughout the United States, 1997. Oncology 2000; 14:371-378.

11. Palmer JS, Worwag EM, Conrad WG, et al . Same day surgery for radical retropubic prostatectomy: Is it an attainable goal? Urol 1996; 47:23-28.

12. Wagner TT, Young D, Bahnson RR. Charge and length of hospital stay analysis of radical retropubic prostatectomy and transperineal prostate brachytherapy. J Urol 1999; 161:1216-1218.

13. Wallner KE. SmartMedicine: How to cut medical costs and cure cancer. Seattle: SmartMedicine Press, 2000.

14. Wodinsky HB, Jenkin RDT. The cost of radiation treatment at an Ontario regional cancer centre. CMAJ 1987; 137:906-909.

15. Yap J, Wallner K, Gray G. Cystourethroscopic findings and long-term urinary function after prostate brachytherapy. Journal of Brachytherapy International 2001;

20

The Future

We are seeing today what seemed more fantasy than reality in the early 1990s: prostate brachytherapy rapidly becoming the treatment of choice for early-stage prostate cancer. Its resurgence initially met with substantial resistance from the fossilized, creatively moribund members of oncologic communities. With mounting evidence confirming its comparable efficacy and acceptable morbidity, even the most mentally sluggish oncologists are jumping on board—brachytherapy is rapidly replacing prostatectomy as the treatment of choice even for younger patients. Prostatectomy, the therapeutic mainstay of the intellectually handicapped, appears poised for its rightful extinction.

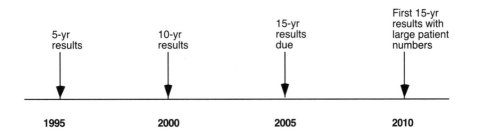

Figure 20-1. Approximate timeline for long-term clinical follow-up of early TRUS implant series.

Early reports, generated by a few brachytherapy enthusiasts, are giving way to a widespread rush of mainstream oncologists. Good—there's plenty more to be done. The primary emphasis in the next five years will likely be on longer follow-up, verification of the relatively favorable morbidity, and standardized quality assurance.

LONGER FOLLOW-UP

The staying power of brachytherapy in prostate cancer treatment will be determined by its ability to eradicate cancer. If longer-term reports show durable biochemical disease-free survival rates, comparable or better than prostatectomy, large randomized trials won't be needed—brachytherapy will simply replace surgery as the treatment of choice.

The longer the follow-up, the more convincing the results appear. Ten-year follow-up, first available in 1997, was a milestone. But for younger patients with life expectancy of 15 years or more, it is not enough. Fifteen-year follow-up will be available in 2003, and will be enough to convince most patients and physicians that brachytherapy is a superior alternative to surgery, even in younger patients. Of course, many oncologists want 20-year follow-up before accepting brachytherapy as *conventional therapy*—but these tend to be the same ones who touted nerve-sparing prostatectomy or 3D conformal external beam radiation as "standard of care" as soon as they were described.

Although early patients will reach 15-year follow-up in 2003, the median follow-up will be only 5 to 10 years. It will take until 2010 to get large series of patients followed beyond 15 years (**Figure 19-1**). And the wait for adequate follow-up will be longer, because the earliest patients did not consistently get the same high-quality implants as those treated more recently. It could take several *more* years to get 15-year follow-up on large numbers of patients with what are now considered optimal implants.

VERIFY FAVORABLE MORBIDITY REPORTS

Early brachytherapy enthusiasts have reported both good tumor control rates and favorable morbidity. Morbidity reports can be substantially influenced by the interpretation and bias of the reporting physician. Nearly all early reports have been compiled by the treating physicians and should be interpreted with caution. They need to be verified or refuted with independent quality of life studies. This is especially so for potency preservation and urinary incontinence, as their evaluation is quite subjective. Independent verifications are coming.

QUALITY ASSURANCE

As is often the case with new techniques, early transperineal brachytherapy results have been presented primarily by enthusiasts in the field, who have dedicated much of their time to perfecting the procedure. Results reported by early enthusiasts may not be representative of what is achieved as the technology and skills are adopted by other, less-specialized practitioners. Better-quality assurance will be needed if brachytherapy is to meet its full potential as a widely available, effective, and relatively cost effective treatment. Fortunately, there is the potential to use medical imaging to evaluate implant quality, to ensure that the technique is carried out properly.

An ideal quality-assurance system would be available in the operating room to verify that an implant has been optimally completed before the operation is terminated. It is easy to visualize such a scenario, probably with some combination of real-time intraoperative CT, MR, or TRUS. Interpretation of intraoperative dosimetry will be complicated by prostatic volume changes at the time of the procedure, but it would offer us more real-time quality assurance than we have now by "eyeballing" the TRUS images and C-arm fluoroscopic views.

TURF BATTLES

One of the recurring points of controversy will be which specialty—urology or radiation oncology—is "in charge" of the procedure. Prostate brachytherapy is a radiation treatment, and it must be overseen by a radiation oncologist. The placement of needles can easily be done by either specialist—both specialties commonly have extensive experience with needle placement for biopsy (urology) or interstitial radiation (radiation oncology). But actual placement of radioactive sources should be performed by a radiation oncologist who understands the physics of radiation and its clinical implications, and is usually the only legally authorized user on the hospital radiation license. Some modification of the planned source placement is frequently necessary due to prostate and source motion during the procedure itself, and a radiation oncologist is capable of intelligently modifying the plan as needed during the course of the implant procedure.

The control issue will probably never be settled completely. It will depend on the vagaries of the politics and personalities of the physicians involved at each institution. Perhaps this is the way it should be, as the level of interest and skill of the specialists involved will vary.

ROOM TO IMPROVE
We still don't know how commonly late treatment failures will occur. There will be some, as they occur after all treatment modalities. If excessive late failures do occur, it will not necessarily spell the end of prostate brachytherapy. Because serious rectal complications are very uncommon with current prescription doses and because limiting the urethral dose with peripheral loading limits the risk of long-term urethral morbidity, the prescription doses can almost certainly be taken higher without undue risk if needed to increase the tumor eradication rate. But considering the high biochemical control rates and high negative repeat biopsy rate, we're not sure that the doses *need* to go higher. In fact, it's possible that current doses could go *lower*, with an equal chance of cure.

TECHNOLOGY READY TO RUN AMOK
Now that brachytherapy has entered the mainstream, there's a rush for manufacturers to supply new technology to improve the procedure. Be careful. This is already a quick, simple procedure with high tumor-control rates and relatively low morbidity. Radiation oncologists are famous for making simple things ridiculously complicated—like 3D external radiation for malignancies such as esophageal cancer or glioblastoma multiforme, when we cannot even agree on what volume should be treated. While technologic advances are central to improving health care, in this current cost-conscious era it will be hard to pass on the cost of superfluous technology to third-party payers unless we can demonstrate better outcomes by legitimate studies.

WE REMAIN BULLISH

We're elated at the burgeoning number of reports confirming high biochemical tumor control rates, acceptable morbidity, and competitive consumer cost of prostate brachytherapy. However, only when we have a quality assurance system in place, and have determined the optimal prescription doses, will we really know the full potential of the modality. Judging from what has been achieved with the present imperfect system, the results should be phenomenal.

Kent Wallner
John Blasko
Michael Dattoli

index